Ecotoxicology and Risk Assessment for Wetlands

Other titles from the Society of Environmental Toxicology and Chemistry (SETAC):

Uncertainty Analysis in Ecological Risk Assessment
Warren-Hicks and Moore, editors
1998

Ecotoxicological Risk Assessment of the Chlorinated Organic Chemicals
Carey, Cook, Giesy, Hodson, Muir, Owens, Solomon, editors
1998

Sustainable Environmental Management
Barnthouse, Biddinger, Cooper, Fava, Gillett, Holland, Yosie, editors
1998

Ecological Risk Assessment Decision-Support System: A Conceptual Design
Reinert, Bartell, Biddinger, editors
1998

Principles and Processes for Evaluating Endocrine Disruption in Wildlife
Kendall, Dickerson, Giesy, Suk, editors
1998

Quantitative-Structure Activity Relationships in Environmental Science-VII
Chen and Schüürmann, editors
1997

Atmospheric Deposition of Contaminants to the Great Lakes and coastal Waters
Baker, editor
1997

Chemically Induced Alterations in Functional Development and Reproduction of Fishes
Rolland, Gilbertson, Peterson, editors
1997

Chemical Ranking and Scoring: Guidelines for Relative Assessments of Chemicals
Swanson and Socha, editors
1997

Ecological Risk Assessment of Contaminated Sediments
Ingersoll, Dillon, Biddinger, editors
1997

Public Policy Applications of Life-Cycle Assessment
Allen, Consoli, Davis, Fava, Warren, editors
1997

Reassessment of Metals Criteria for Aquatic Life Protection: Priorities for Research and Implementation
Bergman and Dorward-King, editors
1997

For information about any SETAC publication, including SETAC's international journal *Environmental Toxicology and Chemistry*,
contact the SETAC Office, 1010 N. 12th Avenue, Pensacola, Florida, USA 32501-3367
T 850 469 1500 F 850 469 9778 E setac@setac.org http://www.setac.org

Ecotoxicology and Risk Assessment for Wetlands

Edited by
Michael A. Lewis
Foster L. Mayer
Rebecca L. Powell
Marcia K. Nelson
Stephen J. Klaine
Mary G. Henry
Gary W. Dickson

Proceedings from the SETAC Pellston Workshop
on Ecotoxicology and Risk Assessment for Wetlands
30 July – 3 August 1995
Fairmont Hot Springs,
Anaconda, Montana

SETAC Special Publications Series

SETAC Liaison
Greg Schiefer
SETAC/SETAC Foundation

Current Coordinating Editor of SETAC Books
C. G. Ingersoll
U.S. Geological Survey

Publication sponsored by the Society of Environmental Toxicology
and Chemistry (SETAC) and the SETAC Foundation for Environmental Education

SETAC PRESS

Cover by Michael Kenney Graphic Design and Advertising
Editing and typesetting by Wordsmiths Unlimited
Indexing by IRIS

Library of Congress Cataloging-in-Publication Data

Pellston Workshop on Ecotoxicology and Risk Assessment for Wetlands (1995 : Fairmont Hot Springs, Anaconda, Mont.)
Ecotoxicology and risk assessment for wetlands : proceedings from the Pellston Workshop on Ecotoxicology and Risk Assessment for Wetlands, 30 Jul–3 August 1995, Fairmont Hot Springs, Anaconda, Montana / edited by Michael A. Lewis...[et al.].
p. cm. -- (SETAC special publications series)
"Publication sponsored by the Society of Environmental Toxicology and Chemistry (SETAC)"
Includes bibliographical references and index.
ISBN 1-880611-16-3 (hardcover)
1. Wetland ecology--Congresses. 2. Pollution--Environmental aspects--Congresses. 3. Ecological risk assessment--Congresses. I. Lewis, Michael A. (Michael Anthony), 1948– . II. SETAC (Society) III. Title. IV. Series.
QH541.5.M3P45 1999
577.68'27--DC21 98-5474
CIP

Information in this book was obtained from individual experts and highly regarded sources. It is the publisher's intent to print accurate and reliable information, and numerous references are cited; however, the authors, editors, and publisher cannot be responsible for the validity of all information presented here or for the consequences of its use. Information contained herein does not necessarily reflect the policy or views of the Society of Environmental Toxicology and Chemistry (SETAC).

International Standard Book Number 1-880611-16-3
Printed in the United States of America
06 05 04 03 02 01 00 99 10 9 8 7 6 5 4 3 2 1

(∞) The paper used in this publication meets the minimum requirements of the American National Standard for Information Sciences—Permanence of Paper for Printed Library Materials, ANSI Z39.48-1984.

Reference Listing: Lewis MA, Mayer FL, Powell RL, Nelson MK, Klaine SJ, Henry MG, Dickson GW, editors. 1999. Ecotoxicology and risk assessment for wetlands. SETAC Pellston Workshop on Ecotoxicology and Risk Assessment for Wetlands; 1995 Jul 30–Aug 3; Fairmont Hot Springs, Anaconda, Montana. Published by the Society of Environmental Toxicology and Chemistry (SETAC), Pensacola, Florida, USA. 398 p.

The SETAC Special Publications Series

The SETAC Special Publications Series was established by the Society of Environmental Toxicology and Chemistry (SETAC) to provide in-depth reviews and critical appraisals on scientific subjects relevant to understanding the impacts of chemicals and technology on the environment. The series consists of books on topics reviewed and recommended by the SETAC Board of Directors and approved by the Publications Advisory Council for their importance, timeliness, and contribution to multidisciplinary approaches to solving environmental problems. The diversity and breadth of subjects covered in the series reflect the wide range of disciplines encompassed by environmental toxicology, environmental chemistry, and hazard and risk assessment. Despite this diversity, the goals of these volumes are similar; they are to present the reader with authoritative coverage of the literature, as well as paradigms, methodologies and controversies, research needs, and new developments specific to the featured topics. All books in the series are peer reviewed for SETAC by acknowledged experts.

The SETAC Special Publications are useful to environmental scientists in research, research management, chemical manufacturing, regulation, and education, as well as to students considering careers in these areas. The series provides information for keeping abreast of recent developments in familiar subject areas and for rapid introduction to principles and approaches in new subject areas.

SETAC would like to recognize the past SETAC Special Publications Series editors:

- T. W. La Point, The Institute of Applied Sciences,
  University of North Texas, Denton, TX
- B. T. Walton, U.S. Environmental Protection Agency,
  Research Triangle Park, NC
- C. H. Ward, Department of Environmental Sciences and Engineering,
  Rice University, Houston, TX

Contents

List of Figures

List of Tables

Foreword

This workshop was a continuation of a series of successful workshops called the Pellston Workshop Series. Since 1977, 31 workshops have been held at Pellston and several other locations to evaluate current and prospective environmental issues. Each has focused on a relevant environmental topic, and the proceedings of each have been published as a peer-reviewed or informal report. These documents have been widely distributed and are valued by environmental scientists, engineers, regulators, and managers because of their technical basis and their comprehensive, state-of-the-science reviews. The workshops in the Pellston Series are as follows:

- Estimating the Hazard of Chemical Substances to Aquatic Life. Held in Pellston, Michigan, June 13–17, 1977. Proceedings published by the American Society for Testing and Materials, STP 657, in 1978.
- Analyzing the Hazard Evaluation Process. Held in Waterville Valley, New Hampshire, August 14–18, 1978. Proceedings published by The American Fisheries Society in 1979.
- Biotransformation and Fate of Chemicals in the Aquatic Environment. Held in Pellston, Michigan, August 14–18, 1979. Proceedings published by The American Society of Microbiology in 1980.
- Modeling the Fate of Chemicals in the Aquatic Environment. Held in Pellston, Michigan, August 16–21, 1981. Proceedings published by Ann Arbor Science in 1982.
- Environmental Hazard Assessment of Effluents. Held in Cody, Wyoming, August 23–27, 1982. Proceedings published in a SETAC Special Publication by Pergamon Press in 1985.
- Fate and Effects of Sediment-Bound in Aquatic Systems. Held in Florissant, Colorado, August 11–18, 1984. Proceedings published in a SETAC Special Publication by Pergamon Press in 1987.
- Research Priorities in Environmental Risk Assessment. Held in Breckenridge, Colorado, August 16–21, 1987. Proceedings published by SETAC in 1987.
- Biomarkers: Biochemical, Physiological, and Histological Markers of Anthropogenic Stress. Held in Keystone, Colorado, July 23–28, 1989. Proceedings published in a SETAC Special Publication by Lewis Publishers in 1992.
- Population Ecology and Wildlife Toxicology of Agricultural Pesticide Use: A Modeling Initiative for Avian Species. Held in Kiawah Island, South Carolina, July 22–27, 1990. Proceedings published in a SETAC Special Publication by Lewis Publishers in 1994.
- A Technical Framework for [Product] Life-Cycle Assessments. Held in Smuggler's Notch, Vermont, August 18–23, 1990. Proceedings published by SETAC in January 1991, with second printing in September 1991 and third printing in March 1994.

- Aquatic Microcosms for Ecological Assessment of Pesticides. Held in Wintergreen, Virginia, October 7–11, 1991. Report published by SETAC in 1992.
- A Conceptual Framework for Life-Cycle Assessment Impact Assessment. Held in Sandestin, Florida, February 1–6, 1992. Proceedings published by SETAC in 1993.
- A Mechanistic Understanding of Bioavailability: Physical-Chemical Interactions. Held in Pellston, Michigan, August 17–22, 1992. Proceedings published in a SETAC Special Publication by Lewis Publishers in 1994.
- Life-Cycle Assessment Data Quality Workshop. Held in Wintergreen, Virginia, October 4–9, 1992. Proceedings published by SETAC in 1994.
- Avian Radio Telemetry in Support of Pesticide Field Studies. Held in Pacific Grove, California, January 5–8, 1993. Proceedings published by SETAC in 1998.
- Sustainability-Based Environmental Management. Held in Pellston, Michigan, August 25–31, 1993. Co-sponsored by the Ecological Society of America. Proceedings published by SETAC in 1998.
- Ecotoxicological Risk Assessment for the Chlorinated Organic Chemicals. Held in Alliston, Ontario, Canada, July 25–29, 1994. Proceedings published by SETAC in 1998.
- Application of Life-Cycle Assessment to Public Policy. Held in Wintergreen, Virginia, August 14–19, 1994. Proceedings published by SETAC in 1997.
- Ecological Risk Assessment Decision Support System. Held in Pellston, Michigan, August 23–28, 1994. Proceedings published by SETAC in 1998.
- Avian Toxicity Testing. Held in Pensacola, Florida, December 4–7, 1994. Co-sponsored by OECD. Proceedings published by OECD in 1996.
- Chemical Ranking and Scoring (CRS): Guidelines for Developing and Implementing Tools for Relative Chemical Assessments. Held in Sandestin, Florida, February 12–16, 1995. Proceedings published by SETAC in 1997.
- Ecological Risk Assessment of Contaminated Sediments. Held in Pacific Grove, California, April 23–28, 1995. Proceedings published by SETAC in 1997.
- Ecotoxicology and Risk Assessment for Wetlands. Held in Fairmont, Montana, July 30–August 3, 1995. Proceedings to be published by SETAC in 1999.
- Uncertainty in Ecological Risk Assessment. Held in Pellston, Michigan , August 23–28, 1995. Proceedings published by SETAC in 1998.
- Whole-Effluent Toxicity Testing: An Evaluation of Methods and Prediction of Receiving System Impacts. Held in Pellston, Michigan, September 16–21, 1995. Proceedings published by SETAC in 1996.
- Reassessment of Metals Criteria for Aquatic Life Protection: Priorities for Research and Implementation. Held in Pensacola, Florida, February 10–14, 1996. Proceedings published by SETAC in 1997.

- Reproductive and Developmental Effects of Contaminants in Oviparous Vertebrates. Held in Fairmont, Montana, July 13–18, 1997. Proceedings to be published by SETAC in 1999.
- Multiple Stressors in Ecological Risk Assessment. Held in Pellston, Michigan, September 13–18, 1997. Proceedings to be published by SETAC in 1999.
- Re-evaluation of the State of the Science for Water Quality Criteria Development. Held in Fairmont, Montana, June 25–30, 1998. Proceedings to be published by SETAC in 1999.
- Criteria for Persistence and Long-Range Transport of Chemicals in the Environment. Held in Fairmont Hot Springs, British Columbia, Canada, July 14–19, 1998. Proceedings to be published by SETAC in 1999.
- Assessing Contaminated Soils: From Soil-Contaminant Interactions to Ecosystem Management. Held in Pellston, Michigan, September 23–27, 1998. Proceedings to be published by SETAC in 1999.

Preface

This volume represents the proceedings of a workshop held from 30 July–3 August 1995 at Fairmont Hot Springs, Montana. The workshop was designed to meet the scientific and regulatory need for current information describing ecotoxicology and risk assessment for wetlands. Professionals from government, industry, and academia were selected to participate based on their expertise on the specific topic to be considered. These workshops have provided an excellent forum for stimulation and exchange of ideas on the technical and scientific issues underlying chemical fate and effects in the environment and overall hazard assessments of chemicals in ecosystems. The organizers and participants of this workshop hope that the current proceedings will be as useful as the previous workshop proceedings to scientists, engineers, and decision-makers concerned with maintaining and reducing the loss of the nation's wetland resources.

Although the organization and objectives of this workshop were similar to some earlier workshops, this is the first workshop to deal primarily with the environmental aspects of an ecosystem rather than with a discrete environmental problem. The proceedings of this workshop is published by the Society of Environmental Toxicology and Chemistry.

—— Michael A. Lewis

Acknowledgments

The Workshop on Ecotoxicology and Risk Assessment for Wetlands and publication of the proceedings were made possible through the financial support of

- The U.S. Environmental Protection Agency,
- The National Marine Fisheries Service,
- The National Biological Survey,
- E.I. Du Pont de Nemours and Company,
- Zeneca,
- Shell Development Company,
- Monsanto Company,
- Ciba-Geigy Corporation, and
- the U.S. Department of Interior, Minerals Management Service.

The content of this publication does not necessarily reflect the position or the policy of any of these organizations or the United States government, and an official endorsement should not be inferred.

The organizers of the workshop want to commend the participants and the discussion group leaders for their enthusiastic commitment to meeting the workshop's goals and for their diligent efforts in the preparation and review of this volume. We are also appreciative of the efforts of the SETAC/SETAC Foundation staff and in particular, Greg Schiefer, Linda Longsworth, and Tanya Shaffer in the planning and on-site implementation of the workshop. Finally, the workshop organizers would like to thank the staff of the Fairmont Hot Springs for their assistance and their hospitality. We also greatly appreciate the valuable assistance of Stacey Hagman, James Blackwell, and Chris Englert in preparing the final manuscript as well as Mimi Meredith's review of the volume for editorial style and format.

Dr. Michael A. Lewis supervised the peer review of this volume as a Special Publication of the Society of Environmental Toxicology and Chemistry. Harry Ohlendorf of CH2M Hill and John Goodrich-Mahoney of EPRI devoted considerable time to provide constructive comment to improve the quality of this volume, and we appreciate their efforts.

About the Editors

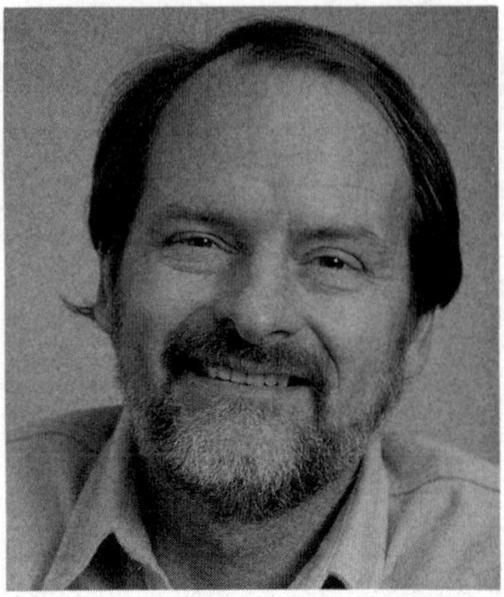

Michael A. Lewis has served as a branch chief and senior scientist with the United States Environmental Protection Agency (USEPA) in Gulf Breeze, Florida. Field validation of laboratory-derived toxicity estimates, estuarine assessments, and phytotoxicity evaluations have been the focus of his 20 years of industrial and governmental experience. Dr. Lewis was the president of a Society of Environmental Toxicology and Chemistry (SETAC) regional chapter and member of the SETAC Board of Directors; he is currently a member of the SETAC Editorial Board. He has chaired numerous programs and sessions at scientific meetings, authored more than 70 papers, and delivered dozens of presentations. Dr. Lewis holds a B.S. in biology, an M.S. in zoology, and a Ph.D. in environmental toxicology.

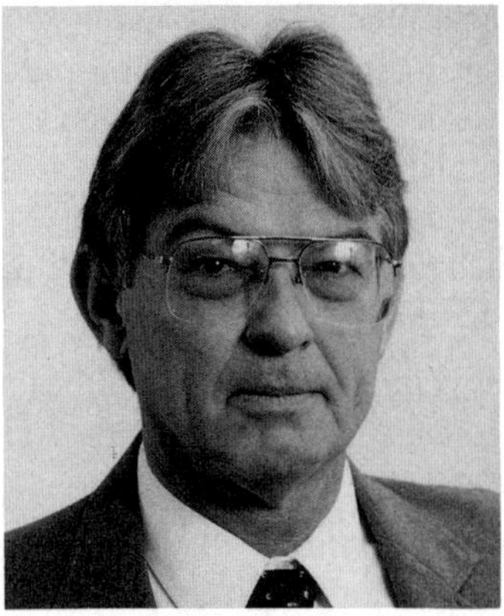

Foster L. Mayer is Senior Research Scientist-Ecotoxicology and Acting Director of the Gulf Ecology Division-NHEERL/ORD, USEPA, Gulf Breeze, Florida. The author of more than 100 papers, Dr. Mayer has participated in international research projects in Sweden and Russia, and he has received 13 awards for outstanding performance and special achievement in research, research management, and technical assistance. He has been an active member of the American Chemical Society, the American Fisheries Society, the American Institute of Fishery Research Biologists, Sigma Xi, the Society of Toxicology, ASTM, and SETAC. He holds a B.S. in biology and chemistry from Southwestern Oklahoma State University and an M.S. in wildlife biology and Ph.D. in toxicology from Utah State University.

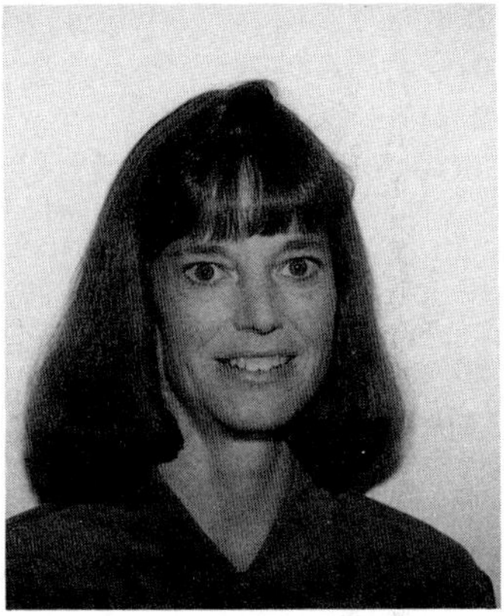

Rebecca L. Powell, formerly a senior research biologist with Monsanto, is a self-employed consultant whose professional memberships include SETAC and the American Society for Testing and Materials (ASTM). She holds a B.S. in biology and an M.S. in soil science. Her interests are concentrated in work with aquatic plants, developing methods for assessing toxicity to emergent macrophytes.

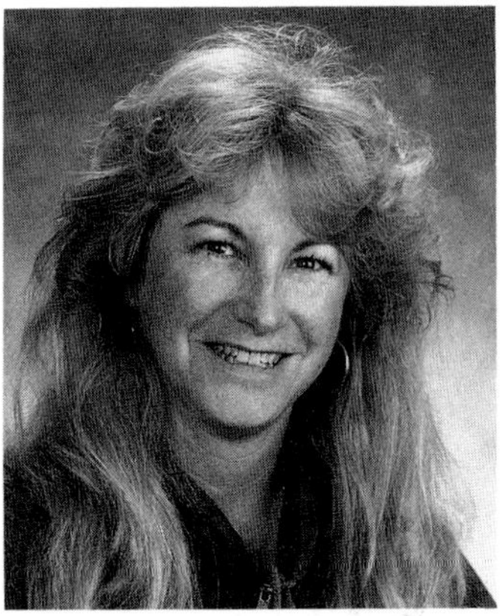

Marcia K. Nelson is the Outreach Coordinator for the Environmental and Contaminants Research Center of the USGS and an environmental scientist and educator with expertise in aquatic toxicology and ecology, environmental education, and public relations. Ms. Nelson earned an MS in biology from Central Missouri State University and continued graduate studies in ecology and pharmacology at the University of Missouri-Columbia. In 1994, her outstanding work performance and promotion of young women in science earned her the Woman of the Year Award from the Missouri Chapter of Women in Government. She has been an active member in ASTM, the Wetlands Society, and Sigma Xi and is currently a member of the SETAC board of directors. Her research interests focus on invertebrate sediment and aquatic macrophyte toxicity test development, acid mine drainage contaminants, and assessment of contaminants in wetlands.

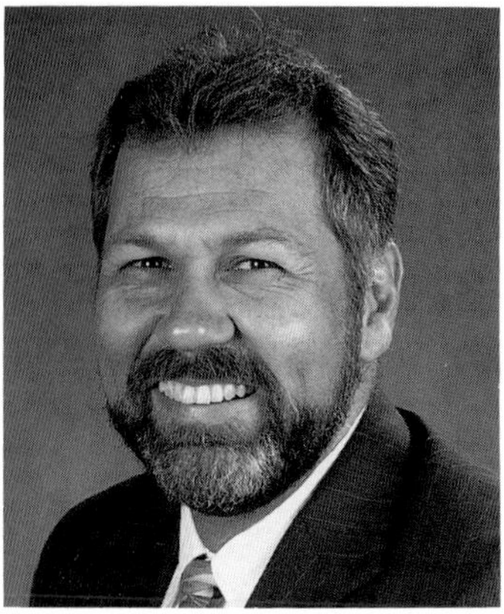

Stephen J. Klaine chairs the Department of Environmental Toxicology and the Institute of Wildlife and Environmental Toxicology at Clemson University. Between 1974 and 1982, he earned a B.S. in biology from the University of Cincinnati and an M.S. and Ph.D. from Rice University. While a professor at Memphis State University, he won research and teaching awards; in addition, he has been a Sigma Xi National Lecturer, won a National Research Council Fellowship, and received a Special SETAC Europe Service Award. Dr. Klaine's special interests include aquatic toxicology, ecological risk assessment, watershed assessment and management, and fate and effects of contaminants in natural and constructed wetlands.

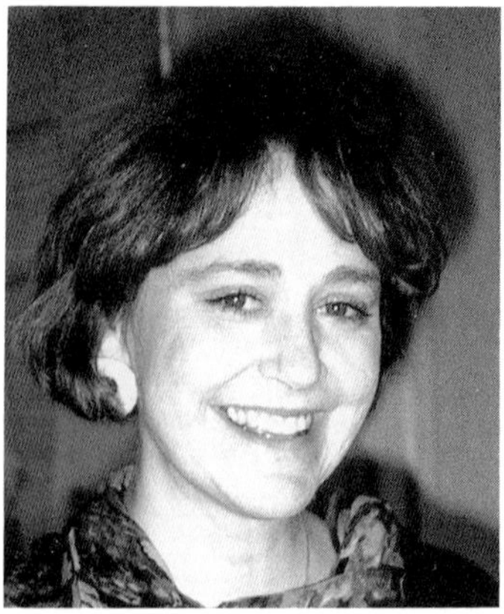

Mary G. Henry is chief of the Ecosystem Health Branch Division of Environmental Contaminants, U.S. Fish and Wildlife Service. A past member of the SETAC Board of Directors, she has also served SETAC as a short course committee chair. In 1974, she received a B.A. in biology from the University of Detroit, followed by an M.S. in environmental health from Purdue University in 1978 and a Ph.D. in animal ecology from Iowa State University in 1984. Dr. Henry is particularly interested in field–laboratory techniques to assess the biological impact of contaminants on natural resources.

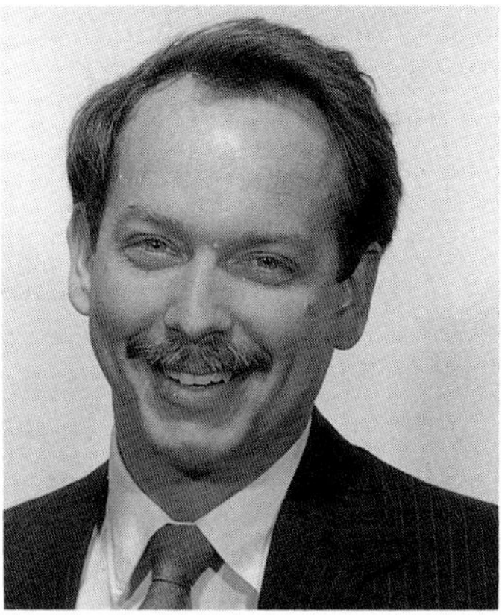

Gary W. Dickson is on assignment as the Global Head of Human Safety for Novartis Crop Protection in Basel, Switzerland. He holds a B.S. in biology from the University of Pittsburgh, an M.S. in biological sciences from Old Dominion University, and a Ph.D. in zoology from the University of Georgia. He has worked in various aspects of the environmental sciences, initially with the U.S. Environmental Protection Agency in Washington DC, followed by a number of positions within the crop protection industry. The Board of Environmental Professionals has designated him a Certified Environmental Professional, and Dr. Dickson is also a Senior Ecologist with the Ecological Society of America. In addition to his environmental pursuits, he is a captain in the U.S. Naval Reserves. Dr. Dickson is a charter member of SETAC and has served on the SETAC Board of Directors. His current interests include the environmental and human risk assessment of crop protection chemicals and management of research and development activities.

List of Attendees and Participants*

G. Ronnie Best
National Biological Service

James T. Blankemeyer
Oklahoma State University

Donald F. Boesch
Center for Estuarine & Environmental Studies

William J. Catallo
Louisiana State University

William Crumpton
Iowa State University

Gary W. Dickson
Ciba Plant Protection

Tom Dillon
EA Engineering

Kenneth R. Dixon
Clemson University

Philip B. Dorn
Shell Development Company

Anne Fairbrother
ecological planning & toxicology

Janis Farmer
BP Oil

Robert P. Gambrell
Louisiana State University

Robert A. Gearheart
Humboldt State University

Jerry F. Hall
Texaco

Judy Helgen
Minnesota Pollution Control Agency

Mary G. Henry
U.S. Fish and Wildlife Service

Donal D. Hook
Clemson University

Thomas Kelsch
U.S. Environmental Protection Agency

Stephen J. Klaine
Clemson University

A. Dennis Lemly
U.S. Forest Service

Michael A. Lewis
U.S. Environmental Protection Agency

Greg Linder
Heron Works Farm

Patrick Masscheleyn
University of Ghent

Foster Lee Mayer
U.S. Environmental Protection Agency

Beverly McFarland
Chevron Research & Technology Co.

William Mckee
U.S. Forest Service (retired)

Douglas Morrison
National Audubon Society

Marcia K. Nelson
U.S. Geological Survey
Biological Resources Division

Peter Nix
EVS Environment Consultants, Ltd.

John H. Pardue
Louisiana State University

* These affiliations were correct at the time of the workshop.

Gary A. Pascoe
EA Engineering, Science, & Technology

Hans G. Peterson
Saskatchewan Research Council

Rebecca Lynn Powell
Monsanto Company

Bruce Pugesek
U.S. Geological Survey
Biological Resources Division

Ramesh Reddy
University of Florida

Curtis J. Richardson
Duke Wetland Center

John H. Rodgers, Jr.
University of Mississippi

Pasquale F. Roscigno
U.S. Department of the Interior
Minerals Management Service

Terrence Salt
U.S. Department of the Interior

Geoffrey I. Scott
National Marine Fisheries Service

Jennifer L. Shaw
Zeneca Ag Products

Ralph G. Stahl, Jr.
E.I. Du Pont de Nemours & Co.

J. Kevin Summers
U.S. Environmental Protection Agency

Russell Theriot
U.S. Army Corps of Engineers

Dennis P. Tierney
Ciba Crop Protection

CHAPTER 1

Introduction

Wetlands such as those shown in Figure 1-1 provide many benefits, including food and habitat for fish and wildlife, water quality improvement, flood protection, shoreline erosion control, and opportunities for recreation and aesthetic appreciation. A number of classification systems are currently used to distinguish major wetland categories in the United States. These categories, based on location, include palustrine (forested wetlands, marshes, and swamps), lacustrine (wetlands bordering lakes), riverine (wetlands bordering rivers and streams), estuarine (salt marshes, mangrove swamps), and marine (intertidal and subtidal vegetation beds). Estimates of the value of these wetlands to commercial and recreational fisheries range from $2,200/acre on the Pacific coast to $10,000/acre on the Florida coast. Because of these values, efforts for wetland preservation have increased during the last decade.

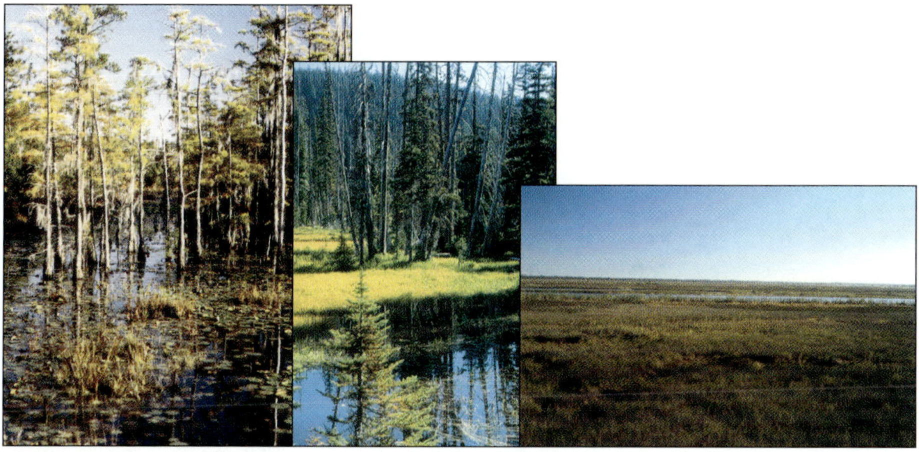

Figure 1-1 Examples of the many types of wetlands in the U.S.

CHAPTER PREVIEW

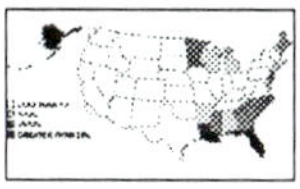

Ecotoxicology and Risk Assessment for Wetlands. Michael A. Lewis et al., editors.

It is estimated that in the 1600s more than 88 million hectares of wetlands existed in the contiguous 48 states; however, by the mid-1980s, wetlands in the lower 48 states were reduced to approximately 41.2 million hectares, the majority of which were located in the southeast (Figure 1-2). Six states have lost 85% or more of their wetlands and 22 have lost 50% or more because of habitat destruction and water quality deterioration (Dahl 1990; Dahl and Johnson 1991). Approximately 18% of aquatic and wetland plant species and as much as 35 to 37% of the fish and amphibian species are at risk.

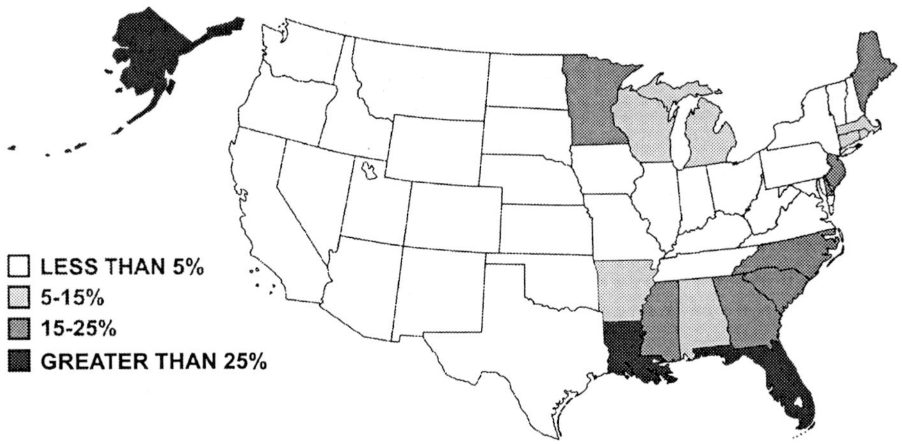

Figure 1-2 Relative abundance of wetlands in the U.S. (adapted from USEPA 1988)

The loss of wetland area continues to occur; the average annual loss is estimated at 183,200 hectares (176,000 hectares of inland wetlands and 7,200 hectares of coastal wetlands). The reasons for this decline and degradation include mining, dredging and draining, energy and urban development, and a variety of point-source and nonpoint-source contaminants. It has been estimated that, as a result of these activities, 65% of wetlands are contaminated with xenobiotic waste or toxic waste materials. The scientific community has begun to determine the impact of these activities and toxic chemicals on wetland fauna and flora and on wetland ecology, but limited information exists. Assessment methods have varied (Danielson 1998), and the database is scattered throughout the scientific literature. For these reasons, a basic understanding of these effects on the trophic levels in wetlands has not yet been achieved. Therefore, there is a need for a comprehensive summary of the current state of the knowledge related to wetland hazard assessments, not only to assist regulatory agencies in establishing protective strategies and restoring wetlands but also to provide direction for future scientific research.

Ecotoxicology and Risk Assessment for Wetlands Workshop Goals

Many workshops have been held during the past 5 years to discuss various issues related to wetland assessment, categorization, and protection. In addition, reviews have been published, such as the 1993 annual review issue of *Environmental Toxicology and Chemistry* (Volume 12, Number 12), which was devoted to wetland ecotoxicology and chemistry. However, at the time of this workshop, few workshops or publications have dealt specifically with contaminant hazard assessment procedures pertaining to wetlands, and fewer still have focused on the overall risk assessment process for these unique ecosystems. Consequently, the Society of Environmental Toxicology and Chemistry (SETAC) sponsored the Pellston workshop Ecotoxicology and Risk Assessment for Wetlands, which was held near Anaconda, Montana from 30 July–3 August 1995, to discuss these issues and to develop a better understanding of the fate and effects of contaminants and other stressors on freshwater and estuarine wetlands. More specifically, the workshop was designed to enable participants to

1) discuss the basic types of freshwater and saltwater wetlands and their unique ecologies and geochemistries,
2) determine the amount of information available concerning the extent of damage to wetland flora and fauna caused by specific contaminants,
3) evaluate the current laboratory and field methodologies used to assess the effects of toxicants, nutrients, and nonchemical stressors on wetland flora and fauna,
4) present case studies that give perspectives on assessments of wetlands' response to different stressors,
5) discuss wetlands ecological risk assessment procedures in general and in the context of current regulations and regulatory issues,
6) discuss the value of constructed wetlands in risk mitigations, and
7) provide recommendations for future research.

Workshop Approach and Workgroups

The workshop consisted of plenary session presentations, discussions by 5 workgroups, a Superfund site visit, and presentation of 4 site-specific studies of wetland ecological risk assessments. The plenary presentations covered discussion topics such as wetland definition, biogeochemical characteristics, effects of contaminants on freshwater and coastal wetlands, wetland regulations, constructed wetlands, and risk assessment strategies.

The 45 workshop participants represented an interdisciplinary mix of individuals from government, industry, academia, and public interest groups. These participants were assigned to the following 5 workgroups, chaired by experts in each field.

1) Biogeochemical processes: William J. Catallo, Wetland Biogeochemistry Institute, Louisiana State University
2) Contaminant fate and effects in freshwater wetlands: A. Dennis Lemly, U.S. Forest Service
3) Contaminant fate and effects in coastal and estuarine wetlands: Donald F. Boesch, University of Maryland, Center for Estuarine and Environmental Studies
4) Regulatory issues and risk assessment: Thomas Kelsch, U.S. Environmental Protection Agency, Office of Wetlands, Oceans and Watersheds
5) Constructed wetlands as a risk mitigation alternative: John H. Rodgers, Jr., University of Mississippi

The 4 case studies of wetland risk assessment and their presenters were as follows.

1) Clark Fork River/Milltown Reservoir Wetland by Greg L. Linder, Heron Works Farm
2) Kesterson National Wildlife Refuge by A. Dennis Lemly, U.S. Forest Service
3) Ecotoxicological Assessment of Nonpoint Source Runoff in a South Carolina Coastal Wetland by Dana B. Finley, Geoffrey I. Scott, James W. Daugomah, and Sean L. Layman
4) Everglades/South Florida by Terrence Salt, U.S. Department of Interior

A brief description of each workgroup's topic appears below.

Biogeochemical processes

Biogeochemical processes are directly relevant to issues in wetland ecotoxicology because the deposition, fate, and effects of toxic materials are influenced by sediment, biota, and water parameters, which in turn are affected by the presence of toxicants. The principal objectives of the Biogeochemistry Workgroup were to review and provide recommendations for further study on the following issues:

1) effects of contaminants and nonchemical stressors on biogeochemical processes in wetlands,
2) relationships of these stressors to the ecological functioning of wetlands and connecting watersheds,
3) linkages between sediment–plant processes and ecological functioning of wetlands,
4) analytical and conceptual techniques for integrating ecological processes, and
5) experimental and analytical techniques for monitoring process outputs from wetlands and evaluating significant changes that may result from contamination.

Important fate and transport processes for toxic organics in wetland systems were outlined, and biogeochemical indicators were evaluated in relation to the effects of contaminants on water quality and biological productivity of wetlands. The biogeochemical functions of wetlands that are used as indicators were divided into microbial, physicochemical, and transport processes.

Contaminant fate and effects in freshwater wetlands

The main objectives of the Freshwater Wetlands Workgroup were to provide a critical review of the topic area, propose new assessment approaches, and recommend future research needs for the following:

1) hazard assessment approaches to wetland ecotoxicology and risk assessment;
2) an ecosystem approach to integrating ecology, hydrology, geomorphology, and wetland soils;
3) application of the ecosystem approach to wetland-specific risk assessment; and
4) evaluation of case studies using the ecosystem approach.

Several important considerations were identified for ecotoxicology and risk assessment in freshwater wetlands. The most fundamental of these was recognizing that most of the remaining freshwater wetlands in the U.S. are altered from their natural state because of changes in hydrology and surrounding land use. In addition, it was necessary to place the risk assessment process into an ecological context. This involved identifying and integrating the principal ecosystem processes (ecology, hydrology, geomorphology, soils) that serve to structure wetlands, while determining contaminant transport, chemical speciation, and biological exposure and effects.

Contaminant fate and effects in coastal and estuarine wetlands

The primary objectives of the Coastal Wetlands Workgroup were to review the topic area, discuss the current scientific knowledge, and recommend needed research. The discussions centered on

1) the characteristics and processes that are unique to or are of unusual importance in coastal and estuarine wetlands, with a focus on contaminant effects and fate;
2) definition of reference conditions, including the consideration of natural variability of physicochemical conditions;
3) use of interpretative models that consider both the direct effects of contaminants and cascading indirect effects;
4) determination of the effects of contaminants on the bioaccumulative potential of populations of important resident and migratory species; and
5) determination of the effects that environmental factors have on storage and release of contaminants and on their bioavailability.

Regulatory issues and risk assessment

The discussions in the Regulatory Issues and Risk Assessment Workgroup centered on identifying regulations pertaining to wetlands and providing a brief explanation of each. The ecological risk assessment process was reviewed in relation to unique aspects of wetlands, and a framework was developed for conducting this process. The applicability of numerical, biological, and narrative criteria to wetlands assessments was also discussed. It was concluded that the ability to utilize the ecological risk assessment approach to address ecotoxicology in wetlands is data-driven, and it is necessary to identify and fill technical data gaps, as well as to develop methods and models to process the data at various spatial and temporal scales. Three new approaches and methods for assessing ecosystem-level effects in the risk assessment process were discussed:

1) establishment of a wetlands biological index of integrity similar in concept to the Index of Biotic Integrity (IBI);
2) development of a multi-endpoint approach, identifying a range of "norms" for each endpoint that will allow a ranking of condition from very poor to excellent without the use of reference or control sites; and
3) derivation of a process-based endpoint approach to the effects portion of risk assessment that would supplement the common measurement endpoints of survival, growth, and reproduction.

Constructed wetlands as a risk mitigation alternative

Detailed discussion points in the Constructed Wetlands Workgroup included a history of wetlands used in a wastewater treatment context and reasons for the movement from use of natural to constructed wetlands for this purpose. Design issues surrounding construction of wetlands were discussed and included hydrological considerations, scale, site selection, cost, maintenance, longevity, capacity, and success criteria. Important scientific issues were stressed, including treatment performance versus ecological compatibility, selection of wetland functions and values to be optimized, classes of chemicals appropriate for treatment, and the regulatory context for dealing with constructed wetlands, along with risk assessment and risk management aspects. In addition to the discussion points, several activities were completed:

1) evaluation of the potential of constructed wetlands for treating point and nonpoint sources,
2) creation of a decision-making support system to aid in implementing constructed wetlands and dealing with risk management issues, and
3) discussion and evaluation of case studies delineating the performance of constructed wetlands.

Workshop Proceedings

The Ecotoxicology and Risk Assessment for Wetlands Workshop was very successful and met its intended objectives. The published proceedings of the workshop include a plenary presentation, reports from the 5 discussion workgroups, and 3 case studies. A synthesis chapter integrates the important aspects of the plenary session, case studies, and workgroups and includes a summary of the recommendations for future research. Overall, this publication provides a scientific and regulatory synthesis of critical environmental information that is essential to assess and prevent any additional decline in wetland resources from anthropogenic contamination.

References

Dahl TE. 1990. Wetlands losses in the United States 1780's to 1980's. Washington DC: U.S. Department of the Interior (USDOI), Fish and Wildlife Service.

Dahl TE and Johnson CE. 1991. Status and trends of wetlands in the conterminous United States, mid-1970's to mid-1980's. Washington DC: U.S. Department of the Interior (USDOI), Fish and Wildlife Service. 28 p.

Danielson TJ. 1998. Wetland bioassessment fact sheets. Washington DC: U.S. Environmental Protection Agency (USEPA), Wetlands Division. EPA/843/F-98/001.

[USEPA] United States Environmental Protection Agency. 1988. America's wetlands, our vital link between land and water. Washington DC: Office of Wetlands Protection. EPA/87/016.

Chapter 2

Plenary Session Presentation: Ecological Functions of Wetlands in the Landscape

Curtis J. Richardson

Wetlands comprise nearly 6% of the earth's land surface and are found at every latitude from the frozen tundra to the tropics. Wetlands link terrestrial and aquatic systems and have a global similarity of water supply such that these lands have water at or near the surface of the ground for much of the year. The massive conversion of wetlands to agriculture, forestry, and urban uses resulted in the loss of 53% (89 million hectares to 42 million hectares) of the wetland habitats in the U.S. during the period from 1780 to 1980 (Dahl 1990). In addition, nearly 65% of the wetlands in the U.S. are contaminated with xenobiotic waste or toxic waste materials that have been dumped near sites draining to these ecosystems (Mitsch and Gosselink 1993; U.S. Environmental Protection Agency [USEPA] unpublished report 1993). Native plants and animals living in wetlands are uniquely adapted to live under conditions of intermittent flooding, lack of oxygen (anoxia), and harsh, often toxic conditions of reduced chemical species (e.g., H_2S rather than SO_4, and Mn^{+2} versus Mn^{+4}). The generic term "wetland" is now used worldwide and includes specific ecosystems known regionally as bogs, bottomlands, carr, fens, floodplains, mangroves, marshes, mires, moors, muskegs, playas, peatlands, pocosins, potholes, reedswamps, sloughs, swamps, wet meadows, and wet prairies. The term "wetlands" is used collectively to describe a great diversity of ecosystems worldwide whose formation and existence is controlled by water. Permanently flooded, deep water areas (generally greater than 2 m) are not considered wetlands. Wetlands form part of a continuous water gradient from the drier upland to the continuously wet, open water ecosystems on the landscape. Thus, the upper and lower limits of a wetland are somewhat arbitrary—a fact causing consid-

Chapter Preview

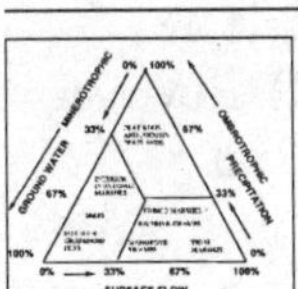

Ecotoxicology and Risk Assessment for Wetlands. Michael A. Lewis et al., editors.
 ISBN 1-880611-16-3

erable problems in the legal determination of what is defined as the wetland area regulated under Section 404 of the 1977 Clean Water Act (CWA). No formal or universally recognized definition of wetlands existed until the U.S. Fish and Wildlife Service (USFWS) in 1979, after years of review, posed the following comprehensive definition (Cowardin et al. 1979):

Wetlands are lands transitional between terrestrial and aquatic systems where the water table is usually at or near the surface or the land is covered by shallow water. Wetlands must have 1 or more of the following 3 attributes:

1) at least periodically, the land supports predominantly hydrophytes (water-loving plants),
2) the substrate is predominantly undrained hydric soil (wet soils), and
3) the substrate is nonsoil and is saturated with water or covered by shallow water at some time during the growing season of each year.

This definition, although comprehensive and useful for the purposes of classification and mapping of wetlands, does not lend itself to the legal definition of wetlands. In 1987, 4 federal agencies (U.S. Army Corps of Engineers [USACOE], USEPA, Soil Conservation Service, and USFWS) collaborated and developed an "accepted" jurisdictional wetland definition which, unlike the USFWS definition, is more restrictive because it must meet all 3 attributes USACOE 1987). In simple terms a jurisdictional wetland must have hydric or waterlogged soils, 50% or more of the dominant plants must be wetland plants, and the water table must be found within 30 cm of the ground surface during 7 days of the growing season.

Wetland Functions

Wetland functions or processes can be placed in 5 ecosystem-level categories: hydrologic flux, productivity, decomposition, biogeochemical cycling, and community and wildlife habitat (Richardson 1994). Because not all wetlands function equally, the importance of each process depends on wetland type. Additionally, these functions and processes are lost once the wetland is drained. The introduction of contaminants or toxic waste materials also greatly alters wetland functions and, in turn, the wetland values that can be derived from these ecosystems. Values ascribed to wetlands include providing habitats for hunting, fishing, waterfowl, timber harvesting, wastewater assimilation, and flood control (Table 2-1). However, there is a lack of understanding that wetland values can be sustained only if ecosystem functions are maintained.

In this paper, wetland functions and values and discussions of the potential effects of contaminant additions on ecosystem functional rates are reviewed. In addition, the potential impacts of introducing hazardous or toxic waste materials are introduced briefly, using selenium and mercury as case examples of how biogeochemical processes in wetlands can affect the availability of these heavy metals.

Table 2-1 Attributes generally reported as functions and values of wetland ecosystems

Wetland Functions

1. Hydrologic flux and storage
   a. aquifer (ground water) recharge to wetland and/or discharge from the ecosystem
   b. water storage reservoir and regulator
   c. regional stream hydrology (discharge and recharge)
   d. regional climate control (evapotranspiration export = large-scale atmospheric losses of H_2O)
2. Biological productivity
   a. net primary productivity
   b. carbon storage
   c. carbon fixation
   d. secondary productivity
3. Biogeochemical cycling and storage
   a. nutrient source or sink on the landscape
   b. C, N, S, P, etc., transformations (oxidation/reduction reactions)
   c. denitrification
   d. sediment and organic matter reservoir
4. Decomposition
   a. carbon release (global climate impacts)
   b. detritus output for aquatic organisms (downstream energy source)
   c. mineralization and release of N, S, C, etc.
5. Community and wildlife habitat
   a. habitat for species
   b. habitat for algae, bacteria, fungi, fish, shellfish, wildlife, and wetland plants
   c. biodiversity

Wetland Values

Value	Functions
1. Flood control (conveyance), flood storage	1, 2[a]
2. Sediment control (filter for waste)	3, 2
3. Wastewater treatment system	3, 2
4. Nutrient removal from agricultural runoff and wastewater systems	3, 2
5. Recreation	5, 1
6. Open space	1, 2, 5
7. Visual-cultural	1, 5
8. Hunting (fur-bearers, beavers, muskrats)	5, 2
9. Preservation of flora and fauna (endemic, refuge)	5
10. Timber production	2, 1
11. Shrub crops (cranberry and blueberry)	2, 1
12. Medical (streptomycin)	5, 4
13. Education and research	1–5
14. Erosion control	1, 2, 3
15. Food production (shrimp, fish, ducks)	2, 5
16. Historical, cultural, and archaeological resources	2
17. Threatened, rare, endangered species habitat	5
18. Water quality	3, 1
19. Water supply	1

[a] Denotes wetland values that are directly related to wetland functions (1–5), or those functions that can be adversely affected by overutilization of values. The order of the numbers suggests which primary function is most directly or first affected.

Source: Richardson 1994. Reprinted with permission from the Society of Wetland Scientists © 1994.

Hydrology

Despite their diversity, all wetlands have one thing in common: their formation, processes, and characteristics are controlled by water. To categorize wetlands on the landscape, it is necessary to analyze the relative proportion of 3 water sources that flow to wetlands—precipitation, groundwater discharge, and lateral surface flow—as well as to determine their topographic position on the landscape (Brinson 1993).

The hydrologic function of wetlands on the landscape is determined by the type (e.g., depressional, riverine, fringe, or fen), topographical position (i.e., proximity to large or small streams or lakes), overall size, and connection to ground water. It is critical to understand the hydrologic relationships of wetlands to water supply on the landscape, because contamination of ground water or downstream areas is often the result of the introduction of pollutants directly into wetlands. Many of these introductions are done intentionally to utilize the biogeochemical processes of wetlands (e.g., oxidation/reduction reactions) to store these pollutants or alter their chemical state to reduce downstream impacts (Kadlec and Knight 1996). However, understanding the importance of the water source to the wetland is critical to understanding the potential effects of chemical introductions to these ecosystems.

The relationship of major wetland types, when scaled according to the relative importance of water sources (Figure 2-1, Richardson 1994), shows that bogs and pocosins are ombrotrophic, receiving their water almost exclusively from rainfall and as such are nutrient poor, or oligotrophic. In contrast, fens, seeps, and some marsh types are controlled by groundwater inputs; these wetlands are minerotrophic, nourished by minerals from the ground and are often more nutrient rich, or eutrophic. Surface-flow-dominated wetland types are very diverse and include swamps, salt marshes, and wetlands found along the fringes of lakes and streams.

The positions of these wetland types relative to each other on the landscape are best displayed when scaled out along axes of both water regime and nutrients (Figure 2-2). The nutrient content of vegetation and soils is lowest in the bogs and increases along the fen, marsh, and swamp gradient. In contrast, the amount of peat formation decreases along this gradient because of increased decay (decomposition) of organic matter (OM) in enriched sites with higher pH and longer dry periods. The biomass of trees in proportion to shrubs in bogs is generally low, but forest species increase to become dominant in swamps. The duration of the hydroperiod (seasonal pattern of water level at or near the surface) ranges from permanently flooded for 12 months in the lacustrine (shallow lake) wetland to between 6 and 9 months in the bogs and as little as 2 weeks in some swamp systems. The seasonal magnitude of water-level change ranges from as little as 0.5 m in bogs to more than 7 m in tropical swamp forest systems. Thus, the amount of rainfall versus surface or ground water can be used to separate the general types of wetlands, bog, fens, marshes, and swamps. The amount of peat formation and tree productivity is related to nutrient content, acidity, and length of time the soil is covered by water.

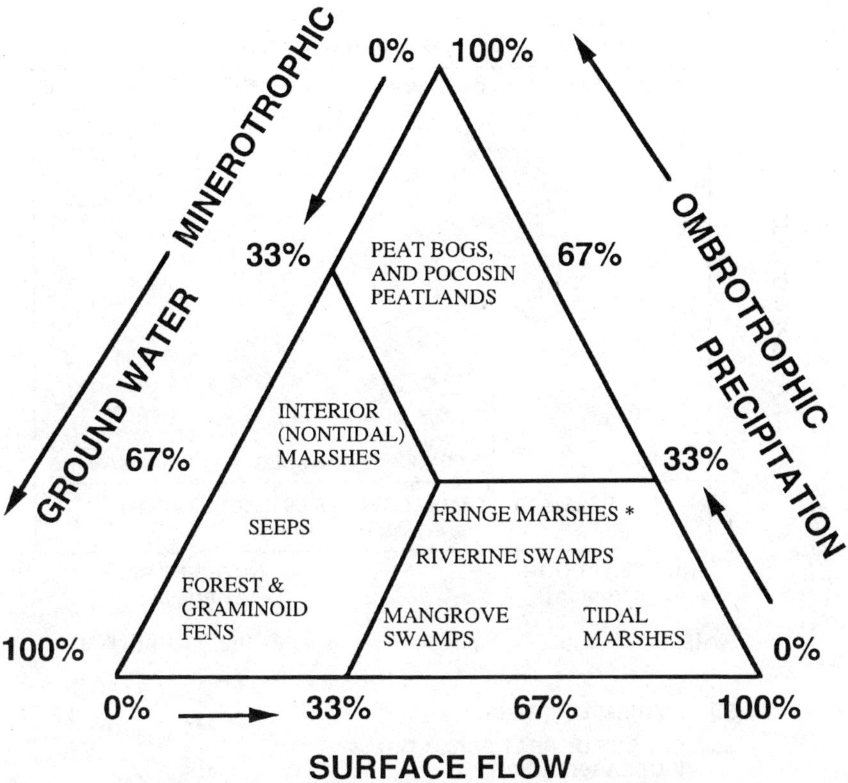

Figure 2-1 Relative importance of water source to major wetland types (modified from Brinson 1993). The percentage of water contributions to a wetland from precipitation, ground water, or surface flow creates different types of wetlands. Ombrotrophic bogs lack groundwater contributions and upstream inflow. Minerotrophic wetlands, such as fens, receive water and minerals from ground water. (*Includes both lacustrine and estuarine marshes.)

Many wetlands, including bogs, pocosins, peatlands, and marshes, function as "water pumps" on the landscape, losing nearly two-thirds of their annual water inputs by evapotranspiration (ET), leaving only 30% or less for annual runoff or groundwater recharge (Figure 2-3a). Prime pothole marshes lose most of their water by ET (Figure 2-3a). Bogs are ombrotrophic, receiving most of their water by rain and losing almost none to ground water (Figure 2-3b). The large portion of annual runoff from raised bogs, where the water table is elevated above the regional water table, is in spring, after the winter snow melt, or after the bog peat has filled with rain because of low winter ET rates. The peat soils of these systems act much like a sponge on the landscape, holding and slowly releasing vast quantities of rainfall when the peat is drier and rapidly giving up water when the sponge is full. Many small kettle-hole bogs of the northern U.S. have no flowing outlets and lose almost all of their water by ET. Because of their size, often 20,000 hectares or more,

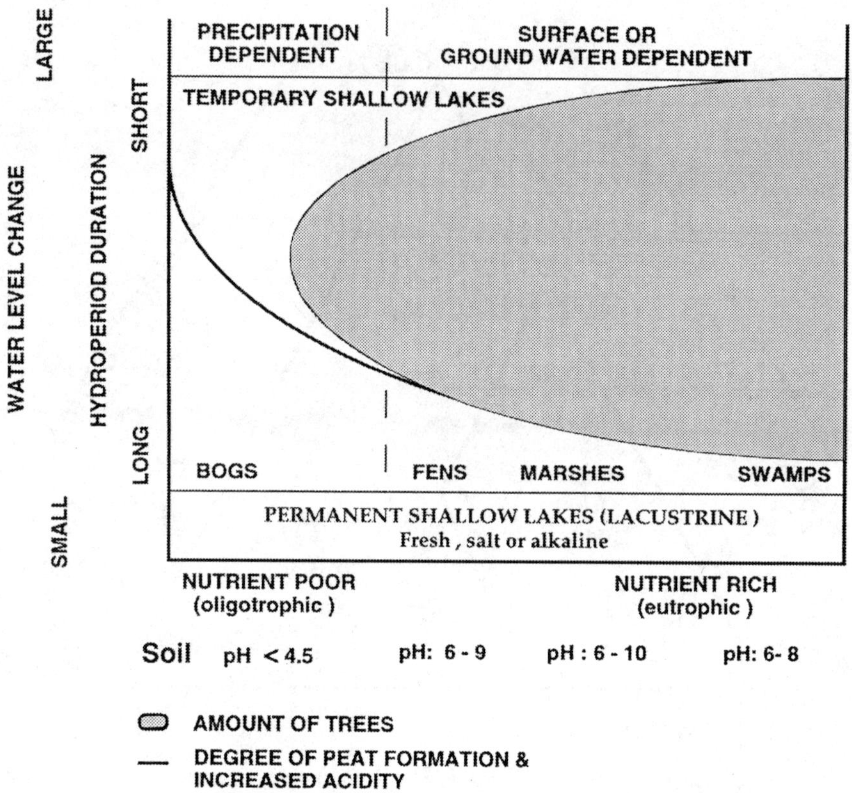

Figure 2-2 Types of wetlands found along gradients of nutrients (X axis) and water regimes (Y axis) (modified from Gopal et al. 1990). Swamps are dominated by trees under both long and short hydroperiods. Water-level changes within wetland types vary from permanently flooded or long hydroperiods and small water-level changes (lacustrine marshes) to those with short hydroperiods and large water-level changes (tropical swamp forests).

pocosins slowly lose water by surface and subsurface runoff, which is then distributed over broad areas to the surrounding lakes, rivers, and estuaries. The proportion of water inflow compared to rainfall varies greatly, with swamps receiving most of their inputs by stream flow (Figure 2-3c). They also gain and lose some water to shallow aquifers beneath them. Swamp stream flow comprises the largest loss, although the water can be held for months and released more slowly than in areas where the vegetation is removed. Fen systems are flow-through systems with runoff often exceeding ET, especially during ice thaw periods in the spring. The annual flow from minerotrophic fens to ground water is very uniform through the year (Figure 2-3d).

Wetlands can be an important source or sink of regional surface and ground water supplies kilometers away from the actual wetland itself. Recent studies (Winter 1989) have shown that the relationship between the regional water table and

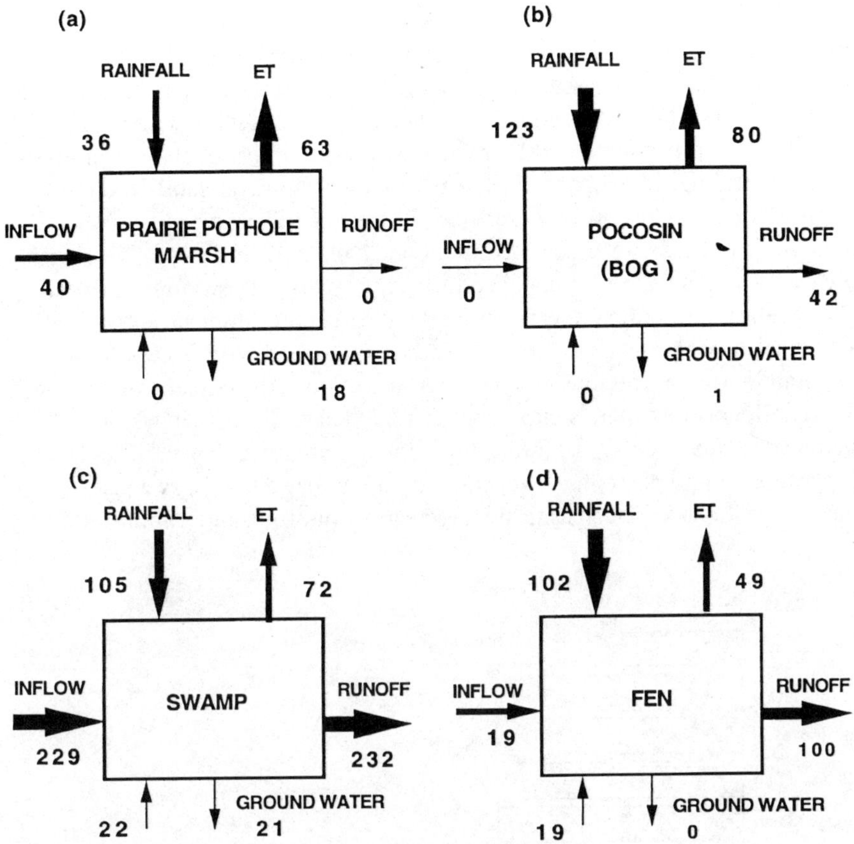

Figure 2-3 Annual water budgets in cm/y for a) a prairie pothole marsh in North Dakota, b) a pocosin bog in North Carolina, c) an alluvial cypress swamp in southern Illinois, USA, and d) a rich fen in North Wales, UK (data from Mitsch and Gosselink 1993 and Richardson 1994.)

wetlands is more complex and dynamic than once thought and that seasonal reversals of groundwater flow often occur among wetlands and between wetlands and lakes. This suggests that the drainage of a wetland in one area or the placement of pollutants in connected areas may have serious consequences for water quality in lakes, ground water, other wetlands, or downstream areas that are not readily evident without detailed hydrologic studies. It has also been demonstrated that peak stream flows are only 20% as large in basins with 40% lake and wetland areas as they are in similar basins with no lake or wetland area. Studies by Johnston et al. (1990) have shown a relationship between the amount of wetland area on the landscape and stormwater flow peaks. These data suggest that when less than 10% of the watershed is in wetlands, significant peak flows occur and contaminants can be easily moved downstream.

Primary productivity

Wetlands are among the most productive ecosystems in the world. Their rates of primary productivity greatly exceed those of grasslands, cultivated lands, and most forests (Figure 2-4). The most productive wetlands are cattail, salt marsh, and reed grass marshes. Their production of above- and below-ground annual plant biomass is double that of sedge marshes or bogs, fens, and muskegs. Grasslands and croplands of the U.S. produce only one-fourth of the fiber of the most productive wetlands, while upland forests produce about one-half. Only the tropical rain forest comes close to matching the primary productivity of mangrove swamps or cattail and salt marshes. This biomass serves as food for a great multitude of both aquatic and terrestrial animals as well as for many species that are endemic to wetlands. Thus, contamination of the soils and biomass, and in turn, the higher trophic levels, with xenobiotics or trace metals may result in a significant decrease in wetland productivity. Because insects, fish, waterfowl, and mammals all depend heavily on marsh plant seeds and plants for food, contamination may also lead to a loss of wetland values (Table 2-1) such as fishing, recreation, hunting, and wildlife habitat.

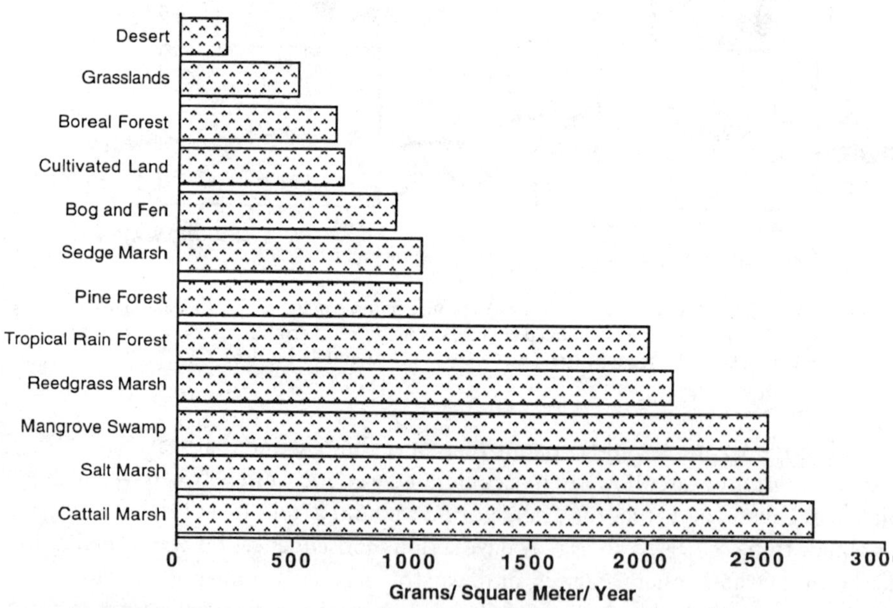

Figure 2-4 Comparison of net primary productivity by ecosystem type (Richardson 1995. Reprinted with permission from Academic Press ©1995.)

Decomposition

A unique feature of wetlands compared to terrestrial ecosystems is that dead plants and animals do not decay as fast, especially in acid peatlands (Chamie and Richardson 1978). The decomposition rate in peatlands is only one-half to one-quarter the rates of the more aerobic uplands (Mitsch and Gosselink 1993). When leaves, stems, and roots die in upland systems, they normally are shredded by macroinvertebrates, earthworms, nematodes, and microbes. The complex OM, which is 45% carbon by weight, usually decays to CO_2 and H_2O within 1 year in terrestrial ecosystems, and the mineral elements are released for new growth. Anaerobic conditions slow the decay rates in wetlands, not only because of a lack of oxygen but also because of low pH, shortages of calcium, and low soil temperatures. These anaerobic conditions also eliminate most of the decomposer organisms like filamentous fungi, and the existing anaerobic bacteria obtain energy by inefficient processes like fermentation. Very reduced soils (i.e., no NO_3 or SO_4 present) release important greenhouse gases like methane and hydrogen as "marsh gas." Normal metabolism is so greatly reduced in wetlands that many of these ecosystems slowly build up peat at 1 to 2 mm/y on average (Craft and Richardson 1993). Moreover, peatlands store vast quantities of carbon and help balance the global carbon cycle (Gorham 1991). The introduction of toxics or waste materials that greatly alter the decomposition process will result in a shift in the balance between wetland productivity and decomposition and, in turn, between the storage and release of carbon as well as other nutrients and metals. For example, it has been shown that the introduction of copper can greatly decrease decomposition and alter the growth of bacteria, algae, and fungi (Mather et al. 1979).

Biogeochemical cycling

One of the main ecological functions of wetlands is their ability to transform, cycle, and act as a sink for nutrients. They have been shown to filter and hold 60 to 90% of the suspended solids and sediments from wastewater additions and agricultural water runoff prior to water discharge into streams and lakes (Richardson and Nichols 1985). Wetlands maintain among the widest range of oxidized and reduced chemical states of all ecosystems because of their periodic flooding and drying cycles. The unique shift from aerobic (free oxygen present) to anaerobic (no free oxygen) soil conditions provides these systems with the ability to process PO_4, NO_3, SO_4, and C and to release gases (N_2O, H_2S, CH_4, CO_2) to the atmosphere, thus affecting biosphere-level problems such as acid rain, global warming, and greenhouse gases. One example of these transformations is shown by the nitrogen cycle (Faulkner and Richardson 1989). Nitrogen transformations are a complex assortment of microbially mediated processes and chemical reactions strongly influenced by the redox status (degree of reduced or anaerobic conditions) of the wetland soils (Figure 2-5). Most flooded wetland soils have a thin, oxidized layer at the surface caused by the proximity to air or higher dissolved oxygen in overlying floodwater. The reduced layer below dominates the soil and lower water-column processes and prevents upland plants, bacteria, and animals from invading these ecosystems because the oxygen required for normal metabolism is lacking. Multiple biotic and abiotic transformations take place in these layers and involve 7 valence states (+5 to –3) and the formation of such oxidized nitrogen species as nitrate (NO_3^-), nitrite

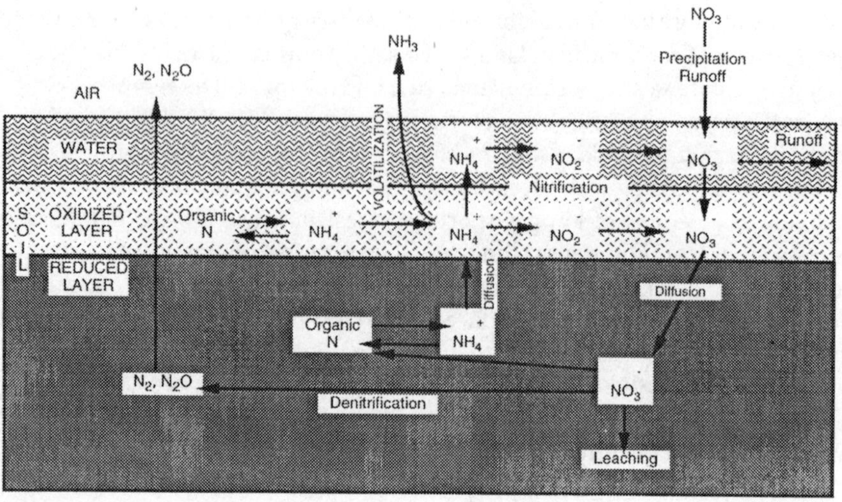

Figure 2-5 Nitrogen transformations in wetlands (reprinted with permission from Faulkner SP, Richardson CJ. 1989. Physical and chemical characteristics of freshwater wetland soils. In: Hammer DA, editor. Constructed wetlands for wastewater treatment. Chelsea MI: Lewis. p 41–72. Copyright CRC Press, Boca Raton, Florida.

(NO_2^-), and nitrogen dioxide gas (N_2O), as well as the reduced ammonium ion (NH_4^+). Organic N is mineralized in both the reduced and oxidized layers to NH_4^+. The thin oxidized zone is where NH_4^+ is oxidized to NO_3^- by bacteria (nitrification). In the reduced layer, NH_4^+ is stable and may be adsorbed to sediment or utilized by plants and microbes for growth. Any NO_3^- that diffuses downward in this zone is denitrified (microbially converted) to N_2 or N_2O and released to the atmosphere as a gas. Thus, wetlands provide one of the key ecosystem processes that keeps N in global circulation. Therefore, the most unique wetland functions may be related to their ability to transform ions, given that these systems maintain the widest range of oxidation/reduction reactions on the landscape. Thus, the biogeochemical process that these systems possess may be used to reduce toxic materials on the landscape, especially in wetlands constructed to optimize varying states of oxidation and reduction. However, any major alteration of these cycles by introduction of toxic materials must be avoided.

An example of one of these toxic problems as related to biogeochemical processing concerns the introduction of heavy metals, salts, and acids to wetlands (Kadlec and Knight 1996). One critical case was the introduction of selenium to the Kesterson National Wildlife Refuge in Merced County, California. Concentrations as high as 300 μg/L of Se were found in agricultural irrigation return flows as compared to average world river Se concentrations of 0.1 μg/L (Ohlendorf et al. 1990). This elevated Se was found in all trophic levels and resulted in significant reductions in aquatic bird reproduction. For example, plants contained about 52.1 mg/kg dry weight (dw) of Se in Kesterson as compared to 0.43 mg/kg dw at the nearby Volta

Wildlife Area, which did not receive agricultural runoff. Bird breast muscle at Kesterson contained concentrations between 10 and 110 mg/kg dw as compared to 2.5 to 13.2 mg/kg dw at Volta (Ohlendorf et al. 1990). The "Kesterson Effect," the bioconcentration of Se in arid wetlands receiving agricultural drainage, is considered a major problem in the western U.S. (Lemly 1993; Lemly et al. 1993). (See Chapter 6 for more details concerning the Kesterson National Wildlife Refuge.)

The global spread of anthropogenic pollutants is becoming an increasingly urgent problem, but in many cases the contaminants of concern are naturally occurring substances whose normal biogeochemical cycles have been disturbed by human activity. Mercury is another such substance whose biogeochemistry has been closely studied because of its great toxic potential; its movement through ecosystems is substantially influenced by microbial processes (Wood 1974). Microbial transformation of inorganic Hg into methylmercury (MeHg) serves as an important pathway for the transfer of this element from soils and water to biota (Winfrey and Rudd 1990; Gilmour and Henry 1991; Saouter et al. 1991). Recent discoveries that sulfur-reducing bacteria are responsible for most Hg methylation in the environment (Compeau and Bartha 1985) suggest that mercury cycling in freshwater wetlands needs to be closely examined even though sulfate-reducers are not generally thought to be important in these systems.

In wetlands characterized by organic soils, Hg is strongly bound to the OM, making it purportedly unavailable for uptake by the aquatic food chain (Zillioux et al. 1993). However, concentrations of MeHg in largemouth bass from the Everglades are the highest in the state of Florida (>3 ppm) (Hand and Friedman 1990) and greater than any concentration of total Hg in fish reported in the National Contaminant Biomonitoring Program of 1976–1984 (Schmitt and Brumbaugh 1990.) Also, mercury accumulation through the food web may have reduced the breeding success of wading birds (Frederick and Spalding 1994; Spalding et al. 1994) and the viability of the endangered Florida panther population (Roelke et al. 1991). Consequently, there is widespread concern that Hg contamination in the Everglades poses a serious hazard, both to the health of the public and to the ecosystem.

The mercury problem in south Florida may be related to

1) increased atmospheric deposition of Hg derived from anthropogenic sources such as urban emissions and burning of crop material (Sengar et al. 1989; KBN Engineering 1992; Patrick et al. 1994; Dvonch et al. 1995),
2) increased Hg in agricultural runoff due to enhanced oxidation of peat soil in agricultural land (Delfino et al. 1993; Stober et al. 1995), and
3) altered microbial and soil biogeochemical processes caused by eutrophication and perturbations of the natural hydroperiod.

Several monitoring studies have been initiated to assess atmospheric deposition and spatial distribution of Hg in soil of the Everglades (Delfino et al. 1993; Rood et al. 1995; Stober et al. 1995). A recent study shows that there is no relationship between methylation-to-demethylation ratios and soil P concentrations, suggesting that eutrophication and agricultural runoff have no effect on net MeHg formation (Vaithiyanathan et al. 1996). However, there is an urgent need to complete further process research with a thorough examination of the mechanisms controlling the transport and transformation of Hg within the Everglades ecosystem, if measures are to be taken to mitigate this problem.

Transformations of Hg in the environment are a key issue in any Hg contamination problem (Figure 2-6). The input of Hg from natural and anthropogenic sources is mostly in the inorganic form, but the Hg found in fish is almost exclusively in the methylated form (Huckabee et al. 1979; Grieb et al. 1990), even though fish do not themselves methylate Hg (Pennacchioni et al. 1976; Huckabee et al. 1978). The amount of MeHg that is available for bioaccumulation is a function of the rate of Hg methylation relative to the rate of methylmercury demethylation. Processes such as reduction, volatilization, adsorption, and precipitation are also important, as they regulate the concentration of ionic Hg, the substrate for methylation (Figure 2-6).

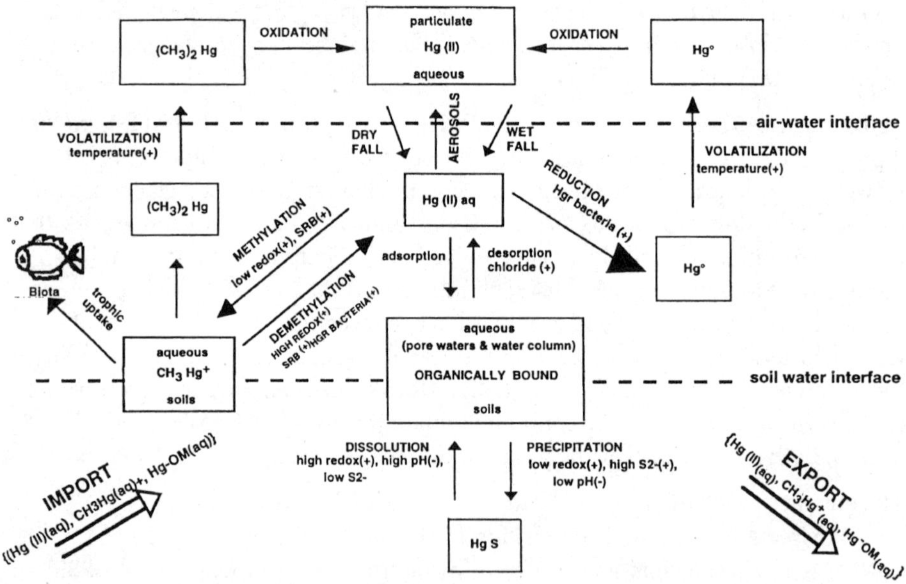

Figure 2-6 Hypothetical model for Hg cycling in wetlands. + indicates that the parameter has a positive effect on the process, while – indicates that the parameter has a negative effect on the process.

The nature of oxidative demethylation and its significance in the biogeochemical cycling of Hg in wetlands needs to be investigated, as the amount of MeHg available for biotic uptake is determined by the balance between methylation and demethylation reactions (Figure 2-6). In addition to bacterial methylation and demethylation of Hg, a number of Hg-resistant bacteria detoxify ionic Hg through the production of volatile elemental mercury (Hg^0) (Figure 2-6). This activity is mediated by the inducible *mer* (mercury resistance) operon and is found in some strains of all eubacterial species tested to date (Silver and Walderhaug 1992). This pathway contributes to the removal of Hg from highly contaminated natural waters where Hg concentrations reach the mg/L levels necessary to induce the *mer* operon (Barkay et al. 1991). However, the significance of this process in natural waters and wetlands with low Hg concentrations is not known. Other possible mechanisms of reduction and volatilization under these conditions are reduction by organic acids produced during photosynthesis (Ben-Bassat and Mayer 1978) and the abiotic reduction of Hg(II) to Hg(I) and the subsequent disproportionation to elemental and ionic mercury (Baltisburger et al. 1979). Reduction of Hg in wetlands most likely is due to the latter 2 mechanisms, as concentrations in the water are too low for *mer* operon induction (Richardson et al. 1995). Thus, the quantification of rates of Hg methylation, demethylation, and reduction/volatilization is a key factor in understanding the fate and transport of Hg in the wetlands environment.

The Hg problem in wetlands is global, as shown by a pattern of high Hg and/or MeHg levels associated with runoff from drained peatlands in Finland, Sweden, and Canada (Simola and Lodenius 1982; Westling 1991). If hypotheses about factors controlling Hg methylation are correct, projected changes in climate and land-use patterns at the global level are likely to exacerbate this problem by

1) increasing oxidation of peat when global climate warms,
2) increasing drainage of peatlands,
3) stimulating of Hg methylators by increasing sulfate deposition as acidic precipitation, and
4) increasing atmospheric deposition of Hg derived from regional industrial sources. Consequently, further research on the effects of heavy metals and materials on wetland functions is desperately needed, and the importance of understanding wetland biogeochemical processes is critical to developing answers to these contamination problems.

Community and habitat

Wetlands are essential breeding grounds, overwintering areas, and feeding grounds for millions of migratory waterfowl, other birds, and mammals. Sixty to seventy percent of the 10 to 12 million ducks that breed annually utilize the prairie pothole region of the U.S. and Canada alone (van der Valk 1989). Rare orchids (*Habenaria* spp.) and unusual insectivorous plants such as sundews (*Drosera* spp.), Venus flytraps (*Dionea muscipula*), and pitcher plants (*Sarracenia* spp.) exist only in wetland habitats. The bottomland hardwood forests and marshes along the meandering rivers and adjacent forested riparian wetlands of the southeast are the winter home of millions of ducks that migrate south from northern and central Canada. These bottomland hardwood forests also provide a habitat for neotropical migrant species. It has been estimated that 150 types of birds and 200 fish species are wetland dependent (Tiner 1984). The furbearers like the North American muskrat (*Ondatra zibethicus*) depend on wetland habitats and food like cattail roots, while other species, such as otter (*Lutra lutra*) and mink (*Luterola lutreola*), heavily utilize these communities. The American crocodile, an endangered species, is now found only in mangroves and the coastal waters of Florida. The rare bog turtle (*Clemmys muhlenbergi*) and Pine Barrens tree frog (*Hyla andersoni*) exist only in a few acid bog and swamp habitats and are threatened by the draining of these wetlands. The diversity of wetland types as well as the variation within each wetland thus provide essential habitats for animals and plants. Additionally, many upland animal species depend on wetlands for water and food, especially during drought periods. Hence, the contamination of wetland ecosystems greatly reduces their community and habitat functions and the derived values of hunting, fishing, and trapping.

Key Questions

Finally, ecologists need to do a better job of quantifying wetland functions and relating them to human values so that we can determine what we will lose when we alter, develop, or contaminate wetlands. The key ecological question that needs to be addressed under any scenario is whether wetland functions have been significantly altered. For example, if water storage in a wetland was the important process on the landscape, then the question becomes "What will it cost to replace that function?" Moreover, if contaminants are added, can the wetland function be replaced at all? Wetland replacement costs are often far higher than either the cost of selecting another area or treatment process or of constructing a new wetland for a specific type of contaminant treatment, thus avoiding natural wetland functional loss that is both ecologically important and economically sound.

References

Baltisberger RJ, Hildebrand DA, Grieble D, Ballintine TA. 1979. A study of the disproportionation of mercury (I) induced by gas sparging in acidic aqueous solutions for cold-vapor atomic absorption spectrometry. *Anal Chim Acta* 111:111–122.

Barkay T, Turner RR, VandenBrook A, Liebert C. 1991. The relationships of Hg(II) volatilization from a freshwater pond to the abundance of mer genes in the gene pool of the indigenous microbial community. *Microb Ecol* 21:151–161.

Ben-Bassat D, Mayer AM. 1978. Light induced mercury volatilization and oxygen evolution in Chlorella and the effect of DCMU and methylamine. *Physiol Plant* 42:33–38.

Brinson MM. 1993. A hydrogeomorphic classification for wetlands. Vicksburg MS: U.S. Army Corps of Engineers, Waterways Experiment Station. Technical Report WRP-DE-4.

Chamie JPM, Richardson CJ. 1978. Decomposition in northern wetlands. In: Good RE, Whigham DF, Simpson RL, editors. Freshwater wetlands: ecological processes and management potential. San Diego CA: Academic Press. p 115–130.

Compeau GC, Bartha R. 1985. Sulfate-reducing bacteria: principal methylators of mercury in anoxic estuarine sediment. *Appl Environ Microbiol* 50:498–502.

Cowardin LM, Carter V, Golet FC, LaRoe ET. 1979. Classification of wetlands and deepwater habitats of the United States. Washington DC: U. S. Fish and Wildlife Service, Department of Interior.

Craft CB, Richardson CJ. 1993. Peat accretion and N, P, and organic C accumulation in nutrient-enriched and unenriched Everglades peatlands. *Ecological Applications* 3(3):446–458.

Dahl TE. 1990. Wetlands losses in the United States, 1780s to 1980s. Washington DC: U.S. Department of the Interior, Fish and Wildlife Service. 21 p.

Delfino JJ, Crisman TL, Gottgens JF, Rood BE, Earle CDA. 1993. Spatial and temporal distribution of mercury in Everglades and Okeefenokee wetland sediments. Final project report. Gainesville FL: Univ. of Florida.

Dvonch JT, Vette AF, Keeler GJ, Evans G, Stevens R. 1995. An intensive multi-site pilot study investigating atmospheric mercury in Broward County, Florida. *Water Air Soil Pollut* 80:169–178.

Faulkner SP, Richardson CJ. 1989. Physical and chemical characteristics of freshwater wetland soils. In: Hammer DA, editor. Constructed wetlands for wastewater treatment. Chelsea MI: Lewis. p 41–72.

Frederick PC, Spalding MG. 1994. Factors affecting reproductive success of wading birds (Ciconiiformes) in the Everglades ecosystem. In: Davis SM, Ogden JC, editors. Everglades: the ecosystem and its restoration. Boca Raton FL: St. Lucie Pr. p 659–692.

Gilmour CC, Henry EA. 1991. Mercury methylation in aquatic systems affected by acid deposition. *Environ Pollut* 71:131–169.

Gopal B, Kvet J, Loffler H, Masing V, Patten BC. 1990. Definition and classification. In: Patten BC et al., editors. Volume I, Wetlands and shallow continental water bodies *S.P.B.* The Hague, Netherlands: Academic Publishing. p 9–15.

Gorham E. 1991. Northern peatlands: role in the carbon cycle and probable responses to climatic warming. *Ecolog Appl* 1:182–195.

Grieb TM, Driscoll CT, Gloss SP, Schofield CL, Bowie GL, Porcella DB. 1990. Factors affecting mercury accumulation in fish in the upper Michigan peninsula. *Environ Toxicol Chem* 9:919–930.

Hand J, Friedman M. 1990. Mercury, largemouth bass and water quality: a preliminary report. Tallahassee FL: Florida Dept. Env. Reg. 28 p.

Huckabee JW, Elwood JW, Hildebrand SG. 1979. Accumulation of mercury in freshwater biota. In: Nriagu JO, editor. The biogeochemistry of mercury in the environment. Amsterdam, Netherlands: Elsevier/North-Holland Biomedical Pr. p 277–302.

Huckabee JW, Janzen SA, Blaylock BG, Talmi Y, Beauchamp JJ. 1978. Methylated mercury in brook trout (*Salvelinus fontinalis*). absence of an in vivo methylating process. *Trans Am Fish Soc* 107:848–852.

Johnston CA, Detenbeck NE, Niemi GJ. 1990. The cumulative effect of wetlands on stream water quality and quantity: a landscape approach. *Biogeochemistry* 10:105–141.

Kadlec RH, Knight RL. 1996. Treatment wetlands. Boca Raton FL: Lewis. 893 p.

KBN Engineering and Applied Sciences, Inc. 1992. Mercury emissions to the atmosphere in Florida. Prepared for Florida Dept. of Env. Reg., Tallahassee FL.

Lemly AD. 1993. Guidelines for evaluating selenium data from aquatic monitoring and assessment studies. *Environ Monit Assess* 28:83–100.

Lemly AD, Finger SE, Nelson MK. 1993. Sources and impacts of irrigation drainwater contaminants in arid wetlands. *Environ Toxicol Chem* 12:2265–2279.

Mather SP, Hamilton HA, Levesque MP. 1979. The mitigating effects of residue fertilizer copper on the decomposition of an organic soil in situ. *Soil Sci Soc* 43:200–203.

Mitsch WJ, Gosselink JG. 1993. Wetlands. 2nd ed. New York: Van Nostrand Reinhold. 539 p.

Ohlendorf HM, Hothem RL, Bunck CM, Marois KC. 1990. Bioaccumulation of selenium in birds at Kesterson Reservoir, California. *Arch Environ Contam Toxicol* 19:495–507.

Patrick Jr WH, Gambrell RP, Parkpian P, Tan F. 1994. Mercury in soils and plants the Florida Everglades sugarcane area. In: Watras CJ, Huckabee JW, editors. Mercury pollution: integration and synthesis. Boca Raton FL: Lewis. p. 609–614.

Pennacchioni A, Marchetti R, Gaggino GF. 1976. Inability of fish to methylate mercuric chloride in vivo. *J Environ Qual* 5:451–454.

Richardson CJ. 1994. Ecological functions and human values in wetlands: a framework for assessing impacts. *Wetlands* 14(1):1–9.

Richardson CJ. 1995. Wetlands ecology. In: Nierenberg WA, editor. Encyclopedia of environmental biology. San Diego CA: Academic. p 535–550.

Richardson CJ, Nichols DS. 1985. Ecological analysis of wastewater management criteria in wetland ecosystems. In: Godfrey PJ, Kaynor ER, Pelczarski S, Benforado J, editors. Ecological considerations in wetlands treatment of municipal wastewater. New York NY: Van Nostrand Reinhold. p 351–391.

Richardson CJ, Vaithiyanathan P, Qualls RG, Barkay T. 1995. Microbial and chemical transformations of mercury in the Florida Everglades: factors controlling rates of methylation and demethylation. A proposal to the U.S. Department of Agriculture.

Roelke ME, Schultz DP, Facemire CF, Sundlof SF, Royals HE. 1991. Mercury contamination in Florida panthers. Tallahassee FL: Technical Subcommittee of the Florida Panther Interagency Committee.

Rood BE, Gottgens JF, Delfino JJ, Earle CD, Crisman TL. 1995. Mercury accumulation trends in Florida Everglades and Savannas Marsh flooded soils. *Water Air Soil Pollut* 80:981–990.

Saouter E, Ribeyre F, Boudou A, Maury-Brachet R. 1991. *Hexagenia rigida* (Ephemeroptera) as a biological model in aquatic ecotoxicology: experimental studies on mercury transfers from sediment. *Environ Pollut* 69:51–67.

Schmitt CJ, Brumbaugh WG. 1990. National Contaminant Biomonitoring Program: Concentrations of arsenic, cadmium, copper, lead, mercury, selenium, and zinc in U.S. freshwater fish, 1976–1984. *Arch Environ Contam Toxicol* 19:731–747.

Sengar CBS, Soni DK, Agarwal AL. 1989. Distribution of mercury in air, soil and vegetation around a coal fired thermal power plant. *Energy Env Monitor* 5:61–68.

Silver S, Walderhaug M. 1992. Gene regulation of plasmid- and chromosome-determined inorganic ion transport in bacteria. *Microbiol Rev* 56:195–228.

Simola H, Lodenius M. 1982. Recent increase in mercury sedimentation in a forest lake attributable to peatland drainage. *Bull Environ Contam Toxicol* 29:298–305.

Spalding MG, Bjork RD, Powell GVN, Sundlof SF. 1994. Mercury and cause of death in great white herons. *J Wildl Manage* 58(4):735–739.

Stober QJ, Jones RD, Scheidt DJ. 1995. Ultra-trace level mercury in the Everglades ecosystem: a multimedia canal pilot study. *Water Air Soil Pollut* 80:991–1001.

Tiner Jr RW. 1984. Wetlands of the United States: current status and recent trends. Washington DC: National Wetlands Inventory, U.S. Department of the Interior, Fish and Wildlife Service. 59 p.

[USACOE] U.S. Army Corps of Engineers. 1987. Corps of Engineers wetlands delineation manual. Vicksburg MS: U.S. Army Engineer Waterways Experiment Station. Technical Report Y-87-1.

Vaithiyanathan P, Richardson CJ, Kavanaugh R, Barkay T. 1996. The relationships of eutrophication to the distribution of mercury and the potential for methylmercury production in the peat soils of the Everglades. *Environ Sci Tech* 30:2591–2597.

van der Valk A. 1989. Northern prairie wetlands. Ames IA: Iowa State Univ Pr. 533 p.

Westling O. 1991. Mercury in runoff from drained and undrained peatlands in Sweden. *Water Air Soil Pollut* 56:419–426.

Winfrey MR, Rudd JWM. 1990. Environmental factors affecting the formation of methylmercury in low pH lakes. *Environ Toxicol Chem* 9:853–869.

Winter TC. 1989. Hydrologic studies of wetlands in the northern prairie. In: van der Valk AG, editor. Northern prairie wetlands. Ames IA: Iowa State Univ Pr. p 16-55.

Wood JM. 1974. Biological cycles for toxic elements in the environment. *Science* 183:1049–1052.

Zillioux EJ, Porcella DB, Benoit JM. 1993. Mercury cycling and effects in freshwater wetland ecosystems. *Environ Toxicol Chem* 12:2245–2264.

Chapter 3

Workgroup I Synopsis: Biogeochemical Processes

William J. Catallo, chair
James T. Blankemeyer, Robert P. Gambrell, John H. Pardue, K. Ramesh Reddy

Biogeochemical processes are directly relevant to wetland ecotoxicology because 1) the deposition, fates, and effects of toxic materials are influenced by sediment parameters and 2) these processes are in turn affected by the presence of toxicants and therefore may serve as indicators of subtle or chronic toxic chemical effects.

The diversity of biogeochemical processes and the associated physicochemical and ecological gradients in wetlands far exceed those found in other ecosystems. Thus, the impacts and reciprocal interactions among these processes, contaminants, and nutrients are of major concern and interest.

Chapter Preview

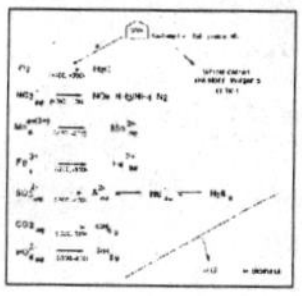

Ecotoxicology and Risk Assessment for Wetlands. Michael A. Lewis et al., editors.

The principal objectives of this workgroup were to review and synthesize, at least generally, elements of the following subjects and provide recommendations for further study:

1) effects of pollution and other physicochemical stress on biogeochemical processes in wetlands,
2) relationships of these effects to the ecological functioning of landscapes,
3) linkages between sediment–plant–microbe processes to ecological functioning of wetlands at different scales,
4) analytical and conceptual techniques for integrating processes and scales, and
5) experimental and analytical techniques for monitoring process outputs from wetlands and evaluating significant changes in these resulting from contamination.

Within these general subject headings, it was the intention of the group to

1) integrate different approaches and disciplines within wetland science (biology, chemistry, ecology, engineering) to describe the importance of central biogeochemical processes at different scales,
2) attempt to relate the results of microcosm and mesocosm experiments to generally accepted ecological process endpoints in wetlands, and
3) relate 1) and 2) to contaminant impacts in wetland ecosystems and landscapes.

It is important to point out that the expertise within the workgroup was diverse, and there was a substantial amount of controversy on the major areas of importance for this document. This applied particularly to the perception of fundamental paradigms and future research needs. Much of this controversy was rooted in the characteristic spatiotemporal scales addressed by participants in their individual study of wetlands. It was sometimes noted that discord on particular issues and approaches actually reflected agreement about basic principles, with difficulties becoming apparent as unfamiliar scales and time frames were addressed. On the other hand, all participants were aware of the pitfalls of upscaling and generalizing: there are too many unknowns for this to be a highly accurate process. All participants agreed that much productive work remains to be done in the area of wetland ecotoxicology, particularly at ecosystem and landscape levels of organization. While this should not supplant or replace basic mechanistic studies of processes, there is a need for these studies to encompass larger scales and more complex interactions than in the past.

In what follows, pertinent terms are defined; wetland functions are described; the biogeochemistry of C, H, O, N, P, S, and various trace metals is summarized; and the interactions between normal biogeochemical processes and organic and inorganic contaminants are discussed. Review of the measurement, interpretation, and geochemical significance of the redox potential (RP) is presented, particularly as it applies to pollutant transformations and fates in wetlands. Next, an attempt is made to integrate these concepts with ecological theory and the results of recent studies at the landscape level. Finally, discussions of emerging techniques in data acquisition and analysis for highly connected ecological processes are presented, along with recommendations for further work.

Terms and Concepts

The following sources are referred to in this section: Hutchinson 1948; Margalef 1963; Odum 1983; Risser et al. 1983; Pimm 1984; Odum 1985; Loucks 1985; Charef and Sun 1990; Ehleringer and Field 1993; Odum 1993; Cantwell and Foreman 1993; Johnston 1994; Schmidt-Nielson 1994; Reice 1994; Catallo 1994; Audi 1995; Likens and Bormann 1995; de Ruiter et al. 1995.

The term "biogeochemical" refers to process interactions between biotic and abiotic compartments of ecosystems that result in transfer or transformation of matter or energy. Hutchinson (1948) used the term specifically to describe "circular causal systems" involving groups of organisms and environmental compartments participating in complex and reciprocal exchanges of energy. In this sense, biogeochemical interactions are differentiated from low order or one-way interactions between ecosystem elements and are characterized by recursive outputs that display distinct, but generally classifiable, behavior in space and time. There is a strong sense of "homoeomerism" in this notion: components of the system or clusters of constitutive processes within it share structural and functional aspects of the whole, and the whole affects the constitutive processes to varying degrees (Audi 1995; Likens and Bormann 1995). A more modern rendering of this notion is found in "fractal" scaling models of environmental structure or function, and this applies to wetland biogeochemical processes, particularly with respect to time dynamics of processes (Charef and Sun 1990; Ehleringer and Field 1993; Odum 1993; Schmidt-Nielson 1994; de Ruiter et al. 1995). Wetland biogeochemical processes reflect networks of biotic interactions that in turn are influenced by physicochemical factors, including temperature, light, tide, climatic, and solar cycles (Odum 1983).

"Ecotoxicology" can be defined operationally as the study of toxic agents in ecological systems with a view toward understanding their significance to ecosystem structure and function (Catallo 1994). This includes the study and resolution of "effects" (at the ecosystem or sub-ecosystem level) and "impacts" (landscape level and above). The study of ecotoxicology involves scaling across broad spatiotemporal scales (e.g., those characteristic of chemical reactions to those of landscape processes) and understanding chronic, low-level effects of contaminants in systems experiencing numerous such as fragmentation and hydrological disruption (Ehleringer and Field 1993).

"Toxic contaminants" are defined here as any natural or anthropogenic chemical introduced to the environment in levels sufficient to cause a deleterious alteration of a biological process. The words "toxicants," "pollutants," "xenobiotics," and "toxic chemicals" are used interchangeably with "contaminants" and are synonymous for the purposes of this chapter. "Eutrophicants" and "nutrients" refer to those essential inorganic chemicals and elements (e.g., NO_3^-, PO_4^{2-}, Fe) that can promote elevated or abnormally sustained biological activity and can cause biological and ecological impacts (e.g., prolonged anaerobiosis, blooms of algae and macrophytes, and accumulation of toxins from these blooms). While usually not directly toxic, eutrophicants can give rise to deleterious biological and ecological events. Further, eutrophication can change the fate and toxicity of pollutants and alter the adaptive or depurative capacities of wetland species and ecosystems.

There is no universally accepted definition of "wetlands" (see Chapter 2). In general, wetlands are areas of emergent land forming the transition zones between uplands and open water, although some wetlands (e.g., potholes) have discrete boundaries and rapid transition zones (Catallo 1994). Wetlands have one or more of the following traits:

1) at least temporarily waterlogged sediment and physicochemical properties reflecting saturation,
2) dominance of plants adapted to saturated soils (hydrophytes), and
3) scarcity of flood-intolerant plants. Although minor in geographical extent (6% of the earth's surface), wetlands have global significance in terms of biotic diversity, productivity, and sediment biogeochemical processes.

These processes are mediated by sediment–microbe–plant assemblages that interact in ways that fit Hutchinson's notion of "biogeochemical" (Hutchinson 1948). Thus, wetland biogeochemical processes have a high degree of "connectance," which is defined as the ratio of actual process interactions (connections) to the total number of possible interactions (Margalef 1963; Pimm 1984; de Ruiter et al. 1995). This means that these assemblages can respond to perturbation in ways that reflect a network of interconnections and can "surprise" investigators who monitor system outputs (Loucks 1985; Odum 1985; Reice 1994). From a statistical perspective, wetland process variables can be characterized as "multiple collinearity," i.e., there is covariance among numerous variables. This introduces significant procedural and analytical difficulties for "bottom-up" experimental designs that seek to isolate and quantify process responses to perturbation such as contamination. These difficulties increase as higher levels of organization are addressed.

"Landscape ecology" refers to the study of reciprocal interactions between ecosystems and the effects of spatial and temporal patterns (mosaics) on ecological processes (Risser et al. 1983; Cantwell and Foreman 1993; Johnston 1994). The notion of landscape encompasses different spatiotemporal scales including

1) ecosystems and patches on the order of kilometers and above and
2) smaller scales within systems showing spatial heterogeneity (e.g., burrowing effects, ecophenic variations).

Landscape ecology attempts to integrate these scales and focus on interactions between elements of a matrix of observables, especially those corresponding to spatially adjacent elements. These approaches require new technologies (e.g., geographic information systems) and analytical methods (e.g., structural equation modeling) to be feasible, and multiple levels of resolution need to be incorporated into experimental designs (Catallo 1994; Johnston 1994). In the landscape approach, observables are related to function by

1) elucidation of fine-scale events (mechanisms) and their relationships to the dynamics and structure of the entire system (functions) and
2) study of the large-scale behavior of the mosaic.

That these large-scale studies can also be mechanistic in the traditional sense has been the subject of some comment (Ehleringer and Field 1993). The extent and nature of connections between elements of the mosaic are fundamentally related to function of the landscape and are critical to the development of structural or functional units that comprise ecosystems. As with individual ecosystems, these landscape mosaics are functionally variable in space and time, and their dynamics reflect interactions among biotic, abiotic, and human processes. Interestingly, the connections between wetlands and other elements of landscapes can be described by a very limited number of geometries (Cantwell and Foreman 1993).

Wetland Functions in Landscapes

The following sources either are referred to or provide further discussion: Turner 1977; Odum 1983; Deegan and Thompson 1985; Browder et al. 1989; Chambers 1992; Catallo 1994; Likens and Bormann 1995;

Wetlands perform major functions in landscapes, including provision of habitat for fish and wildlife; catchment of fertile sediments; purification of runoff and industrial and domestic wastewater; recharge of aquifers; biogeochemical transformation of C, H, N, S, P (including greenhouse gases); and exchanges of chemicals, nutrients, and OM with associated aquatic and upland ecosystems (Odum 1983; Catallo 1994; Likens and Bormann 1995). It has been reported that regional groundwater quality is well correlated with the spatial extent and functional quality of wetlands in the watershed. Similarly, land use patterns and agricultural practices influence C and N processing at the landscape level. In coastal wetlands, the extent of intertidal wetlands (i.e., the water–land interface) rather than the total wetland area is positively related to fisheries production (Turner 1977; Deegan and Thompson 1985; Browder et al. 1989). Decreases in coastal wetland extent and habitat quality have contributed to undesirable changes in estuarine or wetland-dependent coastal fisheries. Over the past few decades, the landings of virtually all estuarine-dependent commercial fish in the Gulf of Mexico, south Atlantic, Chesapeake Bay, and Alaska have declined significantly "...to all-time lows" (Chambers 1992). Similarly, there is evidence of declines in migratory fowl in many areas and deleterious changes in populations of wetland-dependent vertebrates such as amphibians. The reasons for these trends include

1) over-exploitation of commercially valuable target species and increasing levels of by-catch,
2) destruction and fragmentation of wetland habitats that provide the support systems and nurseries for fish and wildlife, and
3) decline of wetland structural and functional quality from acute and chronic inputs of eutrophicants, toxic chemicals and metals, and other wastes (solids, pathogens, atmospheric chemicals, antibiotics).

Understanding and mitigating these processes is a global societal need (Catallo 1994).

Biogeochemistry of Wetlands

Important elemental cycles and methods of measuring wetland biogeochemical processes are given in Table 3-1 and are discussed below.

Oxygen and biogeochemistry of wetlands

The following sources either are referred to or provide further discussion: Armstrong 1975; DeLaune et al. 1976; DeLaune and Pezeshki 1991; Mendelssohn et al. 1995.

In natural and constructed wetlands, levels of dissolved oxygen (DO) in the water column usually remain high and uniform relative to the soil because

1) respiratory oxygen demand is low (there are relatively low densities of heterotrophic aerobes, on the order of 10^2 to 10^4 bacterial cells/mL),
2) algal photosynthesis releases oxygen to the system, and
3) wind action and convection promote turbulent aeration and vertical mixing.

Much higher densities of heterotrophs are found in the sediments (10^4 to 10^7 bacterial cells/g), and these give rise to high oxygen demand. This can result in the development of distinct layers (or "horizons") in the vertical profile:

1) an oxidized or aerobic surface layer where DO is present and aerobic respiration may proceed and
2) an underlying reduced or anaerobic soil layer in which no free oxygen is present and where fermentation and other anaerobic respiratory processes are dominant.

The thickness of an aerobic layer can change as a result of

1) fluctuations in dissolved oxygen in surface water (daily, seasonal),
2) bioturbation,
3) physical mixing (e.g., by tidal or storm flushing), and
4) draining of surface sediments (e.g., lowering of ground water).

Table 3-1 Examples of discrete biogeochemical process measurements

Cycle	Process	Measurement
Carbon	CO_2 fixation [CO_2 to organic matter]	Net primary productivity
	Soil organic matter decomposition	Change in OC, O_2 consumption
	Enzymatic hydrolysis	Extracellular enzyme activity [e.g., cellulase, phenol oxidase]
	Aerobic respiration	CO_2, O_2, and nutrients
	Nitrate reduction	CO_2, NO_3^-, N_2O, and nutrients
	Manganese reduction	CO_2, Mn^{2+}, and nutrients
	Iron reduction	CO_2, Fe^{2+}, and nutrients
	Sulfate respiration	CO_2, S^{2-}, and nutrients
	Methanogenesis	CH_4 and nutrients
	Flux of dissolved species	Dissolved total organic carbon, dissolved organic carbon, SO_4^{2-}, Mn^{2+}, Fe^{2+}, CH_4 in soil pore water and water column
	Plant litter decomposition	Litter bags and dry weight loss
Nitrogen	Ammonification	NH_4-N
	Nitrification	NO_3-N andNH_4-N
	Denitrification	NOc-N and N_2O
	Nitrogen fixation	C_2H_2 assay
	Plant uptake	Plant tissue N and biomass
	Flux of dissolved species	Dissolved NH_4-N and NO_3-N in soil pore water and water column
Phosphorus	Mineralization of organic P	Inorganic P
	Extracellular enzymes	Phosphatase
	Adsorption/desorption	Partition coefficients
	Plant uptake	Plant tissue P
	Flux of dissolved species	Dissolved P and selected cations in soil pore water and water column
Oxygen	Respiration Chemical reduction	Biological oxygen demand/chemical oxygen demand
RP	Microbial and chemical oxidation-reduction	Redox indicators Trace gas measurements Potentiometry at solid electrodes

Many wetland plants have the ability to translocate oxygen through stems and leaves into the root zone (DeLaune and Pezeshki 1991; Mendelssohn et al. 1995). The known mechanisms of oxygen transport in wetland plants are convective flow and diffusion rather than active pumping. In some important grass species, diffusion of oxygen from aerial parts to roots occurs through specialized channels of dead parenchyma called "aerenchyma." Oxygen not reduced during root respiration can diffuse into the adjacent soil, thus creating an aerobic environment at some distance from live root tissues. This "oxidized rhizosphere" can constitute an oxidized volume in an otherwise highly reduced sediment. The oxidized rhizosphere can aid in the oxidation and immobilization of natural and anthropogenic toxicants, including sulfides and reduced forms of Fe and Mn. Further, microbial cells in and near the rhizosphere can exploit gradients and boundaries in redox conditions to perform a wide range of metabolic and ecological processes, including aerobic and fermentative oxidation of soluble organic compounds, fixation of atmospheric N, and nitrification of ammonium N. The maintenance of oxidized rhizospheres in the root zone and the presence of specialized microbial affiliates and symbionts in wetland plants can have important implications in the design of constructed wetlands for wastewater treatment, evaluation of natural wetland structure or function, and functional assessment of restored or affected systems (e.g., bioindicators, mechanistic studies of toxicant transport and metabolism). It is important to note that the oxidized rhizosphere, in conjunction with daily and annual physicochemical cycles, also can influence the magnitude, stability, and reproducibility of measured RPs, as described below.

(See also Armstrong 1975; DeLaune et al. 1976.)

Redox potential

Wetland soils can be characterized by the intensity of soil reduction, which is frequently expressed as the "redox" or oxidation-reduction potential (RP). Conceptually, the RP can be regarded as a relative measure of the chemical potential energy of the system, as determined by the oxidation states of the constituents. Hence, oxidized systems are depleted in high-energy chemical bonds, elements tend to have positive oxidation states (e.g., C (+4), Fe(+3), Mn(+4), S(+6), etc.), and the free energy of the system is low. Reduced systems have chemical constituents with high-energy bonds, elements in lower oxidation states (e.g., C(–4), Fe(+2), Mn(+2), S(–2)) and the free energy of the system is high. In practice, the RP of a soil can be measured by a solid electrode, frequently platinum, gold, or graphite, that can readily accept or donate electrons versus a known reference half-cell electrode, usually the saturated calomel electrode (SCE). Depending on wetland type and intensity of soil reduction, a variety of RP values can be observed in wetland soils (Figure 3-1). The oxidized system will display more positive potentials (lower potential energy) and will tend to accept electrons from suitable donors. Conversely, the reduced system will display more negative values (higher potential energy) and will tend to donate electrons to suitable sinks. In general, the range of RP and its spatiotemporal variability is much greater in wetland soils than in other elements of landscapes including aquatic systems such as lakes and streams, upland forests, and grasslands or agricultural fields (excluding rice paddies). As discussed below, this indicates a fundamental functional aspect of wetlands within landscapes.

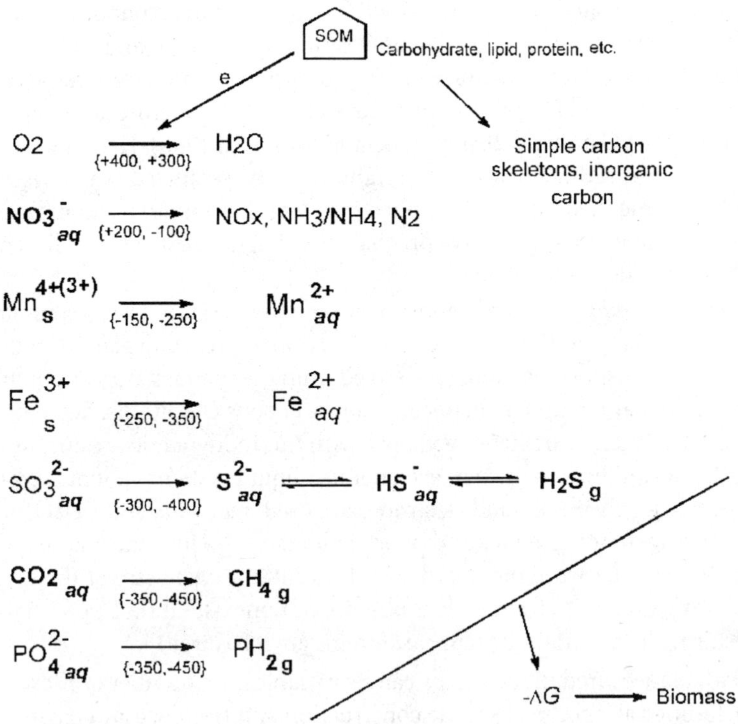

Figure 3-1 Schematic summary of biogeochemical redox reactions. (Values in parentheses are approximate potential ranges in millivolts versus the standard calomel reference electrode at which these reactions occur.)

The RP both reflects and influences chemical and biological processes in many wetland, marine, and freshwater sediments. Much data exist on relationships among measured or inferred redox conditions in sediment–water bulk phases and in

1) biogeochemistry of C, H, O, N, S and numerous trace metals;
2) wetland plant distributions, productivity, and physiological status;
3) microbial and meiofaunal distributions and ecology;
4) transformation and transport of hydrophobic pollutants and trace metals;
5) sediment exchange of radioisotopes; and
6) preservation of "chemical fossils" used in organic chemical source and diagenetic studies.

(See also Baas-Becking et al. 1960; Bohn 1968, 1969, 1971; Bailey and Beauchamp 1971; Howarth and Teal 1980; DeLaune et al. 1981; Howes et al. 1981; Pardue et al. 1989; DeLaune and Pezeshki 1991; Grenthe et al. 1992; Cogger et al. 1992; Meyers and Ishiwatari 1993; Haraguchi 1995; Hudnall et al. 1995; Catallo et al. 1995.)

Other works have related RP to wetland soil function and to taxonomy and ecotoxicology of sediment microbes (Koepfler and Kator 1986; Catallo and Gambrell 1987; Faulkner et al. 1989). Manipulation of redox conditions in dredge materials and other contaminated sediments also may prove to be a viable remediation option for some toxic metals (Gambrell 1994; Catallo and Gambrell 1995). Hence, RP can be considered an integrating or "master" variable in many sediment–water systems. Nevertheless, some theoretical and applied problems have limited the applicability of RP measurements to quantitative predictive or diagnostic work in sediments and water. These include the following:

1) The Nernst equation (a relationship among the measured RP, a standard half-cell potential, and the effective concentrations of reactants and products of electron transport reactions) is derived from the mathematics of equilibrium thermodynamics under chemically homogeneous conditions. Sediment chemical systems are heterogeneous, with thermodynamic conditions usually far from equilibrium. In fact, even defined liquid systems cannot be considered homogeneous if solid electrodes are used: reactions at the electrode surface are heterogeneous and poorly understood. Thus, the mathematical relationship between measured RP values and the chemistry of dissolved constituents in situ frequently is obscure or nonexistent (i.e., potentials resulting from complex chemical systems are measured).
2) RP data measured in sediments can be variable for a number of reasons, including variance in electrode construction and response and passivation of surfaces by oxide or sulfide layers.

With attention to factors such as electrode construction, calibration, and surface chemistry, these and other problems can be minimized in many circumstances, and RP data can provide a general indication of the electrochemical status in the bulk phases of soil and sediments. Research on approaches for measuring and interpreting RP data are of continuing interest. (See also Armstrong 1975; DeLaune et al. 1976; Audi 1995; Mendelssohn et al. 1995.)

The vertical and horizontal distributions of RP and its variability in time reflect the interplay of the

1) supply of readily oxidizable OM,
2) microbial abundance and diversity,
3) sediment characteristics (e.g., clay content, density),
4) hydrological variables (flood-drain periodicities, length of flood or drained conditions),
5) temperature, and
6) plant and detrital properties (e.g., nutrient demand and uptake, meiofauna biomass and activity, rhizosphere characteristics).

In general, the metabolic energy (adenosine triphosphate [ATP] and other biochemical reducing equivalents) derived from respiration in wetland soils is inversely proportional to the degree of reduction of the system (Nicholls and Ferguson 1992). With the exception of small quantities of transient species (singlet O_2, H_2O_2, and OH·), molecular oxygen is the most powerful, stable oxidant found in natural waters. It is exploited as a terminal electron acceptor in respiration because of its high affinity for electrons in comparison with other electron acceptors. Hence, a mole of glucose metabolized under aerobic conditions (i.e., transformed by glycolysis and tricarboxylic acid pathways to CO_2 and H_2O in the presence of oxygen) will provide the larger amount of energy compared to the same mole of glucose metabolized under anaerobic or highly reduced conditions. As a result, metabolic products formed under reducing conditions (e.g., organic acids, sulfides, methane) contain some of the free energy that would have been liberated by aerobic respiration (as indicated above in the discussion of potential energy and oxidation states). These energy-containing products can themselves be used by microbes as substrate and can form the basis of an entire sediment ecosystem (Fenchel 1978). The enormous ecological importance of this system has been discussed in detail in Fenchel 1978 and Giere 1993. (See also Bohn et al. 1985; Valiela 1995.)

pH in wetland soils and water

The pH of a soil refers to the relative degree of acidity or basicity. More formally, pH is defined as the negative logarithm of the hydronium ion activity, as measured using indicators or ion-specific electrodes. A pH of 7.0 (i.e., 10^{-7} M H_3O^+ ion activity) is considered neutral for aqueous systems and is close to characteristic pH of many biological systems (e.g., physiological fluids in vertebrates typically have pH 7.2 to 7.6). Terrestrial soils and surface waters commonly have pH levels from 5 to 9, but depending on parent soil materials and many other factors, terrestrial soil and surfacewater pH values out of this range also are to be expected. Of particular significance for wetland soils is that upon flooding, chemical and microbial processes cause the development of reducing conditions and the soil pH can converge on 7.0. Thus the range of pH values in wetland soils is much narrower than in terrestrial soils in general and narrower than the range found in the soils of the wetland watershed. For example, the pH of both acid and alkaline soils of constructed and natural wetlands tends to converge toward neutrality as a result of reduction reactions and consumption of protons. This pH poising results from the interplay of

1) the increased partial pressure of CO_2 from OM decomposition (resulting in decreased pH) and
2) the chemical and biological reduction of NO_3^-, Mn^{4+}, and Fe^{3+} as oxyhydroxides and of CO_2 (resulting in elevated pH).

It is important to note that when some wetland soils are drained and oxidized, as can occur with impoundments or upland placement of dredged material, the pH of the material can become strongly acidic. Materials can become acidic also as a result of access channels or canals being dug through wetlands and placing the sediment to the side of the newly constructed channel as a “spoil bank.” These acid conditions result from the oxidation of ferrous (reduced) iron-sulfur materials such as pyrite. As an example of the potential for acidic conditions to form, Prasana (1994) stirred a slurry of a coastal Louisiana marsh sediment under argon purging (i.e., anoxic conditions); the pH was 7.3 after 2 weeks. The same sediment material stirred similarly under 1 atmosphere had a pH of 3.5 (Prasana 1994). Gambrell and Patrick (1978) treated a New Jersey marsh sediment similarly and found that the initial pH of near 7.0 decreased to 3.0 after 8 days stirring under air. Further, Catallo (1994) has performed automated time-series RP measurements on brackish marsh soils from an impounded wetland and demonstrated significant periodic RP fluctuations (50 to 300 mV/day) that followed a simulated diurnal tide. This sediment had pH values that varied between 3.5 and 4.7 over the tide cycle, i.e., the pH increased upon flooding and decreased after draining.

Moderately to strongly acidic conditions in disturbed wetland soils can affect microbial activity, contribute to substantial release of metal contaminants, and adversely affect plant growth. Diurnal changes in pH also have been noted, e.g., submerged macrophytes and algae can fix dissolved CO_2 during the day, thus raising the pH values, in some cases to > 10. The pH of the water column then can decrease by 2 to 3 units in the evening when photosynthesis is terminated and respiration increases. These fluctuations can result in profound changes in biogeochemical processes, including microbially mediated nutrient transformations, chemical precipitation-complexation reactions, adsorption reactions, toxicity, partitioning behavior, and water solubility.

(See also Armstrong 1975; DeLaune et al. 1976; Seke 1982; Bohn et al. 1985; Cogger et al. 1992; Lazerte 1993; Likens and Bormann 1995.)

Organic matter turnover and nutrients

Wetlands are characterized by aerobic and anaerobic interfaces in the soil–water column and by the accumulation of slowly decomposing organic matter (OM). Primary production typically exceeds total plant and microbial respiration, resulting in accretion of OM in reduced sediment horizons. In rapidly sedimenting systems, this C is buried and sequestered from high-energy respiration in the aerobic surface layers of the sediment. In wetland systems not receiving large amounts of mineral sediments, plant OM forms much of the surface soil profile, and residues are characterized by refractile polymers (i.e., polyphenols, lignins, and humic acids).

Although wetlands cover about 6% of the earth, their relative importance to the earth's biogeochemical cycles far exceeds their surface area, for they contain 68% of terrestrial soil C reserves and represent a major carbon sink (Kolasa and Pickett 1991; Catallo 1994). Soils and recently deposited plant litter can function as the control center for nutrient regeneration and recycling in wetlands, as well as loci for metal and organic contaminant entrapment, transformation, and transport. Decomposition of OM to a large degree may regulate secondary productivity, productivity of associated aquatic systems, and local water quality.

Ombrotrophic (isolated from anthropogenic nutrients) wetlands are characterized by low external loading of nutrients and relatively closed elemental cycling (Northup et al. 1995). Microbial activity and plant productivity are nutrient limited. Vascular plants, periphyton, and microbial communities are extremely efficient in utilizing and accumulating nutrients through rapid uptake at very low concentrations. Plant litter in these systems generally has high C:N:P ratios, and decomposition of this material results in conditions in which microbial and periphytic communities may out-compete vascular plants for nutrients. The overall turnover rate of high-C:N:P-ratio OM is usually slow, and long-term decomposition may be both C and nutrient limited. Environmental factors such as water-table fluctuations and fire can result in pulsed release of nutrients, which may provide a significant source of plant-available nutrients in low-nutrient systems (Wotton 1988; Mitsch and Gosselink 1993; Devai and DeLaune 1995c).

In eutrophic wetlands, where inputs exceed demand, rapid turnover of C and nutrients and relatively open elemental cycling frequently are observed. In these systems, factors other than nutrients are limiting, and variable degrees of nutrient cycling within the system are observed. Under these conditions, plants, periphyton, and soil microbial communities are less efficient in nutrient utilization, and excess nutrients are shunted or passed out of the system through air (e.g., phosphene gas generation from reduction of ortho- and polyphosphates) and water (e.g., NO^{2-}/ NO^{3-} runoff in surface and ground water). Plant litter generally has low C:N:P, and net mineralization of nutrients during decomposition results in decreased significance of internal cycling by microbes and plants. For example, addition of nutrients to Everglades Water Conservation Area-2a has resulted in a vegetative shift from a sawgrass-dominated system to one dominated by cattails. The continuous supply of nutrients to this system caused increased cattail productivity and a subsequent increase in OM accumulation. Organic matter accumulation was highest in the affected areas and decreased with distance from inflow. Further, the rates of OM turnover and basal respiration in the surface litter layer were found to decrease with distance from inflow. Toxic pollutant effects on sediment microflora and meiofauna also can alter C:N:P cycles in ombrotrophic and eutrophic systems (Catallo and Gambrell 1987, 1995).

Although loading of anthropogenic nutrients can stimulate the growth of aquatic vegetation in wetlands, a significant portion of the nutrient demand in situ may be met through decomposition of OM. The rates of OM turnover and nutrient regeneration are influenced by hydroperiod, OM composition, and supply of mobile oxidants. Similarly, contaminants such as trace metals and toxic organic compounds may be entrained in organic matrices and become available when soil physicochemical conditions change. Tides, seasonal floods, storm events, field runoff events, and fluctuations in the water table can create alternate aerobic and anaerobic conditions, which may stimulate OM decomposition and release of nutrients and pollutants. The presence of oxygen in surface layers and rhizospheres allows for the existence of microeukaryotes (fungi, protozoans), which are critical for decomposition and mobilization of organic C and N. In the presence of added nutrients, increased primary productivity corresponds with increased litter production, and this in turn may give rise to increased soil oxygen demand. Much of the oxygen in the water column is usually consumed in the litter layer, leaving underlying soil anaerobic. Epiphytic algae associated with litter fragments, however, can increase oxygen supply during photosynthetic periods, thus promoting aerobic decomposition. Lack of oxygen production at night can result in anaerobic conditions under which the microeukaryotes become inactive. These diurnal fluctuations in oxygen supply and consumption can have a major impact on several biogeochemical processes in wetlands.

(See also McKey et al. 1978; Seke 1982; Catallo et al. 1996.)

Nitrogen processing in wetlands

Nitrogen is processed in wetlands through N-fixation, mineralization, nitrification and denitrification, ammonia volatilization, plant uptake, and organic N loss as buried sediment OM. Under normal or slightly eutrophic conditions, these processes aid in maintaining low levels of inorganic N in the water column. A significant portion of dissolved organic N is returned to the water column during breakdown of detrital plant tissue or soil OM. A majority of this dissolved and colloidal organic N is resistant to decomposition. Under these conditions, effluent leaving wetlands may contain elevated levels of N in organic form. Depending on the metabolic activity of aquatic bacteria, organic-bound N is mineralized to ammonium N. The rates of conversion, however, depend on the nature of organic N and C/N ratio of the OM and electron acceptor availability. For example, the rate of inorganic N formation from detrital plant matter is influenced by the C/N ratio of the plant tissue, dissolved oxygen concentration of the water, and water temperature. Mineralization processes also occur in the underlying soil, and the ammonium N forms can be

1) subsequently released into the overlying water,
2) accumulated on the soil exchange complex, or
3) assimilated by plants.

Nitrification involves the biological oxidation of ammonium to nitrate. The bacteria involved are chemoautotrophic and use oxygen as their electron acceptor, while ammonium is used as their substrate. In a floating aquatic macrophyte system, nitrification occurs in the water column and in the rhizosphere, with rates limited by oxygen supply. In the absence of oxygen, facultative anaerobic microorganisms utilize nitrate as a terminal electron acceptor during their respiration. During this process, nitrate is reduced to gaseous end products such as nitrous oxide and nitrogen gas. Denitrification can occur in the soil and water column devoid of oxygen and in the anoxic sites of the rhizosphere, provided the energy source (available C) and nitrate are present in these sites.

Plant uptake of N is dependent on the growth rate of the plant and on environmental parameters such as solar radiation and temperature. Nitrogen added to wetlands is present as ammonium, nitrate, and organic N. Wetland plants are capable of assimilating both ammonium and nitrate; however, many aquatic plants appear to prefer ammonium over nitrate, even though both ions are present at the same time. The efficiency of N utilization by aquatic vegetation is highly variable, and is variable among different wetland types. Nitrogen assimilation by herbaceous vegetation is short-term, and the resulting organic N usually is cycled rapidly within the systems. Unlike herbaceous macrophytes, forested wetlands provide long-term storage in the form of woody biomass. However, a significant portion of nutrients stored in the leaves is returned to the forest floor and eventually incorporated into the soil (Stanford and Smith 1972; Northup et al. 1995). Forest litter decomposition is slow; the turnover periods are much longer. Plant uptake can account for 16 to 75% of total N removal in some wetlands (Likens and Bormann 1995).

In addition to plant assimilation, N removal in wetlands is affected by a number of biological, physical, and chemical processes that function in the water, soil, and rhizosphere (Reddy et al. 1978). In studies on the fate of N added to floodwater, mass balances indicated that plant uptake accounted for 13 to 67% of the total N removal, while unaccounted-for N was assumed to be lost through nitrification, denitrification, and NH_3 volatilization. The oxidized rhizosphere of wetland plants has been shown to support nitrification, while the adjacent anaerobic zone supports denitrification. These mechanisms explain overall N loss from wetlands not accounted for by plant uptake alone.

Addition of N to wetlands can also result in spatial gradients in the direction of inflow to outflow. Most of the added N is processed in the areas affected by loading. For example, constructed wetlands used for nitrate removal will have high denitrification rates in soils adjacent to the inflow area as compared to the soils away from the inflow. Addition of nitrate not only builds microbial populations involved in denitrification but also increases the OM production through increased productivity of vegetation. Decomposition of OM in soils increases dissolved NH_4^+ levels in the soil pore water. This can create a concentration gradient between the soil and the overlying water column.

Concentrations of NH_4^+ are usually low in the water column and surface aerobic layer as a result of nitrification. Nitrate diffuses downward, where it undergoes denitrification. This diffusion-limited sequence of nitrification–denitrification is an important ecological function of wetlands, which helps to maintain N balance in the ecosystem.

(See also Bailey and Beauchamp 1971; Patrick and Mikkelson 1971; DeLaune et al. 1976; Reddy and Patrick 1976; Gambrell and Patrick 1978; Smith and Patrick 1983; Kolasa and Pickett 1991; Mann and Lazier 1991; Boar et al. 1993; Mitsch and Gosselink 1993; White 1993.)

Phosphorus movement in wetlands

Phosphorus movement in wetlands and aquatic systems is mediated by plant uptake, microbial immobilization, retention by the underlying soil, and precipitation in the water column. Most P is conserved in wetland systems, but small losses can occur through biogeochemical processes, sediment erosion, dredging, or removal of plants (harvesting). Phosphorus is present in organic and inorganic forms, the latter of which are more mobile between the soil and the overlying water column. Unlike N and C, large amounts of gaseous P are not lost from wetlands through metabolic processes, although there are minor losses from reduction of orthophosphate to PH_2 (Devai and DeLaune 1995a). Hence, wetlands can function as a source or sink of dissolved P. The amount of P retained or released by the soil depends on P concentration of the overlying water, adsorption/desorption reactions, precipitation, mineralization of organic P, and diffusion. It has been shown that inorganic P added at concentrations considerably greater than those present in the interstitial water of wetland soils may be retained by oxides and hydrous oxides of iron and aluminum and by calcium carbonate. At low P loadings, wetlands tend to release rather than retain P.

Several phosphate minerals regulate the solubility of dissolved P in sediment–water systems. These minerals include apatite, hydroxyapatite, fluorapatite, octocalcium phosphate, strengite, vivianite, variscite, and wavellite. It is difficult to attribute the majority of P retention to any one single mineral because wetlands are complex. The following generalities are supportable:

1) in acid soils, P is fixed as Al and ferric phosphates, if the activities of these cations are high;
2) in alkaline soils, P fixation is governed by the activities of Ca and Mg;
3) P availability is greatest in soils with slightly acidic to neutral pH (the pH of wetland soils usually is near 7, and P retention in these systems may be decreased relative to uplands);
4) phosphorus retention and regulation of dissolved P also is controlled by oxidized and poorly crystalline forms of Al and Fe (ferric hydroxide, ferric oxyhydroxide, ferrous hydroxide, and amorphous oxides), and reduction of these oxyhydroxides to more soluble ferrous forms under reduced conditions can decrease overall P sorption relative to oxidized conditions; and
5) in calcareous systems, P released into the overlying water column can be precipitated as Ca mineral bound-P, especially when pH of the flood water is altered diurnally by photosynthetic activities of algae.

The steep gradients in porewater P concentration result in the diffusive flux from soil to the overlying water column, and the P released into the water column is either assimilated by planktonic organisms or precipitated with Ca minerals. In calcareous systems, coprecipitation of P with $CaCO_3$ was shown to be a dominant mechanism involved in the immobilization of soluble P. In the water column where pH fluctuates diurnally, with high values during daytime (photosynthetic activity of algae) and low values during night (respiration by algae and bacteria), P can be precipitated and resolubilized.

(See also Patrick and Mikkelsen 1971; Gambrell and Patrick 1978; Krairapanond et al. 1993; Likens and Bormann 1995; Valiela 1995; Jugsujinda, Krairapanond et al. 1995; Devai and DeLaune 1995b; Crozier et al. 1995; Kludze and DeLaune 1995.)

Sulfur

Sulfur is an essential nutrient for plant and animal nutrition. The relatively low level of sulfur compounds in most terrestrial soils and freshwater wetland systems is sufficient for plant nutrition purposes, and sulfur is rarely limiting for metabolic activities and growth.

In contrast, sulfate (SO_4^{2-}) is the third most abundant ion in sea water, with a concentration of approximately 800 mg SO_4^{2-} S/L. As a consequence, estuarine waters and coastal sediments receive high levels of sulfate-S. When this soluble sulfate encounters strongly reducing conditions, microbial processes transform sulfate to various reduced compounds (e.g., H_2S, CH_3SH, $(CH_3)_2S$, COS) sometimes cumulatively referred to as "sulfides." The ionizable and polar sulfides (i.e., H_2S and COS, respectively) are water soluble, and all are volatile and toxic. In predominantly mineral sediments, much of the dissolved sulfide reacts with soluble ferrous iron, forming insoluble precipitates. Other reactions of S contribute to appreciable levels of organic-bound S, elemental S, and pyrite. Microbial processes combined with alternating oxidation and reduction conditions and rhizosphere processes contribute to the transformations between these chemical forms of S.

Like many other gases that leave wetland sediments as a result of biogeochemical processes, S gases apparently reflect microbiological and plant (macrophyte) variables. Hence, the spectrum of S gases (e.g., concentration ratios and temporal flux changes in H_2S: $(CH_3)_2S$: COS: CH_3SH) observed in different types of wetlands in a landscape would reflect distinct microbe–plant interactions. It would be expected, and has been observed, that S gas ratios are quite different for different wetland types, including those that are closely related (brackish versus salt marshes) but have different vegetative characteristics (dominance of *S. patens* and *J. roemarianus* versus dominance of *S. alterniflora*) (Devai and DeLaune 1994).

(See also DeLaune et al. 1976; Fenchel 1978; Howarth and Teal 1980; Jakobsen et al. 1981; Mendelssohn et al. 1982; King et al. 1982; DeLaune et al. 1983; Smith and Patrick 1983; Pezeshki et al. 1988; Jorgensen 1990; DeLaune and Pezeshki 1991; Giere 1993; Jugsujinda, Krairapanond et al. 1995.)

Biogeochemistry of Contaminants

Transition metals in the environment

Transition metals in the environment may be divided into 2 broad categories:

1) nutritionally essential but toxic in high levels or in certain speciation (e.g., Cu, Zn, Cr, V, Se) and
2) not nutritionally essential and toxic under certain conditions (e.g., Hg, Pb, Cd).

Alkali, alkaline earth, and metalloids (e.g., Cs, Be, As) also can be found, with significantly high concentrations in areas where coal is burned or converted or where fly ash is disposed. Although a comprehensive review of all these elements in sediments would fill a volume, this section will focus on a few illustrative examples of transition metals in both categories mentioned above and provide a general overview of the forms and transformations affecting mobility and biological availability.

All soils and sediments contain many trace and potentially toxic metals as natural constituents. Problems arise when some trace metals are deficient for nutritional purposes (total concentrations are low and in a form that is unavailable) or when elevated concentrations of trace or toxic metals are sufficiently mobile and available to adversely affect plants and animals. Background concentrations can range widely, depending on a number of factors such as sedimentation processes, soil parent material concentrations, and local geochemical activity (e.g., weathering of cinnabar deposits). Usually, it is human activities that cause metal levels to increase in soils and sediments to the point that they present potential health or ecological risks. However, elevated total concentrations of trace and toxic metals do not always result in detectable toxicity to planktonic and benthic organisms or in significant bioconcentration in plants.

A number of specific metal compounds and general chemical forms of metals in soils and sediments differ in their mobility and plant availability. Some of these include

1) dissolved metals that are
    - soluble as free ions (e.g., Cu^{2+}),
    - soluble as inorganic complexes (e.g., $CdCl^{+}$), or
    - soluble as organic complexes (e.g., Zn–[fulvic acid]);
2) exchangeable metals;
3) metals complexed with high molecular-weight, naturally occurring humic materials;
4) precipitated, inorganic metal compounds (e.g., $Pb(CO_3)_2$);
5) metals adsorbed to or occluded with precipitated hydrous oxides;

6) metals precipitated as insoluble sulfide (e.g., NiS); and
7) metals bound within the crystalline lattice structure of primary minerals.

Dissolved metals are the most mobile and plant available (compared to colloidal or precipitated metals). This does not include the broad range of insoluble metals that can be mobilized by microbial and plant siderophores, metallothioneins, and low-molecular-weight cytosine-rich polypeptides (Catallo et al. 1996). Exchangeable metals are those sorbed to the cation or anion exchange complex (CEC and AEC, respectively) on soil surfaces and held there by electrostatic forces. Metals in this form are weakly bound and may be replaced relatively easily by other metal cations and released to the water-soluble forms over micro and meso time scales (i.e., seconds to decades). The relative affinity for exchange sites (or conversely, the difficulty of removal from these sites) on sediments is given by the following lyotropic series (Bohn et al. 1985):

$$H^+ > Na > K \approx NH_4^+ > Cs \approx Mg^{2+} > Ca^{2+} > Ba^{2+} > Al^{3+}(H) \qquad \text{(Equation 3-1).}$$

It is clear from this series that acidic conditions in a sediment can displace metal cations from the CEC and thereby liberate them for assimilation and transport. There is evidence to suggest that rapid (e.g., diurnal) and more extended (seasonal) cycles of RP and pH in alternately flooded and drained systems can give rise to sorption–desorption cycles of these and other metals. Further, it has been shown that some toxic organic chemicals that complex metals in solution (e.g., azaarenes) can be involved in these events, and this constitutes an important transport mechanism for organo-metal complexes in sediments and other compositionally heterogeneous systems (e.g., living cells) (Catallo and Gambrell 1987).

Together, metals in the soluble and exchangeable forms are considered mobile or readily mobilized and potentially bioavailable. On the other extreme of the availability scale are trace and toxic metals bound within the crystalline lattice structure of clay minerals by isomorphous substitution. These metals are essentially unavailable and would become available only as a consequence of mineral weathering, typically over macro time scales (millennia). Between these availability extremes are a number of general chemical forms of metals that are generated in biogeochemical processes and that may be considered potentially mobile and available.

Trace and toxic metals bound with large-molecular-weight OM or humic material are effectively immobilized. There is evidence that some metals are more tightly complexed by soil OM under anoxic or reducing conditions than under upland conditions. As a result of the more efficient mineralization of organic carbon by aerobic microbes, the amount of OM in a dredged sediment material or wetland soil will decrease if disturbed and placed in an upland environment. It has been suggested that the humic materials may become structurally less complex if dredged material is placed upland for disposal purposes (Folsom et al. 1988). With a reduction in total OM, metals that were tightly bound in a sediment later placed upland or disturbed wetland soil that becomes oxidized tend to become less tightly bound over time scales of months to years. The OM in upland soils is also relatively effective in immobilizing metals, thus we do not imply that oxidation resulting from a disturbance of a sediment or wetland soil will cause a major release of metals from soil and sediment OM. However, the release can be significant, as has been shown for Cd, Zn, and Ni.

Precipitated inorganic trace and toxic metal compounds generally include metal oxides, hydroxides, and carbonates. The stability of these inorganic metal compounds is controlled primarily by the pH of the soil–water system. At near-neutral to slightly alkaline pH levels, most metals tend to be effectively immobilized, and the formation of stable precipitates is one major contributing factor. Should pH become moderately to strongly acid over a period of weeks to years, as can sometimes occur when reduced soils or sediments are drained and oxidized, these metals may be released in forms that are more mobile.

Iron oxides and hydroxides and perhaps similar compounds of Mn and Al can effectively adsorb or occlude trace and toxic metals cations. These hydrous oxides of Fe are common in upland soils, in upland-applied dredged materials, and in disturbed wetlands, resulting in oxidation of the soil; they also are found in the thin surface oxidized layer of wetland soils and sediments. Depending on age and degree of crystallinity, these hydrous oxides become unstable under typically reducing, flooded soil conditions. In wetland transition zones and/or where seasonal changes occur in soil flooding, these hydrous Fe oxides may form and dissolve as a function of changing hydrology, consequently immobilizing and releasing metals within the soil on a cyclic basis. For surface soils and sediment materials (the top few mm or so), Fe oxides and hydroxides may be effective in controlling metal retention during flooding and drainage cycles. Giblin et al. (1986) have shown that Fe oxyhydroxides retained metals in the surface sediment of a salt marsh that received trace and toxic metals contained in sewage sludge applications.

In fine-textured, coastal and freshwater marsh soils and sediments, the sulfate becomes reduced to sulfide as it diffuses into strongly reducing interior pore spaces. Though the soluble and volatile hydrogen sulfide gas is formed first, this sulfide quickly reacts with most trace and toxic divalent metals to form highly insoluble metal sulfide precipitates such as FeS, PbS, CdS, CuS, NiS, and ZnS. These sulfide-containing sediments and coastal marsh soils may effectively immobilize trace and toxic metals as sulfides over meso and macro time scales, so long as the environment remains strongly reducing and near-neutral in pH, such as would occur under undisturbed, continuous flooding conditions. Unlike metal–humic material associations, where the release of metals from the OM upon oxidation may be modest, oxidizing sulfide-containing soils and sediments for extended periods will result in loss of all sulfide and subsequent release of all metals from this phase. These released metals then tend to be immobilized by other processes, but perhaps immobilized a little less effectively. Kerner and Wallman (1992) simulated alternate periods of anaerobic and aerobic conditions of an intertidal mud and sand flat sediment in a laboratory study and followed the mobilization of Zn and Cd. Both elements were believed to be removed from pore water by sulfide precipitation during the anaerobic cycles, then released from the sediment solid phase during aerobic cycles. The Zn and Cd release under aerobic conditions was attributed to mineralization of OM and sulfide oxidation.

The redox-influenced soil processes affecting the mobility and bioavailability of trace and toxic metals were first extensively studied in laboratory microcosms, followed by investigation in field studies.

In soils, there is some background level of metals in all of the forms mentioned above. Fortunately, in metals-contaminated soils and sediments, excess metals become primarily associated with these potentially available forms rather than with the readily available soluble and exchangeable forms. The oxidation-reduction conditions associated with upland or wetland soils affect the stability of metals in these potentially available forms. When changes occur in the oxidation status of soils and sediments, transformations of metals occur between the potentially available forms and between the potentially and readily available forms.

Of the potentially available forms of trace and toxic metals, the metal immobilization capacity for some were observed to be more stable under oxidizing conditions typical of upland soils, and other general chemical forms of metals were noted to be more stable under reducing conditions typical of the bulk of sediments or saturated wetland soils. Upon a change in redox status, these metal retention processes tend to be complementary, in that a change from reducing to oxidized conditions (e.g., seasonal drainage of wetlands or upland application of dredged material) or from oxidized to reducing conditions (e.g., seasonal flooding of wetlands or construction of wetlands) does not normally result in a large release of metals from potentially available forms to readily available forms, so long as pH does not change substantially. However, changes in mobility and plant availability are often significant. In dredged materials and wetland soils, pH does sometimes change greatly as a consequence of flooding–drying cycles.

(See also Jenne 1968; Khalid 1980; Feijtel et al. 1988; Catallo 1994.)

Leaching and surface runoff losses of metals

Mesocosm and field research with contaminated dredged materials provides much of the basis for comparing relative effects of soil oxidation-reduction conditions on potential leaching and surface runoff losses. Where contaminated dredged sediments have been placed in upland environments, runoff losses of trace and toxic metals are enhanced over what occurs with uncontaminated sediments similarly placed (Skogerboe et al. 1987; Folsom et al. 1988). Upon initial upland placement of a typically reducing dredged material prior to appreciable oxidation, the metal losses were primarily associated with suspended particulates. This is a physical process and not a biogeochemical process. However, after time for leaching and oxidation, enhanced soluble levels of Cd were noted in the surface runoff, which reflect changing biogeochemical processes in the upland-applied material. Tests showed this would be the case for Cu, Ni, Zn, Pb, and Mn as well, though Cr was not similarly affected. As previously discussed, the acidification of wetland soils or sediments that result from oxidation also results in the greatest losses of soluble metals by surface runoff.

Though dredged materials have received considerable research attention regarding surface runoff, little if any work has been done regarding surface runoff of contaminants with seasonally or other periodically flooded and drained contaminated wetlands.

Once soluble metals enter a wetland, the biogeochemical properties tend to favor retention. For example, greater than 95% of the Pb entering a New Jersey pine barrens watershed was retained by the fine-textured, highly organic soil and vegetation, such that very little of the entering Pb was exported with stream flow from the wetland studied (Turner et al. 1985).

Leaching losses of trace and toxic metals should not be a problem in typical wetlands where water permeability is low and the strongly reducing conditions favor processes that effectively immobilize metals. Again, studies of contaminated dredged material experimentally simulated upland disposal sites and constructed wetland sites provide information that should pertain to the effectiveness of biogeochemical processes in minimizing leaching losses. In a review of this literature, the data were found to support the theory that the biogeochemical processes associated with reducing soils minimize leaching losses of the common divalent trace and toxic metals, compared to the leaching of the same contaminated substrate materials under upland conditions.

Plant availability of metals

The work described above indicated that redox and pH conditions affected the soil biogeochemical conditions influencing chemical availability (release and mobility) of trace and toxic metals. This work led to the question of whether plant uptake of trace and toxic metals would be affected similarly by RP. At first glance, redox effects on plant uptake seem to border the irrelevant because most plants grow either under upland or wetland conditions, but generally not under both. However, a more detailed evaluation of possible important redox effects on plant availability reveals areas where this is relevant. When disposal alternatives are selected for dredged materials, wetland habitat creation and upland applications may both be options. Though there could be species effects on availability and the plant species that would grow on the dredged material would not necessarily be the same as those existing prior to dredging, the question of relative availability of trace and toxic metals under wetland, intertidal, or upland conditions becomes important. Also, there are some plants that thrive in both upland and wetland soil environments, and there are many seasonal wetlands. Thus, the question of redox effects on plant availability becomes important.

A recent review detailed the sequence of research on soil oxidation effects on plant availability of trace metals such as Fe, Mn, Cu, Zn, and the toxic metals (Gambrell 1994). In summary, studies in laboratory microcosms, greenhouses, and field sites have demonstrated that within species that are adapted to both wetland and upland soil conditions, and generally between wetland and upland plant species, trace and toxic metal availability to plants is usually greater under upland (drained and oxidized) soil conditions (Simmers et al. 1981; cf. Catallo et al. 1996).

Metal availability to fish and terrestrial animals

The work on effects of soil oxidation-reduction status on the availability of trace and toxic metals to fish, birds, and terrestrial animals has not been extensive. Again, the relevance of this issue may be questioned at first glance, but it is important in evaluating disposal options for contaminated dredged materials, which may include subaquatic, intertidal, or upland placement.

Folsom et al. (1988) found that Cd was taken up by plants in laboratory and field sites from Black Rock Harbor dredged material in the Field Verification Program for the upland disposal alternative. Kay (1988) noted increased Cd uptake by plants grown in drained, humic (much leaf litter) soil horizons and an accumulation of Cd in the litter layer of an upland dredged material research site planted in poplar trees in The Netherlands. These field data and other data suggest that if plant uptake of metals is enhanced under oxidized conditions, then the potential is increased for metal exposure to terrestrial animals that consume this plant, either directly or indirectly.

Stafford et al. (1991) reported results of contaminant transport where upland, wetland, and aquatic areas were designed into the Times Beach Confined Disposal Facility (CDF). Cottonwood trees accumulated Cd from the upland-applied dredged material, which subsequently accumulated in the leaf litter zone, resulting in increased Cd levels in earthworms at the site. Cadmium levels were elevated somewhat in ducks from the Times Beach site compared to the reference site, but it was stated that likely there are too little data to make conclusions about the distribution of metals in complex food webs.

White and Cromartie (1985) found that Hg and Pb, and especially elevated levels of Cd and Zn (around 800 ppm Zn in the sediments), did not accumulate above background levels in aquatic birds using a CDF that contained elevated levels of these elements during periods of surfacewater ponding; however, Se uptake from the flooded CDF was enhanced.

(See also Jenne 1968; Khalid 1980; Feitjel et al. 1988; Catallo 1994.)

Toxic organic compounds

Organic contaminants can enter wetlands in a number of ways: discharges of untreated or partially treated wastewater; atmospheric deposition; spills; nonpoint source runoff from urban, agricultural, or industrial areas; and drift from aerial application of pesticides. Unfortunately, of the 3 main contaminant groups (i.e., metals, eutrophicants, and organic chemicals) information on fate, biogeochemistry, and transport of toxic organic chemicals in wetlands is not well developed. Major fate and transport processes for these chemicals include sorption to suspended solids in the water column, minerals and high-molecular-weight humic materials in the sediment bed, partitioning to colloidal matter including dissolved organic carbon (DOC), diffusive exchange between the water column and the bed, settling and burial of particulate-bound organics, volatilization, chemical and biological reactions (e.g., biotransformation), direct and indirect redox reactions, humification, and plant or biotic uptake. These processes determine exposure to wetland ecosystems, and understanding these processes is critical to estimating ecological effects.

Attempts to measure these processes usually proceed in laboratory microcosms and mesocosms, or in controlled field situations. The resulting processes commonly are framed in mathematical constructs that are used to develop conceptual or predictive models for fates of organic chemicals in aquatic systems (Table 3-2).

Of these processes, several appear to have specific features in wetlands that may reduce or increase potential effects on ecological endpoints.

1) Sorption of toxic organics is directly related to pH, RP, temperature, and OM content, which can be extremely high in many wetland soils. Higher OM content would therefore reduce soluble concentrations of organic contaminants.
2) Alternatively, high concentrations of organic carbon found in wetlands can provide for sorption and solvation of hydrophobic organics, and this can take the form of a mobile colloidal phase. The end result is a decrease in the sorption onto particles and an increase in the concentration in the pore water or water column. Equilibrium modeling indicates that this process only becomes important for hydrophobic organics such as polychlorinated biphenyls (PCBs), dicholorodiphenyltrichloroethane (DDT), and hexachlorobenzene (HCB). The effect of this partitioning on bioavailability remains an open question.
3) Biotransformation rates of some chemicals may be enhanced in wetlands because of the large, diverse microflora associated with the systems and the wide ranges of RP observed. Reductive dechlorination, for example, is an anaerobic transformation pathway for halogenated organics that can occur in wetlands. In reductive dechlorination, the organic compound serves as an electron acceptor, resulting in the disproportionation of the system and loss of Cl^-. The resulting lower chlorinated metabolites often (but not always) are less toxic, more soluble, and may diffuse through the anaerobic/aerobic interface where they may be mineralized aerobically. Reductive dechlorination reactions are not always beneficial. Dechlorination of some C_2 chlorinated aliphatics proceeds through vinyl chloride as a stable metabolite. Vinyl

Table 3-2 Important fate and transport processes for toxic organics in wetland systems

Process	Equation	Controlling variables
Sorption/desorption	Dissolved fraction = $1/\{1+K_p m + K_{doc}DOC)\}$ DOC-associated fraction = $1/\{1+(1/K_{doc}DOC)+(Kpm/K_{doc}DOC)\}$ Particulate-bound fraction = $1/\{1+(1/K_p m)+(K_{doc}DOC/K_p m)\}$	Organic matter content, DOC concentration, fundamental chemical properties
Transformation: chemical or biological	Zero-order decay equation First-order decay equation Second-order decay equation	RP, pH, microbial populations, UV, temperature
Volatilization	Mass transfer coefficient: $k = K_l He/[He + RT_a(K_l/K_g)]$	Wind speed, fundamental chemical properties
Plant or biotic uptake	Bioconcentration factor (BCF) = concentration in the biota/concentration in the sediment or water compartment	Fundamental chemical properties
Burial	—	Sedimentation rates, irreversible sorption
Sedimentation	Stoke' s Law	—
Diffusive exchange		Porosity, sediment surface roughness
Humification	—	Fundamental chemical properties, extracellular enzyme concentrations

K_p = partition coefficient between water and particles (L/kg)
K_{doc}=partition coefficient between DOC and water
DOC = DOC concentration
m = particulate concentration

chloride is a known carcinogen, while many of its precursors are not. By contrast, biotransformation rates of contaminants (e.g., petroleum hydrocarbons) can be inhibited in reduced, anoxic sediments where aerobic microbial processes are limited.

4) Transport processes can also be affected by wetland features. Dense vegetation over many wetland surfaces will reduce wind speed (and subsequently volatilization). High concentrations of DOC in wetland systems can reduce the concentration of the contaminant in a “true” dissolved state and therefore reduce volatilization. Direct measurement of volatilization of organic compounds in wetlands is limited.

5) Humification or polymerization of organics in sediments is another potentially important fate process in wetlands that has been poorly studied. Extracellular enzymes in sediments can mediate polymerization of organic compounds and enhance their integration to humic materials, where they can be sequestered.

Assimilative capacities of wetlands

Laboratory microcosm and batch studies frequently are used to estimate assimilative capacity rates and equilibrium partitioning relationships. Field studies, in an attempt to confirm or scale-up laboratory results, have also been conducted, but the overall scope has been confined to local point sources or spills (e.g., hazardous waste sites) and no attempt has been made to extrapolate these studies regionally. At the process level, for example, variability in regional biotransformation rates within wetlands is not understood. The scope of these wetland studies contrasts sharply with well-developed budgets of organic chemicals developed for aquatic systems such as the Great Lakes. In these studies, inputs, outputs, and processing of organic compounds such as PCBs have been measured and confirmed at the macro scale. These studies have demonstrated the dominant role of atmospheric exchange in the budget of hydrophobic, semivolatile organic compounds such as PCBs. Few data exist on the role of atmospheric exchange for wetland systems. The common assumption is that organics are introduced to wetlands through point or nonpoint sources in the watershed. It is likely, however, that these inputs occur over a baseline of regional and global inputs from atmospheric sources (Catallo et al. 1995). The role these systems play in regional or global storage and transfer of semivolatiles, for example, is not well understood.

The assimilative capacity of ecosystems can be expressed most simply as

$$c = \beta c_{in} \qquad \text{(Equation 3-2)},$$

where c = the contaminant concentration in the wetland, c_{in} = the input contaminant concentration, and β = the overall assimilation function. This assimilation function consists of 2 components:

$$\beta = q + v_t \qquad \text{(Equation 3-3)},$$

where q = the hydraulic loading rate (water depth/retention time) and v_t = the sum of all the physical, chemical, and biological processes acting on the contaminant. This relationship separates assimilative capacity into its component parts: 1) hydrology and the residence time of contaminants in wetlands and 2) the rates of the assimilation processes themselves. This concept allows sizing of wetlands to meet different assimilation goals. For example, if both sides of the equation are multiplied by the flow rate through the system, Q, the resulting equation can be rearranged to yield

$$\text{required area} = \text{loading rate} / (v_t)(c) \qquad \text{(Equation 3-4)},$$

where loading is in mass/area and c might be a wetland water-quality criterion. This approach can be modified to account for more complex, realistic hydrology and spatially variable process rates. Although it increases in complexity, the fundamental concepts remain the same. Assimilative capacity is determined by both hydrology (residence time) and process rates, many of which can be classified as biogeochemical processes. In other words, a slow biogeochemical process occurring over a long residence time in a wetland can assimilate the same amount of chemical as a fast process with a short residence time.

A simple example of an assimilative capacity calculation may illustrate other points for assimilation of contaminants in wetlands. Fate processes for HCB have been determined in the laboratory and field for a bottomland hardwood forest and freshwater marsh in Louisiana. The components of the process term, v_t, included reductive dechlorination of HCB in sediments, volatilization of HCB from water to air, burial, settling of HCB sorbed to particles, dissolved and DOC-associated HCB recycling from the sediment to the water column, and speciation of HCB in the water column. Overall mass transfer through various assimilation routes was calculated using a modified steady-state modeling framework. When assimilation processes were summed (v_t) for these wetland systems in Louisiana, the bottomland hardwood marsh ($v_t = 131.4$ m/y) exceeded the freshwater marsh ($v_t = 104.5$ m/y) by 25%. This was due to the increased concentrations of DOC in the freshwater marsh, which inhibited a major removal process, volatilization. Highly organic freshwater marshes presumably would be able to assimilate more. Of course, overall assimilation capacity will also depend on hydrological characteristics and physiography of the 2 systems.

Simple assimilation models such as this cannot be mechanistic but can compare the relative impacts of various processes. They serve as a basis for more complex numerical models that have predictive value. The major uncertainties in determining assimilative capacity reside in the determining the process rates under nonequilibrium conditions. Biogeochemical and other processes are spatially and temporally variable. For example, volatilization rates change with wind speed, and biotransformation rates can change together with factors affecting microbial growth.

Biogeochemical indicators of wetland condition

Contaminant loading to wetlands can result in the alteration of several physicochemical properties of soil–water–plant components and rates and pathways of several biogeochemical processes (Koepfler and Kator 1986; Catallo and Gambrell 1987; Catallo 1994; Catallo and Gambrell 1995). In order to evaluate the impact of contaminant loading on wetland biogeochemical functions, it is important to measure the changes in soil–water physicochemical properties, chemical composition of periphyton and plant communities, and relative rates of various biogeochemical processes.

Biogeochemical functions can be used as indicators to evaluate the impacts of contaminants on wetlands. The process endpoints of these functions include

1) microbial transformation rates for C, N, O, P, S;
2) endpoints of microbial-plant assemblages and physicochemical processes (e.g., time dynamics and amplitudes of RP and elemental fluxes, ratios of dissolved and gaseous products of elemental transformations); and
3) microbial and chemical conditions underlying habitat and landscape operation (e.g., habitat usage, health, or reproductive success of macrobiota, input versus output water quality, and chemical signals such as trace gas signatures).

Rates, temporal structure, and chemical fine structure of outputs from biogeochemical processes can be related to measurable physicochemical properties. This seems particularly the case for large-scale (long path or satellite-based) measurements of trace gas efflux from wetlands experiencing different kinds of impacts versus "pristine" systems in unfragmented landscapes, which are uncommon. Individual wetlands apparently have gas signatures that reflect, and to some extent integrate, the physicochemical, hydrological, and biotic variables in situ. Changes in these outputs, with respect to either gas ratios or changes in mass balance for particular gases, can be related both to small-scale impacts at the microbial population level and to large-scale functional alterations of the system. The experimental and statistical handling of these process outputs are directly relevant to the concluding section, which lists research needs.

Ecological Integration

Toxicology, the study of the effects of toxic substances on single organisms (usually humans), provides the structure upon which the science of ecotoxicology is constructed. Ecotoxicology is the study of the effects of toxicants on populations and communities in ecosystems. A variety of effects is determined, which includes, but is not limited to, the following: successional rates; biogeochemical functioning; biological diversity, zonation, and temporal dynamics; photosynthesis and respiration; reproductive behavior and success; community structure; and trophodynamics. Hence, ecotoxicologists must integrate the methods, concepts, and spatiotemporal scales of toxicology, environmental chemistry, systems ecology, and increasingly, statistics and nonlinear dynamical theory.

The introduction of toxicants to ecosystems may produce alterations in the function of one or more of the organisms or biological processes. A recent review of the literature in aquatic and wetland ecotoxicology provided the following general conclusions (Catallo 1994):

1) Wetlands exposed to pollution can behave in ways similar to some terrestrial and aquatic systems: species abundance and diversity can change at least temporarily, energy transfer through food webs can be altered or "shorted,"

biogeochemical processes can be altered but also can act as powerful compensatory mechanisms that buffer the system against progressive functional changes.

2) As pollutant stress increases, major ecological effects can occur, which include decreased species diversity and biomass, changes in P:R budgets, altered trophodynamics, and altered biogeochemical process variables (RP, soil respiration, and elemental transformations). Some of these effects correspond to a tightening of niche volumes. This frequently is a threshold process: in plant and detrital communities, significant effects may be observed only upon introduction of relatively high contaminant levels (or removal of refuge by mixing, tilling, or dredging). At this point, the toxicants can replace natural processes as drivers of biotic variability within the system. The terminus of these events can be a biocenosis that is successionally "primitive," i.e., marked by the removal of diverse specialist communities and by their replacement with smaller numbers of generalists and opportunists at low biomass.

The extension of standard laboratory toxicological results to ecosystems frequently is problematic, and generalizations useful for risk evaluations and comparisons between different wetlands are few. For example, numerous studies on the effects of pollutants (e.g., south Louisiana crude oil) conducted in the same marsh type have provided a range of results, from data indicating no effects on plant and benthic processes to data suggesting significant effects (Wolfe 1977; Bender et al. 1981; Catallo 1994). This appears to be a result not only of controllable variables such as time of year in which the study was conducted but also of intrinsic properties such as historic pre-exposure of the ecosystem to natural oil seepage (Gulf coast wetlands) versus no previous exposure (mid-Atlantic coast wetlands). Similarly, data on toxic metal uptake by *S. alterniflora* frequently are not in agreement (Catallo 1994).

Wetlands are perhaps more complicated from an ecotoxicological perspective than are other ecosystems because

- these systems have highly integrated plant-soil-microbial assemblages that respond to hydrological forces in nonlinear ways;
- the high degree of intercorrelation between plant–microbe–soil variables renders many traditional statistical models ineffective for showing effects or promoting further mechanistic understanding of the system;
- ecosystem process rates can be stabilized by physicochemical perturbations (e.g., pulses), including the introduction of pollutants, and toxicant-mediated effects on sensitive species can be obscured by rapid replacement with tolerant species that perform similar functions; and
- attempts to isolate single variables in microcosms or field settings frequently give adequate pictures of the process elements involved but little or no idea of how this process is integrated and functionalized within the wetland system (Odum 1983).

These and other complexities in wetland ecosystems make the risk assessment process more difficult. For example, the "keystone species" concept has limited utility in some wetlands because functionally equivalent species can replace those removed or impaired by toxicants. Hence, a monitoring scheme using bioindicators might detect impairment or removal of a keystone species due to contaminants only to discover later that flows and transformation rates of elements and energy are functionally unchanged.

Frequently there are reciprocal effects between contaminants and biogeochemical processes: the disposition and fates of toxic contaminants are influenced by biogeochemical variables (e.g., RP), but the presence of the contaminants also can alter biogeochemical processes (e.g., by intoxicating microbial populations). Particularly susceptible to pollutant impacts are those processes mediated by surface-dwelling microbial communities, i.e., those at the water–sediment interface and the oxic–anoxic interface several millimeters below the sediment surface. It has been shown, for example, that bacterial nitrifiers and denitrifiers are susceptible to toxicity from hydrophobic pollutants, and the degree of toxicity can be influenced by grain size and OM composition (Catallo 1994; USACOE 1996). Biogeochemical fluxes of N gases, however, need not reflect this toxicity; other microbes can transform N species in similar ways. Even though the activity of nitrifying bacteria is decreased by contaminants, the total numbers of specific microbial species change very little. These data suggest that monitoring a limited number of biogeochemical process outputs from contaminated sediments (e.g., N gas flux) may be insufficient to detect real toxic effects at the microbial level; other metrics (e.g., microbial activity, speciation, diversity) must be used in addition, and these must be related (upscaled) to functional properties of the system (e.g., N fluxes and speciation in ground and surface waters). Less is known about toxic effects on nitrogen fixation, methanogenesis, denitrification, and sulfide production. Results of microcosm studies have shown that low levels (50 ppm) of more hydrophilic chemicals (aromatic N-, O-, and S- heterocycles) can alter microbial community structure and S processing in situ (Catallo and Gambrell 1995). In general, the microbial communities mediating these processes are found in subsurface sediment horizons (e.g., below 1 cm) and can be sheltered against surface-deposited hydrophobic pollutants. Traditionally, studies showing changes in activity or structure in these communities or their process outputs have used very high levels of toxicants (parts per thousand), sometimes in conjunction with homogenization or other mixing of the sediment.

At the ecosystem level, a large number of ecotoxicological studies have addressed petroleum and hydrocarbon pollution in coastal saline wetlands. These have been copiously reviewed elsewhere (National Academy of Sciences 1975; Wolfe 1977; Teal and Howarth 1984; DeLaune et al. 1990; Catallo 1994). It is notable that the "ecosystem" studies of toxicant effects in wetlands frequently are comprised of lists of species impacts, with no functional entities invoked in the analysis. Some work with plankton responses to trace levels of organic pollutants, and subsequent effects on food chains, has provided interesting results (Mosser et al. 1972; O'Connors et al. 1978; Cole et al. 1979). Further related work will be needed, however, before these data can be interpreted with respect to productivity trends in estuaries and coastal marine systems.

With respect to integrating biogeochemical process responses to chemical loadings with changes in ecosystem function, a comprehensive study was conducted in fresh watersheds containing lakes, streams, and forests (Likens and Bormann 1995). Whole lake and stream studies have provided data on biogeochemical responses to chemical stress that showcase the effects of connectance, compensatory mechanisms, and scrolling of effects and responses at different scales. For example, laboratory and modeling studies of eutrophication suggest that algal blooms in oligotrophic lakes could be limited by low C concentrations. It was found, however, that C gas flux from the atmosphere was sufficient to support the blooms. (This process was prevented in sealed microcosm experiments and omitted from the modeling.) Whole lake studies then revealed that N also could be supplied by the atmosphere (Carpenter et al. 1995). Acidification of lakes showed food chain and organism effects at numerous levels in the system, including invertebrates, fish, and birds. Also observed was a surprising biogeochemical response: pH neutralization by microbial reduction of H^+ (to H_2) and sulfate (to H_2S) that was promoted by the addition of acids (Schindler 1991; Carpenter et al. 1995).

It is clear from the material summarized above that wetland function is mediated by interdependent networks of processes. Processes mediating stability, resilience, and recovery frequently are intertwined with compensatory mechanisms (such as succession of biological functional surrogates) that can obscure important features of the system. Study of these processes in isolation (e.g., in controlled microcosms) can give imprecise or incorrect results, particularly when conclusions are extrapolated to natural ecosystems.

A large part of the scaling problem in wetlands and other ecosystems is the design and implementation of experiments that explicitly address sources of variation in complex systems while remaining tractable in terms of data handling and statistical power. Numerous analytical and statistical techniques are emerging that can help provide quantitative functional data and then render those data in frameworks that are productive for interpretations and further experimental design. An example of an analytical approach that can accommodate a large number of correlated variables and provide quantitative insight to hypotheses and experimental design is described in the section that follows.

(See also Metcalf et al. 1971; LaPoint et al. 1984; Bormann 1985; Gambrell 1989; Pardue et al. 1993.)

Structural Equation Modeling

Structural equation modeling (SEM) encompasses an entire family of models known by many names: covariance structure analysis, confirmatory factor analysis, latent variable analysis, and often linear structural relations (LISREL) analysis. From a statistical viewpoint, SEM is a method that simultaneously estimates a series of dependence relationships. It has its historical ties to multiple regression, factor analysis, and path analysis. SEM combines the capability of studying dependence relations (as with path analysis) with the ability to formulate complex unobserved variables (as in factor analysis). The term "covariance structure analysis" is sometimes applied because the SEM procedure is based on the examination of covariance and correlation matrices.

The basic idea behind SEM is to test whether variables that have been represented by a group of linear equations are related. The logic of the approach can be summarized in the following steps:

1) The model is described in terms (a path diagram or series of equations) that are consistent with the way in which the variables are believed to be interrelated.
2) A computer program solves a series of matrix equations and determines the implications of this postulated model for variances and covariances of the variables.
3) The program tests whether the variances and covariances within the data fit this model.
4) The program lists the results of the statistical testing of the model fit, provides parameter estimates and standard errors for coefficients of equations, and provides diagnostic indices.
5) On the basis of this information, the experimenter decides whether the model is a good one for the data or needs to be modified.

One of the greatest strengths and distinguishing characteristics of SEM is its ability to validate models. The process of testing and evaluating models involves comparisons between an actual covariance matrix derived from data and an implied covariance matrix derived from the model. Hence there is an overt comparison between the conceptual framework of the experimenter and the actual behavior of the data. Another distinguishing feature of SEM is its capacity to simultaneously estimate a series of dependence relationships. From a statistical perspective, this is a substantial advantage over techniques such as multiple regression, where the order in which variables are entered into an equation can have a major effect on the assessment of a variable's importance. In SEM, relationships between structural variables take the form of partial regression coefficients, and their values are independent of the values of other pathways. Further, SEM generally avoids the problems of multiple collinearity among variables, which are common in multiple regression analysis. An additional advantage of SEM over regression analysis has to do with estimation of measurement error: in SEM, when valid indicators are available, they permit the estimation of the measurement error associated with variables in the model. Typically, regression analysis assumes that there is no error associated with observed variables or that error is unimportant in fitting models to data. Theoretical analyses (Bollen 1989; Pugesek and Tomer 1995) have shown that failing to incorporate measurement error into an analysis can lead to bias and distortion of regression estimates as well as to inflated variances.

With this short introduction, it is now possible to briefly introduce the SEM model. Most SEM models include 2 parts, a measurement model and a structural model. The measurement model corresponds to a confirmatory factor analysis model that expresses how the researcher forms the latent (unobserved) variables. Latent variables are formed as composites of observed measured variables that are called "indicators." Hence, latent variables are analogous to factors in factor analysis and residuals in regression analysis; they are not directly observed but are present in the data.

The structural model uses a series of interdependent regression equations to express the causal relationships among latent variables. All relationships, in both the structural and the measurement models, are linear. The coefficients in the equations formulating the structural model are called "path coefficients."

Anderson and Gerbing (1988) advocate a 2-step approach, starting with the measurement model. If the measurement model fits the data well (e.g., a satisfactory confirmatory factor analysis is completed), indicating adequate measurement of the latent variables, the researcher may proceed to fit the structural model. As mentioned above, SEM also provides measures of the variability of each model parameter and individual significance tests for inclusion of each parameter in the model.

Statistical testing and evaluation

Researchers can estimate, test, and evaluate path diagrams such as the one presented in Figure 3-2 using computer programs such as LISREL (Jöreskog and Sörbom 1989). Data about the indicators are collected and used to evaluate the model. Input for the statistical analysis is the variance–covariance matrix or the correlation matrix. The statistical analysis has 2 main functions. One function is to estimate the free parameters (path coefficients, loadings, and error terms) of the model. This function is analogous to the estimation of regression coefficients in a multiple regression analysis. However, coefficients are frequently derived using the maximum likelihood method of estimation (rather than the least squares method used in multiple regression).

The second function of the statistical analysis is to determine how well the model fits the data. Model fit is assessed by comparing the actual variance–covariance matrix generated from the data to a model-implied variance–covariance matrix. Chi-square statistics then can be used to evaluate model fit. The desired result for model

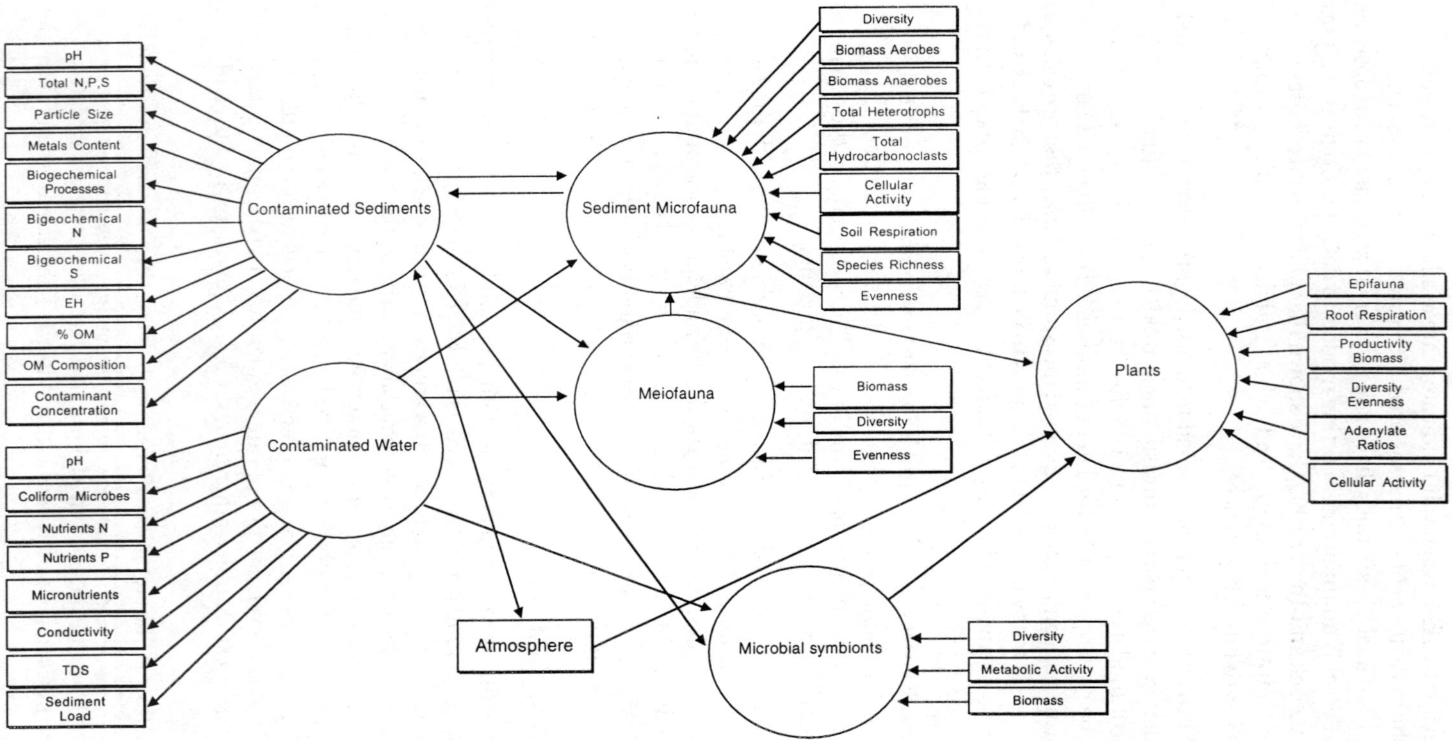

Figure 3-2 Example of a path diagram for an SEM of a wetland ecosystem experiencing contamination. Indicators = rectangles; latent variables = circles. Single-headed arrows relate latent variables to indicators; arrows between latent variables indicate dependence relationships (e.g., a feedback relationship is shown between sediment contamination and sediment microfauna).

acceptance is a nonsignificant chi-square, i.e., there is no detectable difference between matrices generated by the proposed model and those generated by the actual data. In practice, the chi-square test is sensitive to sample size and is generally supplemented with other fit indices (Jöreskog and Sörbom 1989).

Model respecification and modification indices

Ideally, the user of SEM has a strong theory (a conceptualization of how things in the system being measured interact) on which to base proposed models. Models commonly are tentative and entertained as crude approximations. The researcher can use SEM to estimate and evaluate these models and, on the basis of various indicators, can propose a respecification of the model. Estimation proceeds on the newly specified models using the same set of data. If desired, modification indices provided by LISREL can be invoked to guide model respecification. A large (> 4) modification index for a fixed parameter of the model indicates that releasing the parameter to be freely estimated will significantly improve the model. As is shown in Figure 3-2, sediment contamination both affects and is affected by sediment microfauna. Such feedback is common in biological processes, and it is entirely within the capability of SEM to encompass such feedback.

Respecified models such as the one described above should be considered exploratory and in need of further confirmation with additional data. The goal of SEM modeling is to test hypotheses about variable relationships and to gain insight about their relationships through an iterative process of model respecification and confirmation ("tuning"). One of the strengths of SEM lies in the diagnostic tools that it provides to aid the researcher in the evaluation and refinement of knowledge about the system under investigation. Among other things, this can lead to subsequent improvements in experimental design.

Multi-group analyses (stacked models)

It is often of interest to compare samples from different groups or populations, e.g., comparing an undisturbed wetland to one contaminated by toxicants. In these cases, it is possible to estimate a model separately within each group (Figure 3-2). This approach will not, however, answer questions related to the way the model might differ in different populations. This objective can be accomplished using multi-group analyses. In a multi-group analysis, the researcher stacks groups together and estimates a single model simultaneously for all groups. This procedure allows the use of constraints across groups to test for the ways the models differ. If the more constrained model did not fit the data more poorly, the conclusion would be that the 2 groups were invariant.

Additional SEM utilities

Nonlinear path coefficients as well as loadings can be addressed in SEM. Variable interactions can also be modeled in SEM and are analogous to interaction in analysis of variance (ANOVA). In the SEM setting, however, interactions between latent variables are considered. Time series data also can be considered in SEM; such time-dependent models can include lag effects between latent variables and observed variables measured at various time intervals.

(See also Hayduk 1987; Saris et al. 1987; Byrne 1989, 1994; Loehlin 1994; Hair et al. 1995.)

Research Needs

Scientific understanding of the biogeochemical processes in wetlands is not complete. These processes are complex and are affected by a variety of physical, chemical, and biological modifying factors, the effects of which are usually poorly understood. Consequently, there are a variety of research needs; those below are considered to be of the higher priority:

- investigation of the relationship between measured Eh values and the chemistry of dissolved constituents in situ,
- determination of the humification or polymerization of organics in wetland sediments in relation to contaminant fate,
- application of an analytical approach that can accommodate a large number of correlated values (i.e., the simultaneous estimation of a series of dependent relationships, and
- development of studies to encompass larger geographic scales (watersheds) and more complex interactions.

References

Anderson JG, Gerbing DW. 1988. Structural equation modeling in practice review and recommended two-step approach. *Psychological Bulletin* 103:411–423.

Armstrong W. 1975. Waterlogged soils. In: Etherington JR, editor. Environmental and plant ecology. London UK: Wiley. p 181–218.

Audi R, editor. 1995. The dictionary of philosophy. Cambridge UK: Cambridge Univ Pr. 882 p.

Baas-Becking LGM, Kaplan IR, Moore D. 1960. Limits of the natural environment in terms of pH and oxidation-reduction potentials. *J Geology* 68(3):243–284.

Bailey LD, Beauchamp E. 1971. Nitrate reduction, and redox potentials measured with permanently and temporarily placed platinum electrodes in saturated soils. *Can J Soil Sci* 51:51–58.

Bender ME, Hudgins JG, Jordan RA, editors. 1981. Fates and effects of experimental oil spills in an eastern coastal plain marsh system. Final report to the American Petroleum Institute. Washington DC: API.

Bentler PM. 1990. Comparative fit indexes in structural models. *Psychological Bulletin* 107:238–246.

Boar RR, DeLaune RD, Lindau CW, Patrick WH. 1993. Denitrification in bottomland hardwood soils of the Cache River, Arkansas. Vicksburg MS: U.S. Army Corps of Engineers. Wetlands Research Program Technical Report WRP-CP-1. p 1–26.

Bohn HL. 1968. Electromotive force of inert electrodes in soil suspensions. *Soil Sci Soc Am J* 32:211–215.

Bohn HL. 1969. The emf of platinum electrodes in dilute solutions and its relation to soil pH. *Soil Sci Soc Am J* 33:639–640.

Bohn HL. 1971. Redox potentials. *Soil Sci* 112(1):39–45.

Bohn HL, McNeal BL, O'Connor GA. 1985. Soil chemistry. 2nd ed. New York: Wiley-Interscience. 341 p.

Bollen KA. 1989. Structural equations with latent variables. New York: Wiley. 528 p.

Bormann FH. 1985. Air pollution and forests: an ecosystem perspective. *BioScience* 35:434–441.

Browder JA, May LN, Rosenthal A, Gosselink JG, Baumann RH. 1989. Modeling future trends in wetland loss and brown shrimp production in Louisiana using thematic mapper imagery. *Remote Sens Environ* 28:45–59.

Byrne BM. 1989. A primer of LISREL: basic applications and programming for confirmatory factor analytic models. New York NY: Springer-Verlag.

Byrne BM. 1994. Structural equation modeling with EQS and EQS/Windows. Thousand Oaks CA: Sage.

Cantwell M, Foreman RTT. 1993. Landscape graphs: ecological modeling with graph theory to detect configurations common to diverse landscapes. *Landscape Ecology* 8:239–255.

Carpenter SR, Chisholm SW, Krebs CJ, Schindler DW, Wright RF. 1995. Ecosystem experiments. *Science* 269:324–327.

Catallo WJ. 1994. Ecotoxicology of wetland ecosystems. Current understanding and future research needs. *Environ Toxicol Chem* 12(12):2209–2224.

Catallo WJ, Gambrell RP. 1987. The effects of high levels of polycyclic aromatic hydrocarbons on sediment physicochemical properties and benthic organisms in a polluted stream. *Chemosphere* 16(5):1053–1063.

Catallo WJ, Gambrell RP. 1995. Fate and effects of N-, O-, and S- Heterocycles (NOSHs) from petroleum and pyrogenic sources in marine sediments. New Orleans LA: U.S. Department of the Interior, Minerals Management Service. MMS 94-056. 72 p.

Catallo WJ, Schlenker JM, Gambrell RP, Shane BS. 1995. Toxic chemicals and trace metals from urban and rural Louisiana lakes: recent historical profiles and toxicological significance. *Environ Sci Technol* 29(6):1436–1445.

Catallo WJ, Henk W, Younger L, Mills O, Thiele DJ, Meyers SP. 1996. Trace metal uptake by *Pichia spartinae*, an endosymbiotic yeast in the salt marsh cord grass, *Spartina alterniflora*. *Chemistry and Ecology* 13(2):113–131.

Chambers JR. 1992. Habitat degradation and fishery declines in the U.S. In: Bolton S, editor. Coastal wetlands. New York NY: American Society of Civil Engineers. p 46–60.

Charef A, Sun HH. 1990. Time domain analysis of fractal system. *Annual International Conference of the IEEE Engineering in Medicine and Biology Society*. 12:1406–1407.

Cogger CG, Kennedy PE, Carlson D. 1992. Seasonally saturated soils in the Puget lowland II. Measuring and interpreting redox potentials. *Soil Sci* 154(1):50–58.

Cole MA, Reichardt PB, Button DK. 1979. Reversible bioconcentration of monochlorobiphenyls by *Rhodotorula rubra*: correlations with aqueous solubility of substrate. *Bull Environ Contam Toxicol* 23:44–50.

Crozier CR, Devai I, DeLaune RD. 1995. Methane and reduced sulfur gas production by fresh and dried wetland soils. *Soil Sci Soc Am J* 59:277–284.

Deegan LA, Thompson BA. 1985. The ecology of fish communities in the Mississippi River deltaic plain. In: Yanez-Arancibia, editor. Fish community ecology in estuaries and coastal lagoons: towards an ecosystem integration. Ciudad Universitaria, Mexico: Universidad Nacional Autonoma de Mexico. p 35–56.

DeLaune RD, Gambrell RP, Pardue JH, Patrick, Jr. WH. 1990. Fate of petroleum hydrocarbons and toxic organics in Louisiana coastal environments. *Estuaries* 13:72–80.

DeLaune RD, Patrick WH, Brannon JM. 1976. Nutrient transformations in Louisiana salt marsh soils. Baton Rouge LA: Louisiana State University, Center for Wetlands Resources. Louisiana Sea Grant Publication No. LSU-T-76-009.

DeLaune RD, Patrick WH, Casselman ME. 1981. Effect of sediment pH and redox conditions on degradation of benzo(a)pyrene. *Mar Poll Bull* 12(7):251–253.

DeLaune RD, Pezeshki SR. 1991. Role of soil chemistry in vegetative ecology of wetlands. *Trends Soil Sci* 1:101–113.

DeLaune RD, Smith DJ, Patrick WH. 1983. Relationship of marsh elevation, redox potential, and sulfide to *Spartina alterniflora* productivity. *Soil Sci Soc Am J* 47:930–935.

de Ruiter PC, Neutel A-M, Moore JC. 1995. Energetics, patterns of interaction strengths, and stability in real ecosystems. *Science* 269:1257–1260.

Devai I, DeLaune RD. 1994. Changes in reduced gaseous sulfur compounds collected in glass gas sampling bulbs. *Analytical Letters* 27(12):2403–2411.

Devai I, DeLaune RD. 1995a. Evidence for phosphine production and emission from Louisiana and Florida marsh soils. *Org Geochem* 23:277–279.

Devai I, DeLaune RD. 1995b. Formation of volatile sulfur compounds in salt marsh sediment as influenced by soil redox condition. *Org Geochem* 23:283–287.

Devai I, DeLaune RD. 1995c. Light hydrocarbon production in freshwater marsh soil as influenced by soil redox conditions. *Water, Air, and Soil Pollution* 84:1–8.

Ehleringer JR, Field CB, editors. 1993. Scaling physiological processes: leaf to globe. San Diego CA: Academic Pr. 388 p.

Faulkner SP, Patrick Jr. WH, Gambrell RP. 1989. Field techniques for measuring wetland soil parameters. *Soil Sci Soc Am J* 53:883–890.

Feijtel TC, DeLaune RD, Patrick Jr WH. 1988. Biogeochemical control on metal distribution and accumulation in Louisiana sediments. *J Environ Qual* 17:88–94.

Fenchel TM. 1978. The ecology of micro and meio benthos. *Ann Rev Ecol Syst* 9:99–121.

Folsom Jr BL, Skogerboe JG, Palermo MR, Simmers JW, Pranger SA, Shafer RA. 1988. Synthesis of the results of the field verification program upland disposal alternative. Vicksburg MS: U.S. Army Engineer Waterways Experiment Station. Technical Report D-88-7.

Gambrell RP. 1989. Environmental pollution in Louisiana lakes and bayous: selected case studies. *The Cancer Quarterly* 2(4):19–23.

Gambrell RP. 1994. Trace and toxic metals in wetlands: a review. *J Environ Qual* 23:883–891.

Gambrell RP, Patrick Jr WH. 1978. Chemical and microbiological properties of anaerobic soils and sediments. In: Hook DD, Crawford RMM, editors. Plant life in anaerobic environments. Ann Arbor MI: Ann Arbor Science. p 375–423.

Giblin AE, Luther III GW, Valiela I. 1986. Trace metal solubility in salt marsh sediments contaminated with sewage sludge. *Estuarine, Coastal, and Shelf Science* 23:477–498.

Giere O. 1993. Meiobenthology: the microscopic fauna in aquatic sediments. Berlin, Germany: Springer-Verlag. 328 p.

Grenthe I, Stumm W, Laaksuharju M, Nilsson AC, Wikberg P. 1992. Redox potentials and redox reactions in deep groundwater systems. *Chemical Geology* 98:131–150. Amsterdam, The Netherlands: Elsevier Science.

Hair JF, Anderson RE, Tatham RL, Black WC. 1995. Multivariate data analysis. 4th ed. Englewood Cliffs NJ: Prentice Hall. 745 p.

Haraguchi A. 1995. Seasonal changes in oxygen consumption rate and redox properties of floating peat in a pond in central Japan. *Wetlands* 15(3):242–246.

Hayduk LA. 1987. Structural equation modeling with LISREL. Baltimore MD: Johns Hopkins Univ Pr.

Howarth RW, Teal JM. 1980. Energy flow in a salt marsh ecosystem: the role of reduced inorganic sulfur compounds. *Am Nat* 116:862–872.

Howes BL, Howarth RW, Teal JM, Valiela I. 1981. Oxidation reduction potentials in a salt marsh: spatial patterns and interactions with primary production. *Limnol Oceanogr* 26:350–360.

Hudnall WH, Tiarks AE, Waddell WC, Patterson WB. 1995. Soil water relationships within the long-term forest management plots. In: Selim HM, Brown WH, editors. Proc. Conf. Environ. Iss. USFS, Louisiana. LSU Agricultural Center, 24–25 Jul 1995. p 85–89.

Hutchinson EG. 1948. Circular causal systems in ecology. *Annals New York Academy of Sciences* 50:221–246.

Jakobsen P, Patrick Jr WH, Williams BG. 1981. Sulfide and methane formation in soils and sediments. *Soil Science* 132:279–287.

Jenne EA. 1968. Controls of Mn, Fe, Co, Ni, Cu, Zn concentrations in soils and water: the significant role of hydrous Mn and Fe oxides. In: Baker RA, editor. Trace inorganics in water. ACS Advances in Chemistry Series Vol. 73. p 337–387.

Johnston CA. 1994. Cumulative impacts to wetlands. *Wetlands* 14:49–55.

Jöreskog KG, Sörbom D. 1989. LISREL 7: A guide to the program and its application. Chicago IL: SPSS.

Jorgensen BB. 1990. A thiosulfate shunt in the sulfur cycle of marine sediments. Science 49:152–154.

Jugsujinda A, DeLaune RD, Lindau CW. 1995. Influence of nitrate on methane production and oxidation in flooded soil. *Commun Soil Sci Plant Anal* 26(15&16):2449–2459.

Jugsujinda A, Krairapanond A, Patrick Jr WH. 1995. Influence of extractable iron, aluminum, and manganese on P-sorption in flooded acid sulfate soils. *Biol Fertil Soils* 20:118–124.

Kay SH. 1988. Mobility of soil contaminants in an ecosystem of trees growing on dredged material. Rotterdam, the Netherlands: The Broekpolder. TNO Report No. R 88/488.

Kerner M, Wallman K. 1992. Remobilization events involving Cd and Zn from intertidal flat sediments in the Elbe Estuary during the tidal cycle. *Estuarine, Coastal, and Shelf Science* 35:371–393.

Khalid RA. 1980. Chemical mobility of cadmium in sediment-water systems. In: Nriagu JO, editor. Cadmium in the environment. New York NY: Wiley. p 258–304.

King GM, Klug MJ, Wiegert RG, Chalmers AG. 1982. Relation of soil water movement and sulfide concentration to *Spartina alterniflora* production in a Georgia salt marsh. *Science* 218:61–63.

Kludze HK, DeLaune RD. 1995. Gaseous exchange and wetland plant response to soil redox intensity and capacity. *Soil Sci Soc Am J* 59:939–945.

Koepfler ET, Kator HI. 1986. Ecotoxicological effects of creosote contamination on benthic microbial populations in an estuarine environment. *Toxic Assess* 1:465–485.

Kolasa J, Pickett STA, editors. 1991. Ecological heterogenerty. New York NY: Springer-Verlag.

Krairapanond A, Jugsujinda A, Patrick Jr WH. 1993. Phosphorus sorption characteristics in acid sulfate soils of Thailand: effect of uncontrolled and controlled soil redox potential (Eh) and pH. *Plant and Soil* 157:227–237.

LaPoint TW, Melancon SM, Morris MK. 1984. Relationship among observed metal concentrations, criteria, and benthic community structural responses in 15 streams. *J Water Pollut Control* 56(9)1030–1038.

Lazerte BD. 1993. The impact of drought and acidification on the chemical exports from a minerotrophic conifer swamp. *Biogeochemistry* 18:153–175.

Likens GE, Bormann FH. 1995. Biogeochemistry of a forested ecosystem. 2nd ed. New York NY: Springer-Verlag. 159 p.

Loehlin JC. 1994. Latent variable models. Hillsdale NJ: Lawrence Erlbaum. 304 p.

Loucks OL. 1985. Looking for surprise in managing stressed ecosystems. *BioScience* 35:428–432.

Mann KH, Lazier JRN. 1991. Dynamics of marine ecosystems. Oxford: Blackwell Scientific. 400 p.

Margalef R. 1963. On certain unifying principles in ecology. *Am Nat* 97:357–374.

McKey D, Waterman PG, Gartlan JS, Struhsaker TT. 1978. Phenolic content of vegetation in two African rain forests: ecological implications. *Science* 202:61–64.

Mendelssohn IA, Kleiss BA, Wakeley JS. 1995. Factors controlling the formation of oxidized root channels: a review. *Wetlands* 15(1):37–46.

Mendelssohn IA, McKee KL, Postek MT. 1982. Sublethal stresses controlling *Spartina alterniflora* productivity. In: Gopal B, Turner RE, Wetzel RG, Whigham DF, editors. Wetlands ecology management. Jaipur, India: National Institute of Ecology and International Scientific Publications. p 223–242.

Metcalf RL, Sangha GK, Kapoor IP. 1971. Model ecosystem for the evaluation of pesticide biodegradability and ecological magnification. *Environmental Science and Technology* 5(8):709–713.

Meyers PA, Ishiwatari R. 1993. Lacustrine organic geochemistry: an overview of indicators of organic matter sources and diagenesis in lake sediments. *Org Geochem* 20(7)867–900.

Mitsch WJ, Gosselink JG. 1993. Wetlands. 2nd ed. New York NY: Van Nostrand Reinhold. 722 p.

Mosser JL, Fisher NS, Wurster CF. 1972. Polychlorinated biphenyls and DDT alter species composition in mixed cultures of algae. *Science* 176:533–535.

National Academy of Sciences. 1975. Petroleum in the marine environment. Washington DC: National Academy of Sciences.

Nicholls DG, Ferguson SJ. 1992. Bioenergetics 2. New York: Academic Pr. 253 p.

Northup RR, Yu Z, Dahlgren RA, Vogt KA. 1995. Polyphenol control of nitrogen from pine litter. *Nature* 37:227–229.

O'Connors HB, Wurster CF, Powers CD, Biggs DC, Rowland RG. 1978. Polychlorinated biphenyls may alter marine trophic pathways by reducing phytoplankton size and production. *Science* 201:737–739.

Odum HT. 1983. Ecological and general systems. Niwot CO: Univ. Pr. Colorado. 644 p.

Odum EP. 1985. Trends expected in stressed ecosystems. *BioScience* 35(7):419–422.

Pardue JH, DeLaune RD, Patrick WH, Whitcomb JH. 1989. Effect of redox potential on fixation of ^{137}Cs in lake sediment. *Health Phys* 57(5):781–789.

Pardue JH, Masscheleyn PH, DeLaune RD, Patrick Jr WH, Adrian DD. 1993. Assimilation of hydrophobic chlorinated organics in freshwater wetlands: sorption and sediment-water exchange. *Environ Sci Technol* 27(5):875–882.

Patrick Jr WH, Mikkelsen DS. 1971. Plant nutrient behavior in flooded soil. In: Dinauer RC, editor. Fertilizer technology and use. Madison WI: Soil Science of America.

Pezeshki SR, Pan SZ, Delaune RD, Patrick Jr WH. 1988. Sulfide-induced toxicity: inhibition of carbon assimilation in *Spartina alterniflora*. *Photosynthetica* 22(3):437–442.

Pimm SL. 1984. The complexity and stability of ecosystems. *Nature* 307:321–326.

Prasana M. 1994. Trace and toxic metal chemistry of redmud being considered for wetland restoration [master's. thesis]. Baton Rouge LA: Louisiana State Univ.

Pugesek BH, Tomer A. 1995. Determination of selection gradients using multiple regression versus structural equation models (SEM). *Biometrical Journal* 37:449–462.

Reddy KR, Patrick WH. 1976. Effect of frequent changes in aerobic and anaerobic conditions on redox potential and nitrogen loss in a flooded soil. *Soil Biol Biochem* 8:491–495.

Reddy KR, Patrick WH, Philips RE. 1978. The role of nitrate diffusion in determining the order and rate of denitrification in flooded soil: I. Experimental results. *Soil Sci Soc Am J* 42(2):268–272.

Reice SR. 1994. Nonequilibrium determinants of biological community structure. *Amer Scientist* 82:424–435.

Risser PG, Karr JR, Forman RTT. 1983. Landscape ecology: directions and approaches. Champaign IL: Illinois Natural History Survey. 16 p. Illinois Natural History Survey Special Publication Number 2.

Saris WE, Satorra A, Sörbom D. 1987. The detection and correction of specification errors in structural equation models. In: Clogg CC, editor. Sociological methodology. Washington DC: American Sociological Assn. p 105–130.

Schindler DW. 1991. Whole lakes experiments at the experimental lakes area. In: Mooney HA, editor. Ecosystem experiments. New York NY: Wiley. 296 p.

Schmidt-Nielson K. 1994. How are control systems controlled? *American Scientist* 82:38–44.

Seke H. 1982. Organic materials in aquatic ecosystems. Boca Raton FL: CRC Pr. 201 p.

Simmers JW, Folsom Jr BL, Lee CR, Bates D. 1981. Field survey of heavy metal uptake by naturally occurring saltwater and freshwater marsh plants. Vicksburg MS: U.S. Army COE Waterways Expt. Sta. Tech. Rep. EL-81-5.

Skogerboe JG, Lee CR, Price RA, Brandon D, Hollins G. 1987. Prediction of surface runoff water quality from Black Rock Harbor dredged material placed in an upland disposal site. Vicksburg MS: U.S. Army COE Waterways Expt. Sta. Miscellaneous Paper D-87-1.

Smith CJ, Patrick WH. 1983. Nitrous oxide emission as affected by alternate anaerobic and aerobic conditions from soil suspensions enriched with ammonium sulfate. *Soil Biol Biochem* 8:491–495.

Stafford E, Simmers A, Rhett JW, Glenn R, Brown CP. 1991. Interim report: collation and interpretation of data for Times Beach Confined Disposal Facility, Buffalo NY. Vicksburg MS: U.S. Army Engineer Waterways Experiment Station. Miscellaneous paper D-91-17.

Stanford G, Smith SJ. 1972. Nitrogen mineralization potential of soils. *Soil Science Society of America, Proceeding* 36:465–472.

Teal JM, Howarth RW. 1984. Oil spill studies: a review of ecological effects. *Environ Management* 8:27–44.

Turner RE. 1977. Intertidal vegetation and commercial yields of penaeid shrimp. *Trans Amer Fish Soc* 106(5):411–416.

Turner RS, Johnson AH, Wang D. 1985. Biogeochemistry of lead in McDonalds Branch Watershed, New Jersey Pine Barrens. *J Environ Qual* 14:305–314.

[USACOE] U.S. Army Corps of Engineers. 1996. Grain size and total organic carbon effects on benthic organisms. Vicksburg MS: U.S. Army Engineer Waterways Experiment Station. EEDP-01-37.

Valiela I. 1995. Marine ecological processes. 2nd ed. New York NY: Springer-Verlag. 686 p.

White DH, Cromartie E. 1985. Bird use and heavy metal accumulation in waterbirds at dredged disposal impoundments, Corpus Christi, Texas. *Bulletin of Environmental Contamination and Toxicology* 34:295–300.

White TRC. 1993. The inadequate environment. Nitrogen and the abundance of animals. Berlin, Germany: Springer-Verlag. 425 p.

Wolfe DA. 1977. Fates and effects of petroleum hydrocarbons in marine organisms and ecosystems. New York: Pergamon Pr. 478 p.

Wotton RS. 1988. Dissolved organic material and trophic dynamics. *Bioscience* 38:172–177.

Chapter 4

Workgroup II Synopsis: Contaminant Fate and Effects in Freshwater Wetlands

A. Dennis Lemly, chair
G. Ronnie Best, William G. Crumpton, Mary G. Henry, Donal D. Hook, Greg Linder, Patrick H. Masscheleyn, Hans G. Peterson, Terrence Salt, Ralph G. Stahl, Jr.

Pollution ecology is one of the few disciplines in biology that grew out of a societal need to fix a problem. The research community was forming questions as well as simultaneously developing methods, both toxicological and analytical, to address the questions in a cultural framework that demanded immediate answers.

Aquatic toxicologists wrestled with pollution issues as they developed. By establishing basic methods and sorting out different responses between ecosystem compartments, an assessment philosophy emerged that enabled us to better investigate contaminant impacts (Mount and Brungs 1967; Mount and Stephan 1967).

Chapter Preview

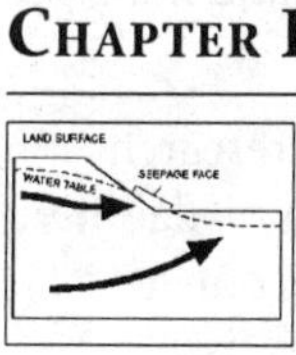

Ecotoxicology and Risk Assessment for Wetlands. Michael A. Lewis et al., editors.
 ISBN 1-880611-16-3

More recently developed disciplines, such as sediment evaluation and ecological risk assessment, have benefited from the early investment of scientists who guided the development of aquatic toxicology. Some of the basic philosophical tenets were in place, and as a consequence, these more recent disciplines developed at a faster rate than those established earlier. Even in instances where the foundation was not a good "fit," it provided a starting point from which modifications could be made, increasing the chances that conceptual or methodological mistakes might be few in number or avoided altogether.

Research on wetlands did not originally focus on toxicology. Wetlands research has long been conducted by aquatic ecologists, hydrologists, waterfowl biologists, botanists, limnologists, etc., many of whom were interested in the structure, function, and biota of different types of wetlands. Management values have also figured into the equation. In the U.S., for example, federal and state agencies manage wetlands for migratory birds, endangered species, bait production, and flood control, just to list a few management values driving research. Water quality improvements resulting from implementation of Sections 402 and 404 of the Clean Water Act (CWA) have had a positive effect on wetland management. In addition, the Comprehensive Environmental Response, Compensation, and Liability Act (CERCLA) and the Federal Insecticide, Fungicide, and Rodenticide Act (FIFRA) also affect many aspects of wetland management. Nongovernment entities such as sportsman groups and conservation organizations also work to protect and manage wetlands.

Unfortunately, there is often a large "disconnect" between the wetlands research community and the risk assessment community regarding wetland data availability and its interpretation. There is a smaller, but nonetheless important disconnect between aquatic toxicology and risk assessment groups. When factors in risk assessments are dealt with as uncertainties, sometimes it is due to a lack of awareness that data exist outside the contaminant realm.

One of the most fundamental oversights in risk assessment is the failure to recognize that most of the remaining freshwater wetlands in the U.S. are altered from their natural state because of changes in hydrology and surrounding land use. For example, surface- and groundwater extractions and diversions for urban and agricultural water supply have affected the hydrology of many wetlands and changed their water quality, vegetation, and animal life (Thompson and Merritt 1988; Lemly 1994). Development of wetlands for other land uses has fragmented large wetland complexes into small remnant wetlands that cannot maintain their original function in water storage and supply or as habitat for biota (Frayer et al. 1989; Moore et al. 1990). Dredging and channelization for navigational purposes have disrupted the hydrologic balance necessary for riparian wetlands to effectively intercept and moderate flows and water quality degradation associated with stormwater and agricultural runoff (Lowrance et al. 1984; Philips 1989; Richardson 1994; Culotta 1995). These physical alterations constitute a chronic stress that influences the way wetland ecosystems respond to new or added stress. On a regional and national scale, physical alterations are having a far greater impact on the integrity of wetlands than are chemical and biological threats.

In addition to recognizing and understanding that most freshwater wetlands have already been altered to some degree, it is necessary to place the risk assessment process into an ecological context. This involves identifying and integrating the principal ecosystem attributes (ecology, hydrology, geomorphology, soils) that serve to structure these wetlands and determine contaminant transport, chemical speciation, and biological exposure and effects. This chapter presents an ecosystem-based approach for evaluating impacts and risks to freshwater wetlands from chemical, biological, and physical stressors.

Major external factors such as climate, geomorphology, and soils determine the base conditions in which wetland ecosystems operate (Figure 4-1). Regional climate influences not only temperature, which mediates many biological processes within the ecosystem, but also the amount, form, and timing of precipitation. How these climatic variables are expressed in the landscape depends in significant part on regional and local geomorphic setting and soils. Of particular importance to wetlands is the way in which these external factors interact with internal wetland processes to determine the risk setting, i.e., the transport, fate, and effects of contaminants or other stressors (Figure 4-2). Wetlands provide a critical link between uplands and aquatic systems (streams, rivers, and lakes) whether the connection is across the surface or through the ground water (Figure 4-3). It is this critical linkage that in part determines the importance of wetlands as biogeochemical filters or transformers buffering flows from uplands to aquatic systems. In addition, it is this critical linkage that often places wetlands at risk and makes them an important component of many toxicological evaluations.

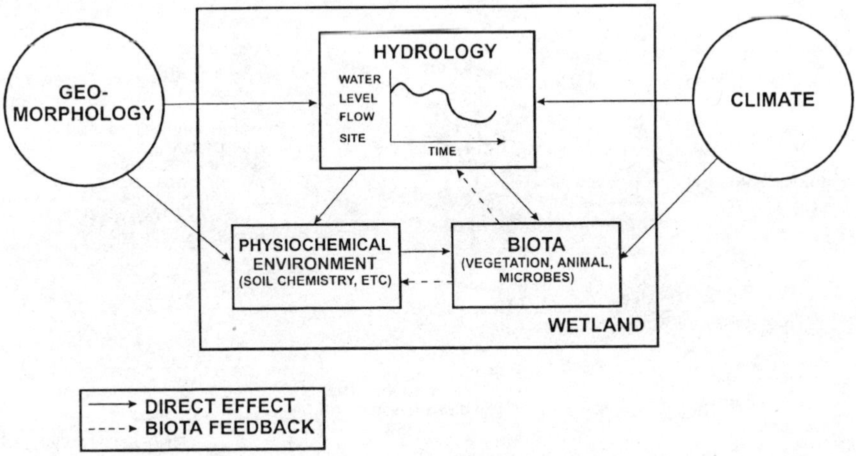

Figure 4-1 Major external factors that determine the baseline conditions in which wetland systems operate

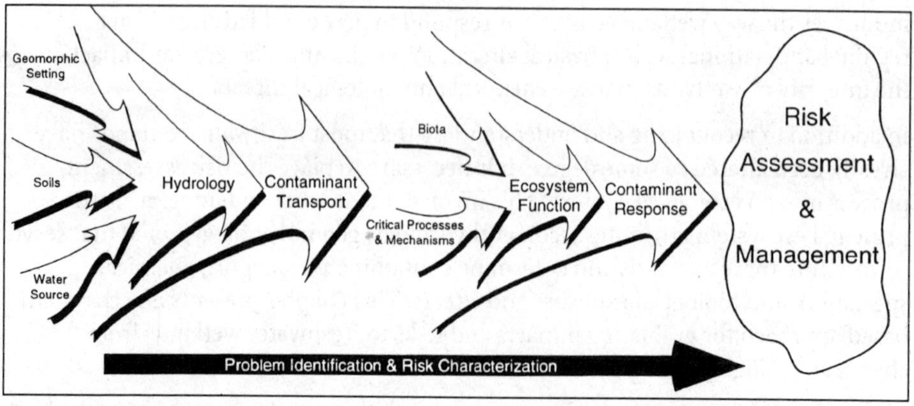

Figure 4-2 Interaction of external factors and internal processes that determine the risk setting (potential for transport of and impacts from stressors) for wetlands

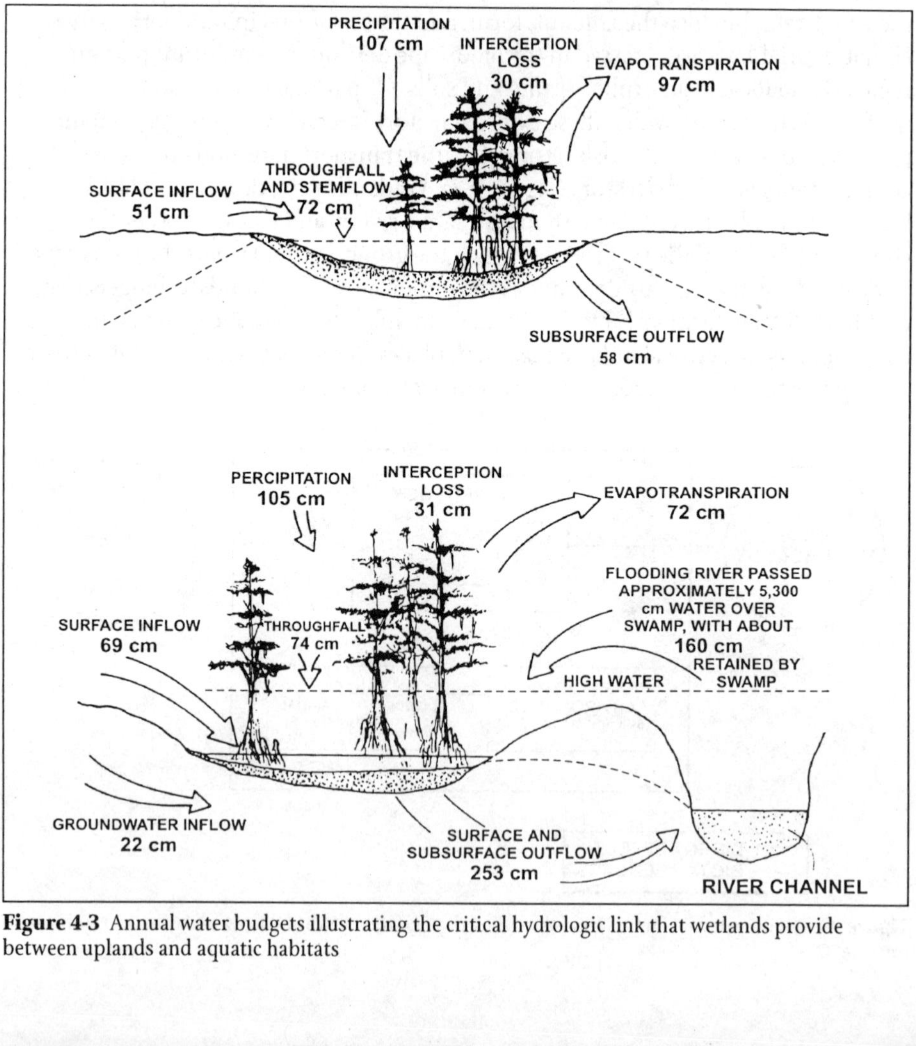

Figure 4-3 Annual water budgets illustrating the critical hydrologic link that wetlands provide between uplands and aquatic habitats

The complex interaction of external controlling factors on wetland ecosystems, when coupled with the diverse array of internal interactions, has led to a myriad of wetland types throughout North America and the world (Table 4-1). Wetlands vary from infrequently inundated, isolated, depressional wetlands (such as some prairie potholes, Playa lakes, and vernal ponds) to large, spatially complex landscape systems (such as the Everglades, Okefenokee Swamp, and the Great Dismal Swamp). The proportion of the landscape dominated by wetlands varies from areas such as Florida and Louisiana, where wetlands are significant features in the landscape, to other areas such as the north-central section of the U.S., where wetlands represent only a small portion of the landscape.

Table 4-1 Major types of wetlands in the United States (from NRC 1995)

Wetland type	Distribution and hydrology	Major vegetation
Freshwater marsh	Widespread; seasonal to permanent flooding	Grasses, sedges
Tidal salt or brackish marsh	Intertidal zones; semidiurnal to fortnightly flooding	Salt-tolerant grasses and rushes
Prairie pothole	Northern plains states; temporary to permanent flooding; fluctuating water levels	Grasses, sedges, herbs
Fen	Associated with mineral-rich water; permanently saturated by flowing water	Sedges, grasses, shrubs, trees
Bog	Abundant in recently glaciated regions; precipitation is the principal source of water	Sphagnum moss, shrubs, trees, desmids
Swamp	Prolonged saturation and flooding	Cypress, gum, red maple

Current Practices in Risk Assessment for Freshwater Wetlands

Through various sources of regulatory guidance, wetlands risk assessment may be pursued in either a qualitative or quantitative manner (Pascoe 1993). Wetlands may be characterized hydrologically by following an engineering practice or by an analysis of physical structure (Brinson 1993). Alternatively, with respect to risk, wetlands may be characterized in an ecological or biological context, which generally yields a focus on soils and vegetation or wildlife (Federal Interagency Committee for Wetland Delineation [FICWD] 1989). For ecological risk assessments for wetlands, these independent approaches have infrequently been fully integrated into the risk assessment process as it is currently practiced.

Risk assessment for wetlands may focus on noncontaminant as well as contaminant issues (Leibowitz et al. 1992; Pascoe and DalSoglio 1994). In practice, physical, chemical, and biological stressors generally impact wetlands simultaneously. In evaluating the role of these stressors, various issues must be resolved during the problem formulation and risk characterization phases of the ecological risk assessment process (USEPA 1992, 1998). To ensure that the risk assessment meets the risk manager's goals, management and policy input must be clearly stated prior to the risk analysis activities associated with exposure and ecological effects assessment. Problem formulation includes the resolution of interrelated questions on data interpretation (performance-based versus criteria-based practices) and the distinctions among risk analysis (complete process), risk assessment (determining risk), and risk management (dealing with risk).

Performance-based and criteria-based practices

Performance-based practices are those that specify design-focused evaluation of wetlands; for example, a naturally occurring or constructed wetland may be considered an effective remediation measure if it decreases heavy metal concentrations in mine tailings runoff by 80%. Criteria-based evaluation practices frequently assess the wetland water quality function by some numeric value developed as a consequence of a regulatory objective; for example, water discharged from a remediation wetland must meet the drinking water standards for heavy metals. Evaluations of wetlands may integrate these concepts to varying degrees (Hammer 1990) with the regulatory context that may be associated with the risk assessment. Regardless of the data sources being used in the risk assessment (e.g., historic data or data derived from designed studies), technical data collections must be applied within the data quality objectives that are developed from either performance-based or criteria-based needs.

Functions versus values and threats versus impacts

The relationships among risk assessment and risk management activities relative to wetlands may be markedly different, especially within the context of a technical characterization of wetland "functions" versus a more risk assessment-like consideration of wetland "values." The roles these potential differences play in evaluating "threats" and "impacts" of anthropogenic activities on wetlands are subsequently dependent upon clear distinctions being given to all these terms.

Wetlands generally are considered to have functions related to hydrology, water quality, and habitat. Hydrologic functions are generally characterized by capacity and input, which may define a wetland as a water source or water sink. Water quality functions are generally focused on physical (e.g., sedimentation and stabilization) or chemical (e.g., denitrification or contaminant removal) characteristics of surface water and ground water within the wetland. Habitat functions of wetlands may be nested with subsets of functions related to biological processes such as decomposition, biological productivity, and biogeochemical processing, but these all directly reflect the biological components of wetland structure (Adamus and Stockwell 1983; Adamus et al. 1987; Brinson 1993). For example, wetland vegetation clearly is critical and plays a major role in maintaining biodiversity and species-critical functions such as reproduction, feeding, and dispersal. Wetland values refer to the benefits obtained by society from wetland functions; for example, wetland values would include flood control and the economic benefits derived from that wetland function (Kentula et al. 1992; Richardson 1994). While the distinction between functions and values is not without technical disagreement, wetland functions are relatively easy to address within risk analysis, but wetland values are better characterized as assessment endpoints wherein societal and policy influences become critical to their definition.

For wetland risk assessments, these terms from wetland science and related wetland assessment disciplines must be clearly defined and distinguished as assessment endpoints or measurement endpoints, if the wetland scientist and risk assessor are to communicate effectively with resource managers. Similarly, the concepts of threats and impacts to wetlands must be established within an ecological risk setting. Within a risk assessment context, threats are considered sources of undesirable disturbance or activities associated with potential adverse effects (Kentula et al. 1992), while impacts are anthropogenic activities (planned or unplanned) or sources that are associated with effects that resource managers may characterize as "adverse." Risk management objectives must be adequately characterized in order to clearly identify measurement endpoints that will distinguish (or eliminate from further analysis) differences between wetlands at risk and their reference environments. In order to develop cost-effective risk analysis programs, the concepts of function and value as well as threat and impact must be consistently defined by wetland scientists and those in the risk assessment community. Wetland risk assessors and managers must clearly define assessment endpoints to ensure that their risk assessment needs are supported by the measurement endpoints that drive the technical activities of ecosystem sampling and measurement (USEPA 1992).

Procedures for assessing and evaluating wetlands

Technical activities that support wetlands evaluation have been developed by state and federal governments (Table 4-2). These technical activities include guidance designed with wetlands as a chief focus or consider components within wetlands that make the guidance equally amenable to the wetland evaluation process (e.g., biological assessment methods for evaluation of surface water). The U.S. Army Corps of Engineers (USACOE) and U.S. Environmental Protection Agency (USEPA) have both developed guidance for evaluating wetlands. Similarly, the Natural Resource Conservation Service (formerly Soil Conservation Service [SCS]) has developed procedures for identifying wetlands for compliance with the "Swampbuster" provision of federal wetland conservation legislation (FICWD 1989). Similar technical approaches developed by states are also available and may be applicable when the assessment activities fall under the jurisdiction of state regulatory offices

Table 4-2 A relative comparison of the applicability of technical approaches to risk or risk-related wetland assessment

Guidance	Risk analysis			Risk characterization			
	Problem formulation	Exposure assessment	Effects assessment	Integration	Uncertainty analysis	Risk summary	Ecological significance
Wetland delineation	+	–	+	+	–	–	+/–
Hydrogeomorphic classification	+	–	+/–	+	–	–	+/–
Wetland evaluation technique	+	–	+	+	–	–	+/–
Avian richness evaluation method	+	–	+	+	–	–	+/–
Synoptic wetland assessment	+	–	+/–	+	–	+/–	+/–
CERCLA risk assessment	+	+	+	+	+	+	+
Natural resource damage assessment	+	+	+	+	+	+	+

+: step explicitly included in process
–: step not explicitly included in process
+/–: step can be included depending upon case-specific implementation

(Adamus 1993a, 1993b). While the methods and guidance summarized in the following sections are not exhaustive, they are representative of the technical methods that are currently available.

Wetland delineation

The Federal Manual for Identifying and Delineating Jurisdictional Wetlands (FICWD 1989) was the first effort to bring together the 4 federal agencies that had primary responsibility for oversight of wetland management or enforcement of wetland regulations (USEPA, U.S. Fish and Wildlife Service [USFWS], USACOE, and SCS). Support for this manual was withdrawn in 1991 by Congress and since that time, USEPA, USACOE, and USFWS have agreed to accept the 1987 manual developed by the USACOE for delineating wetlands. The Natural Resources Conservation Service has developed its own manual to deal with lands that fall under the Farm Bill, a specific federally legislated funding and assistance authorization. The 1982 USACOE manual provides technical guidance to establish physical boundaries of wetlands and uses the following definition (USACOE 1982):

> Those areas that are inundated or saturated by surface or ground water at a frequency and duration sufficient to support, and that under normal circumstances do support, a prevalence of vegetation typically adapted for life in saturated soil conditions. Wetlands generally include swamps, marshes, bogs, and similar areas.

Assessment of the status of wetlands has been assigned to the USFWS by Congress. They inventory wetlands periodically, make maps of wetland areas nationwide, and make reports directly to Congress. However, their definition of wetlands does not fit precisely that of the jurisdictional definition (Hook 1993).

Currently, wetland delineations are a critical part of the wetland assessment and monitoring process. Depending upon the intensity and the data quality objectives associated with any designed wetland evaluation, various levels of effort determine the extent to which a wetland is characterized. Jurisdictional wetland delineations completed following guidance from the interagency manuals currently available (USACOE 1987) include evaluations of soils (hydric soils), vegetation, and hydrology as part of the regulatory process under the Comprehensive Wetlands Act. These methods of evaluation may be pursued with various levels of efforts, which have been categorized as screening, intermediate, and advanced applications. For soils, screening-level evaluations may be pursued using existing data; alternatively, a field survey may be conducted to collect site-specific data focused on the soils occurring in and around a wetland at risk. Similarly, vegetation may be evaluated within the bounds set in the study's design, which may include a cursory review of existing vegetation data for the wetland or an exhaustive field survey wherein a thorough identification and mapping of all plant species is accomplished as part of the delineation effort. In completing the hydrology evaluation within a wetland delineation, it should be noted that hydrologic characteristics are the least exact and most difficult to establish in the field, primarily because of the temporal variations (daily, annual, and seasonal) in water levels. In general, the 1987 delineation manual considers wetland hydrology present when soils are saturated to the surface or inundated sometime during the growing season for 7 or more consecutive days. The geomorphic setting influences the interpretation of soil saturation; hence, the drainage class of the soils must be clearly identified.

Hydrogeomorphic classification

In addition to the wetland delineation process, USACOE and wetland scientists supporting their Waterways Experiment Station (Vicksburg, MS) are developing a procedure for assessing the functions of wetlands that may be useful in the risk assessment process for wetlands (Brinson 1993).

Wetland ecosystems in the U.S. occur under a wide range of climatic, geologic, geomorphic, and hydrologic conditions. This diversity of conditions makes the task of assessing wetland functions difficult because not all wetlands perform functions in the same manner or to the same extent across the U.S. To simplify the assessment process, USACOE has found it useful to classify wetlands into groups that function similarly. Classification narrows the focus on the functions of a particular type of wetlands and the characteristics of the ecosystem and landscape that influence these functions.

The classification procedure summarized below is intended primarily for evaluating the ability of wetlands to perform specific functions. The benefits of classification are a faster and more accurate assessment procedure, which supports the USACOE regulatory program mandated by Section 404 of the CWA. With this regulatory application in mind, hydrogeomorphic (HGM) classification can be used:

1) to compare project alternatives,
2) to compare pre- and post-project conditions for determining impacts or mitigation success,
3) to provide guidance for avoiding and minimizing project impacts, and
4) to determine mitigation requirements.

Hydrogeomorphic classification is modular in its design, and when compared to the risk assessment framework, its hierarchical format should make it easily adaptable to a variety of wetland risk assessment needs, including planning and management of various regulatory situations that involve the assessment of wetland function.

Wetland functions are the actions that are naturally performed by wetlands which result from the interactions among the structural components of a wetland—such as soil, detritus, plants, and animals—and the physical, chemical, and biological processes that occur in wetlands. A process is a sequence of steps leading to a specific end; for example, from a biological perspective, the microbially mediated process of denitrification occurs in many wetlands and leads to a relatively simple wetland function of nitrogen removal. Complex functions resulting from the interaction of structural components and multiple physical processes can also be identified; for example, the physical processes of overbank flooding, reduction of water velocity, and the settling of suspended particulates interact with physical structures and result in the wetland function of particulate retention.

Hydrogeomorphic classification categorizes or groups wetlands on the basis of 3 fundamental characteristics: geomorphic setting, water source, and hydrodynamics. At the highest level of the classification, wetlands fall into 1 of 5 basic HGM classes: depression, slope-flat, riverine, fringe, and extensive peatland.

Hydrogeomorphic classification's hierarchical design can be applied at a regional level to narrow the focus of the classification. For example, ecoregions identified by Omernik (1987), Bailey (1994), or Bailey et al. (1994) may be used as the next filter in the classification scheme. These ecoregions are defined in part by climatic, geologic, physiographic, and other criteria and provide a convenient starting point for applying the classification at a regional level. Within a region, any number of regional HGM subclasses can be based on landscape factors such as geomorphic setting, water source, soil type, and vegetation. While the number of regional subclasses depends in part on the objectives established early in the assessment process, within an ecoregion the number of wetland subclasses will reflect the diversity of condition in a region. Regional subclasses provide a scale that optimizes the assessment process within the context of the USACOE regulatory program for Section 404 of the CWA.

The assessment procedure applies the concepts of HGM classification, functional capacity, reference domain, and reference wetlands. These concepts fit well within the risk assessment framework outlined by USEPA (1992, 1998) and occur within the HGM procedure as 3 phases: characterization, assessment, and application.

The characterization phase includes the

1) definition of assessment objectives;
2) characterization of the proposed project, the wetland ecosystem, and landscape context;
3) screening for "red flag" features;
4) identification of wetland assessment areas within the project area on the basis of HGM classification; and
5) physical separation and potential project impacts.

Clearly, these elements of the characterization phase of HGM classification are consistent with the elements found in the problem formulation phase of the ecological risk assessment framework. These elements occasionally have been considered in wetlands risk assessments that were completed prior to the development of HGM classification, but clearly current guidance should make that process more readily available to the risk assessment community (Brinson 1993).

The assessment phase of the HGM procedure measures the ability of a wetland to perform in terms of "functional capacity." Functional capacity is based on structural components and physical, chemical, and biological processes of the wetland. Depending upon the function, functional capacity and the extent to which it is displayed depend upon interactions between the wetland and the surrounding environment. For example, consider the floodwater storage function performed by some wetlands and the concept of functional capacity. A wetland's inherent capacity, or the theoretical capacity of a riverine wetland to store a volume of overbank floodwater in this example, depends on structural as well as physical characteristics that determine the wetland's storage capacity; however, the functional capacity, or actual amount of floodwater stored in the wetland, depends on the ability of the watershed to generate overbank floods, the state of soil saturation, and the timing of overbank floods. Watershed characteristics such as the size of the watershed, the intensity and duration of precipitation in the region, runoff coefficients of the watershed, and the location of control points in the stream above and below the wetland will influence the wetland's functional capacity, which could differ significantly from its inherent capacity.

Functional capacity of a wetland is described by the functional capacity index (FCI), which is a ratio of the functional capacity of a wetland under an existing or predicted condition to the functional capacity of a wetland under "attainable conditions." Attainable conditions are defined as the conditions under which the highest, sustainable level of functional capacity is attained across the suite of functions that wetlands in a reference domain naturally perform. The "reference domain" is simply the group of wetlands for which an FCI is developed. The reference domain normally is a regional HGM subclass, but depending on assessment objectives, it could be composed of a larger or smaller number of subclasses and geographic extent. For example, if the assessment objective is to compare a subclass of wetlands in the watershed, the reference domain would include all wetlands in the subclass in the watershed. Attainable condition, or the highest sustainable level of functional capacity, would ideally occur in wetlands that occur within landscapes that have not been subject to anthropogenic disturbance associated with long-term effects. When undisturbed wetlands and landscapes do not exist or cannot be reconstructed from historical data, attainable condition is assumed to exist in the wetland ecosystems and environments that have been subject to the least amount of anthropogenic disturbance.

Functional capacity indices are based on an assessment model that defines the relationship between the ecosystem- and landscape-scale variables and functional capacity. The condition of a variable is measured directly or indirectly using indicators that correspond to specific variable conditions. Variables are assigned an index ranging from 0.0 to 1.0, based on the relationship between variable condition and functional capacity in the reference domain that is established using reference wetlands. A "reference wetland" is a group of wetlands that represent the range of conditions that exist in wetland ecosystems and their landscapes in the reference domain. The range of conditions include those resulting from natural processes (succession, channel migration, erosion, and sedimentation) and anthropogenic disturbance.

Reference wetlands and their environments serve as the basis for scaling and calibrating variables in assessment models. The relationship between variable condition and functional capacity in the reference domain is established using empirical data, expert opinion, best professional judgment, or a combination of these options. The relationship is formalized by using logical rules or equations to derive an FCI ranging from 0.0 to 1.0. An FCI of 1.0 corresponds to the level of functional capacity that exists under attainable conditions for the reference domain, while an FCI of 0.0 reflects the absence of functional capacity. Functional capacity indices then provide measures of a wetland's capability to perform a function, relative to similar wetlands in the region.

As a result of the wetland assessment process, FCIs can subsequently be applied in various ways during the application phase. Functional capacity units (FCUs) can be calculated by multiplying an FCI by the area of wetland it represents. Once the functional capacity of a wetland area is expressed in terms of FCUs, a number of the comparisons critical to regulatory permit review processes can be made; for example, comparing the same wetland area at different points in time (e.g., pre/post project conditions), comparing wetlands in the same HGM class at the same point in time, and comparing wetlands in different HGM classes at the same point in time.

Wetland evaluation technique

Various monitoring programs have focused on wetlands, and these monitoring and evaluation programs have developed technical methods that are amenable for use in assessing risk. Monitoring activities are used to account for temporal influences that may change risk through time (e.g., seasonal influences on exposure). While various qualitative and quantitative approaches to wetlands monitoring have been developed, these can be grouped into categories based largely on their geographic focus, i.e., the extent of spatial coverage ranges from the individual site to the watershed. Methods designed for application to individual sites, like those considered in the wetland evaluation technique (WET) and its various modes of implementation (Adamus et al. 1987), are focused on qualitative and quantitative approaches to wetland assessment for relatively small spatial areas.

The WET assesses wetland function in terms of social significance, effectiveness, and opportunity and uses predictors of wetland function, i.e., physical, chemical, or biological processes. These are similar, if not identical, elements common to risk assessment as it is presented in current guidance. The WET and similar approaches are generally qualitative but may reflect a limited amount of field investigation as part of their contribution to wetland risk assessment. Wetland functions routinely evaluated in WET include

- groundwater recharge,
- nutrient removal,
- sediment retention,
- groundwater discharge,
- nutrient transformation,
- toxicant retention,
- floodflow alteration,
- production export,
- aquatic biodiversity,
- sediment stabilization,
- wildlife biodiversity, and
- recreation and heritage.

From an ecological perspective, WET and similar methods do not measure community structure directly but assume community structure or wetland function on the basis of habitat structure (Adamus et al. 1987). While WET is generally focused on individual wetlands, it considers larger landscape associations, including watershed, topographic, and vegetation features, to develop qualitative estimates of wetland function and condition. These estimates take the form of ratings of high, moderate, or low for each function (except recreation), and in conjunction with a habitat suitability rating for fisheries, wildlife, and waterfowl, yield an evaluation for the wetland at risk. Within a given ecoregion, these qualitative estimates could be compiled to develop thresholds that could discriminate between each of the general categories of risk. While these methods are intended for individual wetlands (of limited spatial coverage), WET or similar methods have been applied to extensive wetlands characterized by many wetland types in a complex landscape. Many state regulatory agencies have applied wetland evaluation methods within their particular ecoregional setting, and as such, these methods may be available for use in wetland risk assessment (Roth et al. 1993).

Habitat evaluation procedures and their applications to wetlands

Evaluation of wetland habitats for wildlife relies on methods developed by the USFWS as habitat evaluation procedures (HEPs) (USDOI 1980). Habitat evaluation procedures use individual species models identified by habitat suitability index (HSI) models to generate a composite of key species within a habitat, but only a limited number of HSI models are available for application to wetland risk assessment. While past criticism has focused on HEP's species-level orientation as opposed to a community-level orientation, its application to wetlands risk assessment should be considered, especially if regulatory drivers fall along single-species lines (e.g., threatened or endangered species in critical wetland habitats). Given criticisms of HEP and similar assessment methods, alternative technical methods are being developed, including community-level metrics focused on bird community structure.

Avian richness evaluation method

The avian richness evaluation method (AREM) is one of the first rapid methods to be developed for assessing biodiversity (Adamus 1993a, 1993b). Without requiring extensive user knowledge of birds, it comprehensively addresses wetlands bird diversity and can be modified to predict diversity of other animal groups. The AREM does the following:

1) assigns a score to each evaluated wetland, which represents the number of bird species that could occur in the wetland multiplied by an estimate of the suitability of the wetland for each species;
2) creates a list of species likely to occur in the evaluated wetland that can be combined with lists predicted for other wetlands to identify minimum combinations of wetlands that will provide habitat for all bird species in an area; and
3) tallies the number of species likely to occur in the evaluated wetland and their particular characteristics, e.g., neotropical migrants, uncommon species, or

game species. If they desire, users can assign scores to these characteristics and use them as weights in deriving the wetland score.

The AREM was developed because some available methods (such as WET) assign scores or ratings to wetland wildlife habitat without showing for which species a wetland has been rated high or low. Knowledge of species composition is essential if one wishes to maintain biodiversity at a regional level. For example, knowing the species composition allows one to avoid sanctioning the loss of a wetland containing many narrow-niched, regionally uncommon species in exchange for creating or enhancing a wetland with a perhaps identical number of species, but whose species are mere generalists.

The AREM is intended to be used in the same situations in which HEP is now used and can be applied in addition to, or in lieu of, HEP. A problem with HEP is that the scores it assigns are based on assessments of habitat suitability for only a few presumed indicator species. Many users have noted that the subjectivity of selecting indicator species biases the results, and scientists have widely questioned the validity of assuming that 5 to 10 species can represent the needs of the usual 50 to 100 species that are present at a site. Moreover, few of the HEP species models adequately address habitat needs either at a landscape level or during nonbreeding periods, and HEP assessments are often time-consuming.

The AREM can be used to assist and document resource decisions in the following ways:

1) Performing mitigation calculations. Agencies currently spend time "cover-typing" lands that will be altered or restored where compensatory mitigation has been deemed necessary. This consists of measuring various categories of habitat before a project and estimating any shifts in area that will occur among categories as a result of the project. Areas in each cover-type category that are believed to exist both before and after the project are multiplied by coefficients, determined through the use of HEP, that indicate the suitability of each category for selected species during both time periods. In this manner, net change in habitat suitability, at least for a few selected species, is predicted. Where wetland and riparian cover types are the habitats that are expected to change, AREM might be used in lieu of (or in addition to) HEP to calculate the habitat suitability coefficients of impacted or restored areas. If nonwetland cover types are also present, AREM could be adapted as described above.
2) Diagnosing impaired wetland quality. Where wetlands are officially considered by agencies to be "waters of a state," or where they exist within certain public trust lands (e.g., national wildlife refuges), a legal need sometimes exists to determine the degree to which wetland quality has been impaired. Avian richness evaluation models alone cannot determine this, but they can assist. For example, they are useful for diagnosing the presence of contamination problems by defining which species of birds should be present in a

wetland having a particular habitat structure. If properly designed surveys then fail to find the predicted species, it raises a possibility that nonphysical (e.g., chemical) factors unmeasured by AREM are discouraging wetland use.

3) Selecting appropriate indicator species. By defining which species to expect in particular types of wetlands, AREM can assist resource personnel in selecting indicator species that are the most appropriate for monitoring water quality or physical habitat suitability. Selecting appropriate indicator species is crucial to the proper use of HEP as well as to the development of biocriteria for wetland protection and the accurate monitoring of wetland contamination.
4) Targeting habitat enhancements. Active management of wetlands will usually be most effective when it focuses on improving conditions for species with low species habitat scores, while maintaining conditions suitable for species with high species habitat scores. In combination with other considerations, AREM can be used in this manner to suggest habitat features whose enhancement will support the largest variety of species overall or of species having a particular attribute.
5) Establishing wildlife-based classification of wetland habitats. Wetland types are commonly defined by their vegetative communities. Wildlife communities or individual species also can be useful primary or secondary features in classifying wetlands for scientific or administrative purposes. Avian richness evaluation models can assist such classifications by predicting bird species associated not only with vegetation but also with other environmental factors. Statistically defined, wildlife-based classes of wetlands could be identified by applying AREM to a probabilistic sample of wetlands in a region.
6) Optimizing biodiversity protection. Agencies and conservation groups sometimes have opportunities to purchase or trade properties to enhance regional biodiversity. When biological survey data from the subject properties are lacking, AREM can be applied (during any season) to the properties to predict their avian richness, which is often the largest terrestrial component of a region's vertebrate biodiversity. Richness estimates then can be calculated from the lists of predicted species pooled from multiple wetlands to determine which combination of wetlands is likely to support the greatest species richness. This estimate can be focused further by applying constraints related to land ownership, species characteristics, management costs, or other factors. As such, AREM can provide a complimentary, local refinement of the gap analysis approach currently used for ecosystem management and biodiversity planning at state and regional levels by the National Biological Service.

To date, AREM has been applied to only one ecoregion (the Colorado Plateau), but it was designed for easy adaptation elsewhere. Depending on the situation, the up-front investment required to adapt AREM to another region is probably on the order of 0.1 to 0.5 full time equivalent (FTE), and perhaps double that if field validation is also desired. Adaptation requires the focused involvement of a professional field ornithologist or expert bird naturalist who is experienced in nonstatistical approaches to building habitat models. The adaptation process first requires a comprehensive review of appropriate local literature, followed by construction and encoding of preliminary models, modification of the field questionnaire, interviews with local avian experts at several habitat sites, and final revision of models and the questionnaire. The optional validation process requires selecting survey sites, conducting faunal surveys, data entry, and data analysis. Once AREM has been adapted for an ecoregion and/or habitat type, evaluations of most sites can be completed in less than 30 minutes and are usually not season-dependent. No computer programming expertise is required to adapt the existing AREM software.

Synoptic approach to wetland risk assessment

As indicated in the previous section, wetland risk assessment may occur at various geographic scales, ranging from individual sites to larger watershed coverages where multiple individual sites may be embedded in the larger landscape, or alternatively, a single complex wetland may exist over a large spatial area (e.g., the Florida Everglades and the bayous of Louisiana). While approaches to each scale should be consistent, the level of effort required for each extreme—individual site versus watershed level—precludes identical methods being successfully employed to characterize these wetland features.

A synoptic approach to wetland risk assessment is generally focused on larger spatial coverages, e.g., ecoregions or states, and focuses on cumulative impacts as opposed to single occurrence events. From the spatial perspective, the synoptic approach differs from WET in its routine application to wetland evaluation. Nonetheless, the synoptic approach may be applicable within a risk assessment context, if one were considering a highly heterogeneous landscape characterized by numerous embedded wetland types or developing a landscape-level risk assessment. Relative to WET, the synoptic approach to wetland risk assessment requires more cursory data input, which reflects in part the greater spatial coverage of the assessment method.

The synoptic approach is designed for use by states and at ecoregion levels and is intended to relate cumulative impacts to wetlands among areas in these larger geographic scales. It is not designed to make these relative comparisons within small spatial scales where WET may be more applicable (Adamus and Stockwell 1983; Adamus et al. 1987). The synoptic approach consists of 5 steps or phases (Leibowitz et al. 1992) (Table 4-3), but from a technical perspective, the definition of synoptic indices and the selection of landscape indicators are critical to the wetland risk assessment completed using the synoptic approach.

Overall, synoptic indices are those actual functions and values within the landscape of interest, while the landscape indicators are the actual data used to represent those

Table 4-3 Steps in conducting a synoptic approach to wetland risk assessment

Steps	Inputs
Define goals and criteria of the assessment	Define assessment objectives Define intended use Assess accuracy needs Identify assessment constraints
Define synoptic indices	Identify wetland types Describe natural setting Define landscape boundary Define wetland functions Define wetland values Identify significant impacts Select landscape subunits Define combination rules
Select landscape indicators	Survey data and existing methods Assess data adequacy Evaluate costs of better data Compare and select indicators Describe indicator assumptions Finalize subunit selection Conduct pre-analysis review
Conduct assessment	Plan quality assurance and quality control Perform map measurements Analyze data Produce maps Assess accuracy Conduct post-analysis review
Prepare report of synoptic assessment	Prepare user' s guide Prepare assessment documentation

indices. In general, 4 generic indices are the focus of the synoptic approach—wetland function, wetland value, functional loss, and replacement potential—but each application of the synoptic approach will require that a specific set of functions be identified. Defining wetland functions and values in each synoptic assessment will require an understanding of the interactions among wetlands and the regional landscapes. In practice, each of these elements of the synoptic approach is dependent upon the particular goals and constraints acknowledged in the initial step of the process in which risk assessor and risk manager define goals and criteria of the synoptic assessment. Each step of the synoptic assessment process requires multidisciplinary inputs, which will include technical information such as identification of specific wetland types found in the area of concern and descriptions of natural settings, as well as definitions of wetland values which may be more policy-related than technical.

Methods applicable to National Pollution Discharge Elimination System permit process

For surface waters (including inland fresh water or near-coastal estuarine and marine waters), an integrated strategy consisting of both biological and chemical data requirements has been applied by regulators and the regulated community to protect water quality beyond the technology-based requirements in the CWA. One method for measuring the biological effects of toxic effluents released to wetlands is whole effluent testing. The USEPA and the states have used the data derived from effluent testing to assess compliance with water quality standards and to establish the National Pollution Discharge Elimination System (NPDES), which sets permit effluent limitations necessary to attain and maintain those standards. Technical guidance documents designed to support the NPDES process are available and should be consulted as part of the wetland risk assessment process. Specific guidance for the application of these tools to wetlands focuses on the integration of chemical and biological approaches for evaluating water quality; chemical, physical, and biological testing requirements; use of data; setting of effluent limitations; and monitoring. For wetlands in particular, the Technical Support Document (TSD) for Water Quality-based Toxics Control (USEPA 1991b) would be applicable. The revised TSD provides an explanation of the technical support for whole effluent testing and gives detailed guidance on development of water quality-based permit limitations for toxic pollutants.

In its application to wetlands risk assessment, the effluent testing approach to toxics control for the protection of aquatic life involves the use of acute and chronic tests to measure the toxicity of wastewaters. Whole effluent toxicity tests typically use standardized, surrogate freshwater or marine plants, vertebrates, or invertebrates to measure the aggregate toxic effect of an effluent. An acute whole effluent test is typically a test of 96-h or less in duration, in which lethality is the measured endpoint. A chronic whole effluent test is typically a longer-term test, in which sublethal effects such as fertilization, growth, and reproduction can be measured in addition to lethality. Again, numerous technical guidance documents have been published that focus on these methods, and their potential application to wetland risk assessment, especially at the organismic level of biological organization, has been demonstrated (Warren-Hicks et al. 1989; USEPA 1989; Linder, Bollman et al. 1991; Linder et al. 1994).

Given the policy implications of the NPDES process, various biological assessment methods and applications developed as surfacewater monitoring tools are available "as is" or in modified form for a wetland evaluation, e.g., index of biological integrity (IBI), index of community integrity, and rapid bioassessment protocols (Warren-Hicks et al. 1989). This section briefly describes various methods and, within a risk assessment context, measurement endpoints that can be used in field surveys of wetlands. Approaches available for wetland assessments—be those qualitative or quantitative—consist of methods commonly used to monitor periphyton, plankton, macroinvertebrates, and fish in a variety of aquatic habitats. Measurement endpoints consist primarily of direct and derived measures of population and community structure, such as relative abundance, species richness, and indices of community organization (e.g., USEPA 1973, 1987; Plafkin et al. 1988; APHA 1992).

Risk assessment practices associated with CERCLA and similar regulations

Risk assessment activities pursued under CERCLA, or "Superfund," have become increasingly well documented since the Superfund Amendments and Reauthorization Act was promulgated in 1986, and the CERCLA process for conducting ecological risk assessments at contaminated sites has been summarized in numerous publications. When implemented for wetlands, the ecological risk assessment approach completed under CERCLA (Figure 4-4) is clearly rooted in the USEPA framework approach (1992, 1994c, 1997).

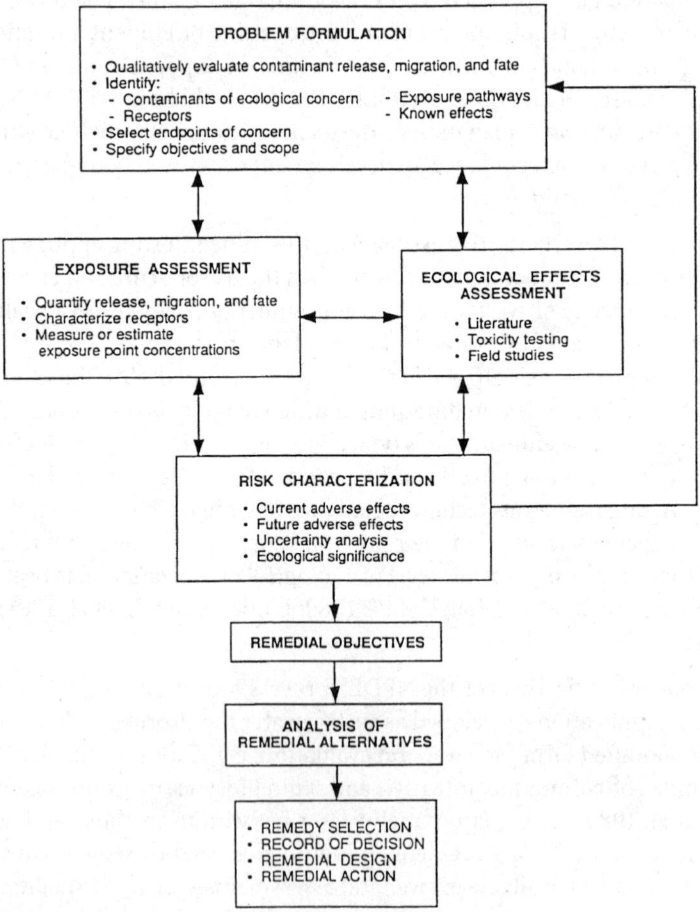

Figure 4-4 Ecological risk assessment approach used in CERCLA or Superfund investigations

In planning ecological risk assessments for wetlands, 4 steps should be fully described to ensure that data sufficient for management needs are available for the decision-making process. As indicated in Figure 4-4, these include problem formulation, exposure assessment and ecological effects assessment (the "analysis phase"), and risk characterization.

Problem formulation

Early in problem formulation, plans should be developed to address the site-specific requirements for a qualitative ecological risk evaluation. These steps in problem formulation are generally identified as

1) qualitative evaluations of contaminant releases, migration, and fate;
2) identification of contaminants and receptors of ecological concern;
3) identification of exposure pathways; and
4) selection of ecological endpoints of concern.

These steps should be carried out within an ecoregional setting; then, within a landscape setting, habitat can be used as an integrating unit for the overall process (e.g., habitat provides an ecological setting to evaluate contaminant effects associated with multiple wetlands in a particular ecoregion).

The outcome of the problem formulation phase for a qualitative ecological risk evaluation often takes the form of conceptual models, which should capture a specific set of objectives designed to address questions driving the risk assessment process (e.g., public concerns, natural resource issues) and should define the scope of the assessment required to answer these questions.

Ecological effects and exposure assessment

Following the problem formulation phase and the identification of environmental resources at risk at any wetland, an ecological effects assessment should then be completed parallel to an exposure assessment in the analysis phase of the ecological risk evaluation. Within the framework process, these parallel efforts will be accomplished through a review of existing information and an extensive survey of local experts familiar with the wetland and surrounding landscape. These parallel efforts are critical first steps in assessing contaminant risks once problem formulation is complete. The exposure assessment that tracks a parallel course to the ecological effects assessment considers in detail the release, migration, and fate of contaminants of potential ecological concern (COPECs). Depending upon the existing information, the exposure assessment should more fully characterize the COPECs, as well as the ecological receptors, beyond their initial consideration in the problem formulation phase. When available within the habitat setting established in problem formulation, estimates of exposure point concentrations should also be fully characterized.

To evaluate wetland risks, an ecological effects assessment should include

1) a review and summary of historic data, as well as comparative data gathered from peer-reviewed literature and surveys of local experts;
2) a review and summary of adverse biological and ecological effects associated with chemicals and radionuclides potentially of concern; and
3) a collection of the existing field survey information for the wetland (e.g., monitoring data on wildlife or previous wetland evaluations).

Risk characterization

From some perspectives, an ecological risk assessment may be considered an integrated evaluation of biological effects, derived through measurements of exposure and toxicity. From an ecotoxicological perspective, however, exposure and ecological effects assessments are complex, interrelated functions that yield estimates of risk associated with environmental contaminants in various matrices sampled at a site. Within the risk characterization phase of a qualitative evaluation of ecological risks, the outputs from the exposure and ecological effects assessments are integrated. In screening-level efforts, the integration relies heavily on strength-of-evidence arguments developed on the basis of the existing information for the facility or site. While screening-level efforts and comprehensive studies supporting the more quantitative applications of the ecological or ecotoxicological risk assessment approach differ with respect to levels of effort involved with their development (e.g., time or budget constraints), risk characterizations within any ecological risk assessment should include:

1) an evaluation of current and potential adverse biological or ecological effects,
2) an identification of the uncertainties associated with the risk characterization, and
3) an evaluation of the ecological significance associated with the contaminants or the physical disturbances associated with contaminant-related facility or site management.

In the past, risk assessments for wetlands under CERCLA were often completed as part of groundwater and soil contamination evaluations completed within the risk assessment process for a particular site; such efforts, however, may not capture the characteristics of the wetland within an ecological context. For example, groundwater evaluations completed in lacustrine, palustrine, or riverine wetlands frequently provide data sufficient for the groundwater risk assessment but may inadequately characterize the ecological context within which the ground water occurs.

As one approach to risk assessment for wetlands, guidance under CERCLA was designed to be flexible and implemented with varying degrees of effort, depending upon the landscape setting of the wetland at risk. The ecological risk assessment activities could range from being qualitative yet extensive efforts consistent with the current state of the science to comprehensive projects requiring multidisciplinary teams of applied ecologists, research scientists, and hydrologists (see Warren-Hicks et al. 1989; USEPA 1989, 1991a, 1992, 1994a). The planning and implementation of an ecological risk assessment based upon an integrated approach for terrestrial and freshwater habitats will be discussed briefly in this section, with particular focus being given to the approach as it relates to wetlands located in various ecoregions throughout the United States.

Regardless of the regulatory and political settings, from a technical perspective, wetland habitats at risk may be evaluated using an integrated approach for ecological risk assessment that has been developed and built upon a framework originally designed for hazard assessment (Warren-Hicks et al. 1989; Suter 1991). An integrated or "ecological triad" approach evaluates risk on the basis of biological and physicochemical data in their ecological contexts (Pascoe and DalSoglio 1994; Pascoe et al. 1994; Linder et al. 1994) to evaluate risks. Whenever possible, quantitative tools are used to describe these relationships. Simply stated, the elements within the ecological triad integrate biological (including toxicological), physical, and chemical (including contaminants) information within an ecological framework (Figure 4-5). In addition to risk-driven questions (e.g., acute or chronic effects) related to chemicals or radionuclides, the analysis of risks to biological resources and ecological systems also considers indirect effects associated with contaminant exposures. Noncontaminant-related effects like physical alteration of habitat are regarded equally with contaminant effects in the integrated ecological triad approach, especially when remediation, restoration, or land-use alternatives are evaluated within the context of ecological risk.

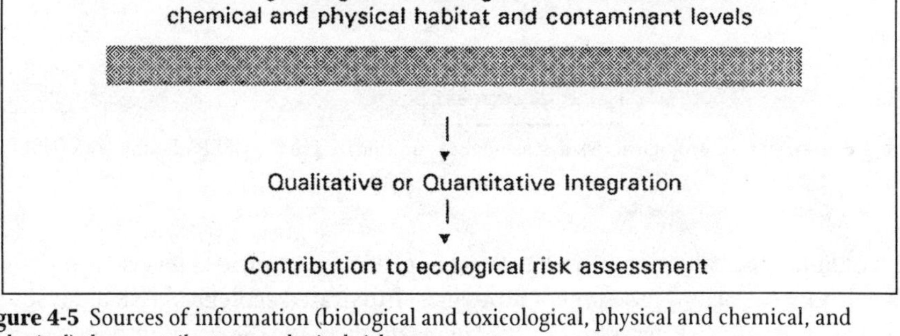

Figure 4-5 Sources of information (biological and toxicological, physical and chemical, and ecological) that contribute to ecological risk assessment

In order to implement any ecological risk assessment, the existing regulatory guidance available from federal and state governments must be considered early in the project's organization (USEPA 1986, 1991a, 1992, 1997, 1998). For ecological risks in wetlands, the CERCLA approach is consistent with the framework document (Figure 4-6; USEPA 1992) and may be considered an integrated evaluation of ecological effects and exposure (USEPA 1991a). Within an ecological assessment, qualitative risk evaluations should consider physical, chemical, and biological interactions associated with contaminant exposures in various environmental media, e.g., soils and surface water.

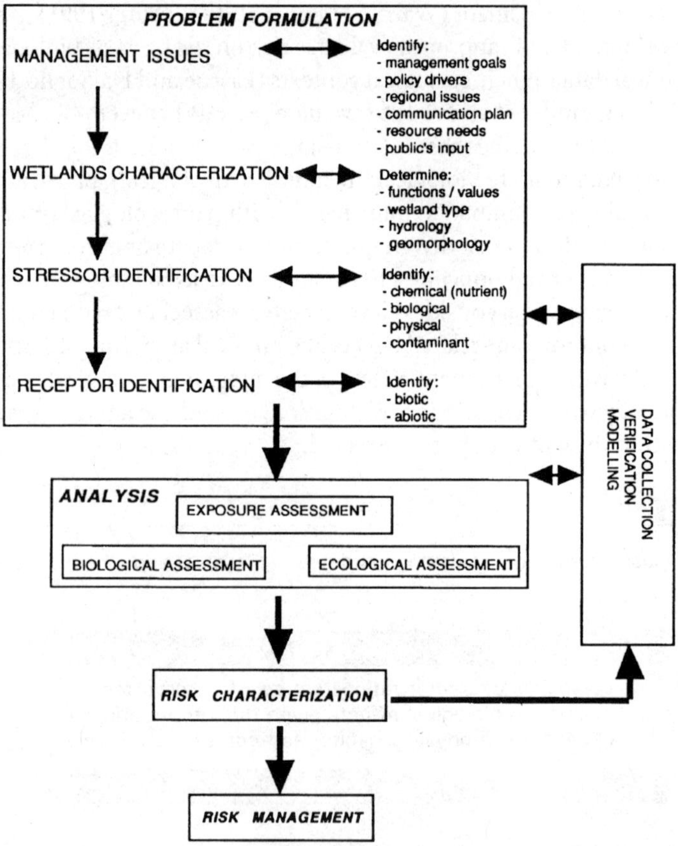

Figure 4-6 Overview of ecological risk assessment as summarized in the USEPA Framework (USEPA 1992)

Such a qualitative evaluation of risk may be approached at various levels of effort and according to various assessment strategies. Integrated ecological risk analyses supporting wetland risk assessments are increasingly being designed under CERCLA, especially if endangered species, critical habitats, or relatively large spatial scales are of concern. Depending upon the level of effort required to satisfy the data quality objectives for any particular wetlands, integrated ecological risk assessment activities may use

1) a "desktop" analysis of existing literature and reports,
2) a screening-level analysis, or
3) an integrated field and laboratory evaluation.

As suggested by their names, these particular risk assessment activities represent different levels of effort that are comparable to those supported through wetland guidance from the interagency manual (FICWD 1989) as well as in the developing HGM assessment process. When a fully integrated ecological risk analysis is completed for wetland risk assessments, a technically adequate data collection may be fully developed from the existing regulatory guidance and then incorporated into the risk assessment process.

Wetland risk evaluations then may range from qualitative desktop to preliminary screening efforts to comprehensive integrated field and laboratory investigations. The level of effort and implementation of the evaluation should directly reflect the data quality objectives and scope of the study that has been identified early in the problem formulation phase of the risk assessment process (USEPA 1991a, 1992, 1997, 1998). Regardless of the level of effort, chemical-based and toxicity-based approaches to risk evaluations have made significant contributions to ecological risk assessment (Parkhurst et al. 1989). From an ecological perspective, the strengths of each strategy may be combined to evaluate ecological effects and exposure within a risk assessment setting. For wetlands, exposure and ecological effects assessments are interrelated functions that will yield qualitative estimates of hazard and risk associated with environmental contaminants in various matrices sampled at a site. In the process developed for wetlands impacted by hazardous waste sites, a qualitative but extensive screening-level effort may be pursued. These initial efforts rely on existing data and include a survey of the available literature for the wetland at risk (e.g., historic wetland-specific and comparative data regarding exposure and ecological effects), as well as gathering information available through local experts familiar with historic and current status of the wetland. Ideally, if critical data gaps are apparent or more detailed information are needed to enhance risk characterizations following initial screening studies, comprehensive studies involving designed field and laboratory investigations could then address these potential sources of uncertainty (Linder, Bollman et al. 1991).

Natural resource damage assessment and habitat equivalency analysis

Wetlands, as highly valued natural resources, may be considered in the natural resource damage assessment (NRDA) process, particularly when their functions become impaired and their values subsequently decreased. In response to the Oil Pollution Act of 1990 (OPA), the National Oceanic and Atmospheric Administration (NOAA) and other natural resource trustees (e.g., USFWS, National Park Service, and tribal governments) have developed guidance documents (e.g., USFWS 1992) on aspects of the NRDA process that may benefit the wetlands risk assessment process as it develops.

There are 3 phases of an NRDA:

1) The preassessment phase in its simplest characterization requires that the trustees determine whether an incident has occurred (under OPA, the release of oil to the environment) and whether to pursue restoration planning.
2) The restoration planning phase has its central focus on the evaluation of information on potential injuries and the application of that information to an evaluation of the need for and type of restoration.
3) The restoration implementation phase is designed to ensure that the trustees implement the developed restoration plan.

The phases of the NRDA process consider questions that are not unlike those of the risk assessor and risk manager working under CERCLA. At this time in the development history of the NRDA regulatory process, the available guidance documents suggest that the technical support for risk assessment and NRDAs will be very similar. The activities currently included in the NRDA process drive the technical support toward this similarity.

Within the restoration planning phase, the current NRDA practice addresses 2 issues:

1) a primary restoration that evaluates alternative actions proposed to return the injured resources and services to baseline or reference states, including a natural recovery option and
2) a compensatory restoration in which actions are evaluated to compensate the environment and public for the resource or services lost from the date of the incident to the recovery of the injured resources.

The type and scale of compensatory restoration is related to the type and scale of primary restoration selected, and the scaling of appropriate compensatory-restoration alternatives is primarily achieved on a service-to-service comparison of services lost as a result of the incident. When service-based cost assessment is not feasible or appropriate to the incident, compensatory restoration may also be determined through a cost analysis of lost services and gains from the compensatory restoration (see Federal Register 1995).

As in ecological risk assessment, public participation is integral to the NRDA process, particularly because that public input shapes policy in many instances. The timing and extent of public involvement in the NRDA process, and the type of documents produced at various stages of the process, fit the scope and scale of the incident in a manner distinct from yet analogous to CERCLA. In part, this stems from the past development of technical guidance by the Department of the Interior (USDOI) for assessing natural resource damages resulting from hazardous substance releases under CERCLA and the CWA. The CERCLA regulations originally applied to natural resource damages resulting from oil discharges and hazardous substance releases. When proposed guidance is finalized under the OPA, it will supersede that currently in place for oil spill and other incidents that fall under its regulatory umbrella.

Wetland risk assessments could also benefit from the existing guidance established under the National Comprehensive Plan (NCP) for response to an incident and, similarly, could provide procedures and technical documents by which trustees could better determine appropriate restoration of injured natural resources and services (FEMA 1992). Natural resources such as wetlands are valued in terms of the services or ecological functions that they provide to other natural resources or the public, and as a result, wetlands would be potential trust resources. From an NRDA perspective, such services could be classified as

1) ecological services, or the physical, chemical, and biological functions that one natural resource provides for another (e.g., provision of food, protection from predation, nesting habitat, biodiversity); and
2) public services, or the functions that natural resources provide for the public (e.g., fishing, hunting, nature photography, education, access).

Value, as proposed for an NRDA action under OPA (Federal Register 1995), represents the amount of other goods that an individual will give up in order to obtain a good or the amount an individual will accept in order to forego the good. The total value of a natural resource or service includes direct-use values (e.g., values individuals derive from consuming or viewing a natural resource) and passive-use values (values not linked to direct use, e.g., the value individuals derive from knowing a natural resource exists). In many contexts, particularly in markets, value is represented in terms of units of currency, the commonly accepted form of exchange. However, value also can be measured in other units, including units of a resource service. In this proposed rule (Federal Register 1995), value can be measured in either units of resource services or dollar amounts. While regulatory and legal definitions may yield subtle but significant differences, values that are the focus of an NRDA and those in the HGM, WET, or synoptic approach to wetland evaluation appear similar upon initial inspection.

From a strictly technical position, the processes of wetland assessment for an NRDA and for a CERCLA are very similar. For example, potential categories of injuries include adverse changes in survival, growth, and reproduction; health, physiology, and biological condition; behavior; community composition; ecological processes and functions; physical and chemical habitat quality or structure; and services to the public, which are not unlike assessment and measurement endpoints in the risk assessment process outlined in the framework document (USEPA 1992). Although injury often is thought of in terms of adverse changes in biota, the definition of injury proposed under OPA is broader. Injuries to nonliving resources (e.g., removal of oiled sand on a beach) as well as injuries to resource services (e.g., lost use associated with a fisheries closure to prevent harvest of tainted fish, even though the fish themselves may not be injured) may be considered.

Determining exposure in an NRDA under OPA means determining whether natural resources came into contact with the oil from an incident. Early determination of exposure during the preassessment phase should focus on those natural resources or services that are most likely to be affected by an incident. In a manner similar to the analysis phase in risk assessment, an NRDA for a wetland impacted by an oil spill must determine whether the natural resource came into contact, either directly or indirectly, with the discharged oil. Exposure in an NRDA is broadly defined to include not only direct physical exposure to oil but also indirect exposure (e.g., injury to an organism as a result of a foodweb disruption).

Documenting exposure is a prerequisite to determining injury, except for response-related injuries and injuries from substantial threats of discharges. Evidence of exposure alone may not be sufficient to conclude that injury to a natural resource has occurred (e.g., the presence of petroleum hydrocarbons in oyster tissues may not, in itself, constitute an injury). Exposure can be demonstrated with either quantitative or qualitative methods. As with other elements of the NRDA process, selection of approaches for demonstrating oil exposure will depend on the type and volume of discharged oil, the natural resources at risk, and the nature of the receiving environment. For example, chemical analysis of oil in sediments, alone, may not be adequate to conclude that a benthic organism was otherwise exposed to the oil. Likewise, the presence of petroleum in fish tissue, alone, may not be adequate to link the exposure to the discharge because metabolism of the oil may blur the chemical characterization. The combination of the 2 approaches may, however, demonstrate exposure. As in the ecological triad applied in the risk assessment for the wetlands at Milltown Reservoir (see Chapter 5), exposure analysis should typically include field observations or measurements, laboratory exposure studies, transport and fate modeling, and a search of the literature. As proposed, the NRDA process emphasizes that these procedures may be used alone or in combination, depending on the specific nature of the incident. The trustees must determine the most appropriate approach to evaluating exposure on an incident-specific basis.

As in ecological risk assessment, pathway analysis is a critical component in the injury assessment phase of an NRDA. In a wetland, for example, pathways would include movement and exposure to oil through the water surface, water column, sediments (including bottom, bank, beach, floodplain sediments), ground water, soil, air, direct accumulation, and food-chain uptake. Pathway analysis includes field investigations, laboratory studies, modeling, and the reviewing literature. Again, the current practice emphasizes that these procedures may be used alone, or in combination, depending on the specific nature of the incident. The most appropriate approach to determine whether a plausible pathway exists would vary on an incident-specific basis.

To determine whether an injury resulted from a specific incident, a plausible pathway linking the incident to the injury would have to be identified, but similar to exposure, the existence of a pathway between source and target is not sufficient to conclude that injury has occurred (e.g., demonstrating that prey species are oiled can be used to document that a plausible pathway to a predator species exists, but such data do not, by themselves, demonstrate that the predator species is injured). Pathway determination can include evaluation of either

1) the sequence of events by which the discharged oil was transported from the incident and came into direct physical contact with the exposed natural resource (e.g., oil transported from an incident by ocean currents, wind, and wave action directly oils shellfish) or
2) the sequence of events by which the discharged oil was transported from the incident and caused an indirect impact on a natural resource and/or service (e.g., oil transported within a wetland by wind and wave action causes reduced populations of bait fish, which in turn results in starvation of a fish-eating bird; or, oil transported from an incident by currents, wind, and wave action causes the closure of a fishery to prevent potentially tainted fish from being marketed).

Pathway determination does not require that injured natural resources or services be directly exposed to oil. In the example provided above, fish-eating birds are injured as a result of decreases in food availability. However, trustees must always determine the existence of a plausible pathway relating the incident to the injured natural resource or service, even if the injury is not caused by direct exposure to oil.

As evidenced by the discussion of exposure and pathway analysis within an NRDA, the technical methods employed for wetland risk assessment could be identical to those supporting the NRDA process. Often, however, the language differences between NRDA and CERCLA confound an otherwise technically similar support function. Under NRDA, for example, injury quantification is the process by which trustees determine the degree and spatial or temporal extent of injuries, which supports the selection of appropriate restoration alternatives. Under CERCLA, this process does not include restoration activities. For NRDA, trustees may pursue one or more of several different conceptual approaches to injury quantification, which may be quantified in terms of

1) the degree and spatial or temporal extent of injury to a natural resource,
2) the degree and spatial or temporal extent of injury to a natural resource with subsequent translation of that change to a reduction in services provided by the natural resource, or
3) the amount of services lost as a result of the incident.

Within the context of injury quantification, the extent of injury may be expressed in terms of percent mortality; proportion of a population, species, community, or habitat affected; extent of oiling; availability of substitute services; or the spatial and temporal extent of the injury. Quantification of the total losses of wetland habitat injured by oil could be obtained by estimating the

1) total number of acres of severely oiled wetland in which vegetation is totally killed,

2) natural recovery time for severely oiled wetland,
3) total number of acres of moderately oiled wetland in which vegetation is not completely killed but the wetland has lower levels of productivity, and
4) natural recovery time for moderately oiled wetlands.

This information could then be combined to quantify the total number of "acre-years" of wetland injury to scale restoration actions.

An analysis of natural recovery, or the return of injured natural resources and services to baseline in the absence of restoration activities, may include evaluation of factors such as degree and spatial or temporal extent of injury, the sensitivity of the injured natural resource or service, reproductive potential, stability and resilience of the affected environment, natural variability, and physicochemical processes of the affected environment.

While it is beyond the scope of the present discussion to provide a detailed technical document to support either NRDA or CERCLA ecological risk assessment for wetlands, many of the technical methods applicable to the NRDA process—especially the injury and restoration assessment phases—are currently available and being used in wetland risk assessment (see section "Methods and endpoints for wetlands" and Table 4-4).

Table 4-4 Representative technical references for aquatic and sediment biological test methods for evaluating risks in wetland habitats

Test matrix	Target biota	Reference
Freshwater	Vascular plants	Wang 1991; ASTM 1997a
Freshwater/marine/estuarine	Algae and vascular plants	Swanson et al. 1991; ASTM 1997a
Freshwater	Aquatic vertebrates and invertebrates	USEPA 1990; Weber 1993; ASTM 1997b
Marine	Marine or estuarine invertebrates and vertebrates	Weber 1993; Klemm et al. 1994; Chapman et al. 1995; ASTM 1997b
Freshwater sediments	Epifauna, infauna, and vertebrates	USEPA 1994b; ASTM 1997b
Marine/estuarine sediments	Epifauna, infauna, and vertebrates	ASTM 1997b

For injury assessments for wetlands, whenever practicable, procedures should be chosen that provide information of use in determining the restoration appropriate for that injury, and frequently a range of assessment approaches, from simplified to more detailed, should be considered. In general, more detailed assessment procedures may include, alone or in any combination,

1) field investigations,

2) laboratory methods,
3) model-based methods, and
4) literature-based methods.

Technical support for evaluating primary and compensatory restoration is also consistent with many of the technical procedures currently available for wetland risk assessment. Within a NRDA, trustees have the discretion to include a compensatory-restoration action as well as a primary restoration action in their restoration alternatives. Here, a scaling of compensatory-restoration actions may be appropriate. For example, in a wetland restoration action under an NRDA, a service-to-service approach may be appropriate and, in many ways, very similar to a wetlands mitigation analysis. Here, under a service-to-service approach to scaling, the appropriate quantity of replacement services is determined by obtaining equivalency between lost and replacement services after discounting appropriately for differences in habitat value. As currently proposed, trustees must use the service-to-service approach for evaluating alternatives that provide services that are of the same type and quality and are subject to comparable resource scarcity and demand conditions as those lost. This proposed "habitat equivalency analysis" has been developed by NOAA in response to OPA and is intended to be applied to the NRDA process when lost resource services are primarily of indirect human use, e.g., species habitat or biological resources like wetlands. Habitat equivalency analysis, then, may be used to scale restoration projects that replace entire habitats, e.g., wetlands, that support multiple species or that replace individual species that provide a variety of resource services. To ensure that the scale of the compensatory-restoration project does not over- or undercompensate the public for injuries incurred, the trustees must establish an equivalency between the present value of the quantity of lost services and the present value of the quantity of services provided by the compensatory-restoration project over time.

Trustees may use any reliable method for calculating interim lost value. Where a site-specific application of one of these valuation methods does not meet the reasonable cost criterion, the trustees may consider estimating interim lost value by using benefits transfer. The choice of approaches in a particular context will depend upon the types of injuries and the type of services provided by the compensatory-restoration alternative. Trustees should consider using similar methods for measuring the value of the lost services and the value of the services provided by the compensatory-restoration alternatives. If different valuation methods are used, then trustees should take steps to ensure that the variation in methods does not introduce bias.

To evaluate restoration, monitoring activities may be incorporated into the NRDA process. As in the monitoring tasks that are frequently included in CERCLA ecological risk assessments, monitoring plans within the NRDA process should address study design elements such as duration, frequency of monitoring required to evaluate progress and success, the intensity of sampling required to detect success or the need for corrective action, and monitoring of a control or reference site to determine progress and success. To evaluate success of restoration actions, performance criteria may be developed which evaluate structural, functional, temporal, and other goals. For example, an agreement to create new marsh habitat as compensation for marsh impacted by oil could be described by performance criteria including the number of acres to be created, the location, the elevation of new habitat, the species to be planted and details for planting, such as density, and the time frame in which identifiable stages of the project should be completed.

Strengths and limitations of current risk assessment approaches for wetlands

From a technical perspective, each of the regulatory-associated practices considered above may be compared relative to the steps outlined in the USEPA framework approach (Figure 4-6). In a strict sense, no one method is best nor was any originally developed for wetlands risk assessment. Each has been molded, however, to assure their implementation for risk assessments mandated by law and regulation. In many respects, each approach summarized in this section, as well as those not included in this discussion (but available from many states and other federal agencies), requires technical support from wetland scientists, ecotoxicologists, and applied ecologists. Each approach identified in Table 4-2, for example, includes guidance for reviewing existing information for the risk assessment process or, alternatively, for designing and completing studies or surveys to address questions identified in the early phases of the risk assessment process. Similarly, each approach recognizes the importance of evaluating ecological effects, although the linkages between stressors (especially chemical stressors) and ecological effects are more thoroughly explored in some implementation plans than others. For example, explicit guidance for evaluating exposure is poorly described in some strategies for evaluating wetlands, but these guidance documents are also better developed for an analysis of physical stressors that may have impacted a wetland as a consequence of changes in land-use practice, e.g., synoptic wetland assessment versus CERCLA risk assessments. Shared limitations among all approaches include problems associated with interpreting existing information within a risk context, especially in comprehensive risk assessments that rely on statistical methods. Here, for example, data quality issues cut across all approaches, and regardless of the risk strategy employed, each shares problems related to inter-study comparisons and their interpretations, data pooling, and statistical issues related to encountered data.

Overall, the strengths and limitations of each approach considered here, as well as other approaches addressing similar risk-related questions, reflect the policy and management issues that are critical to the process, as noted in the USEPA Framework (1992, 1998). The technical support tools available for ecological risk assessment are numerous (see, e.g., "Methods and endpoints for wetlands," this chapter). But to ensure that the best available state-of-the-science is implemented to support wetlands policy and management, clear lines of communication must exist among the policy, management, and scientific professionals involved in the risk assessment process, and the risk assessment must take in all relevant ecological information for the site.

The Ecosystem Approach: Integrating Ecology, Hydrology, Geomorphology, and Soils of Wetlands

Abiotic characteristics of freshwater wetlands

Freshwater wetlands represent a host of ecosystems that have an abundance of surface water some time during most years (Hook 1993). Beyond this common thread, they vary greatly in characteristics. Local climatic conditions, geomorphology, and hydrodynamics have acted over time and are still acting to create the diverse and dynamic nature of these ecosystems.

The purpose of this general overview of the relationship of abiotic factors to wetland characteristics is to point out how they can be used to quickly identify those generic functional traits that should be addressed in a wetland-specific risk assessment. However, these are general guidelines, and each site must be examined closely to determine whether expected conditions actually exist. If the information is used in this context, it should prove helpful in focusing ecological and biological risk studies on relevant issues.

Climate

For wetlands to occur, there must be excess water. It generally comes as runoff from upland drainage areas. A simple form of the water balance equation is

$$dS = P - ET - R \quad \text{(Equation 4-1)},$$

where dS = storage, P = precipitation, ET = evapotranspiration, and R = runoff. In wetlands, ET tends to dominate this equation, and during some periods of the year, ET may exceed P so that no water is available for runoff. When $R > 0$, water runoff occurs either by overland flow and/or subsurface flow and may collect in depressions, thereby creating wetlands. Such climatic data generally are available through state and federal agencies, and they provide valuable clues as to the temporal nature of wetlands within a region (Figures 4-7a, b). Note that at Caribou, ME, R usually exceeds 0 from August through April (Figure 4-7a). Thus, one would expect the wetlands to be highly evident during dormant growth periods and less so during the growing season. In contrast, at Fort Lauderdale, FL, runoff exceeds outputs from March through November; thus, wetlands are apt to be most evident in this area during the summer months or growing season (Figure 4-7b).

Geomorphology

Geomorphology is the landscape position or geomorphic setting that accommodates the runoff and storage of water (Brinson 1993). As a consequence, geomorphology

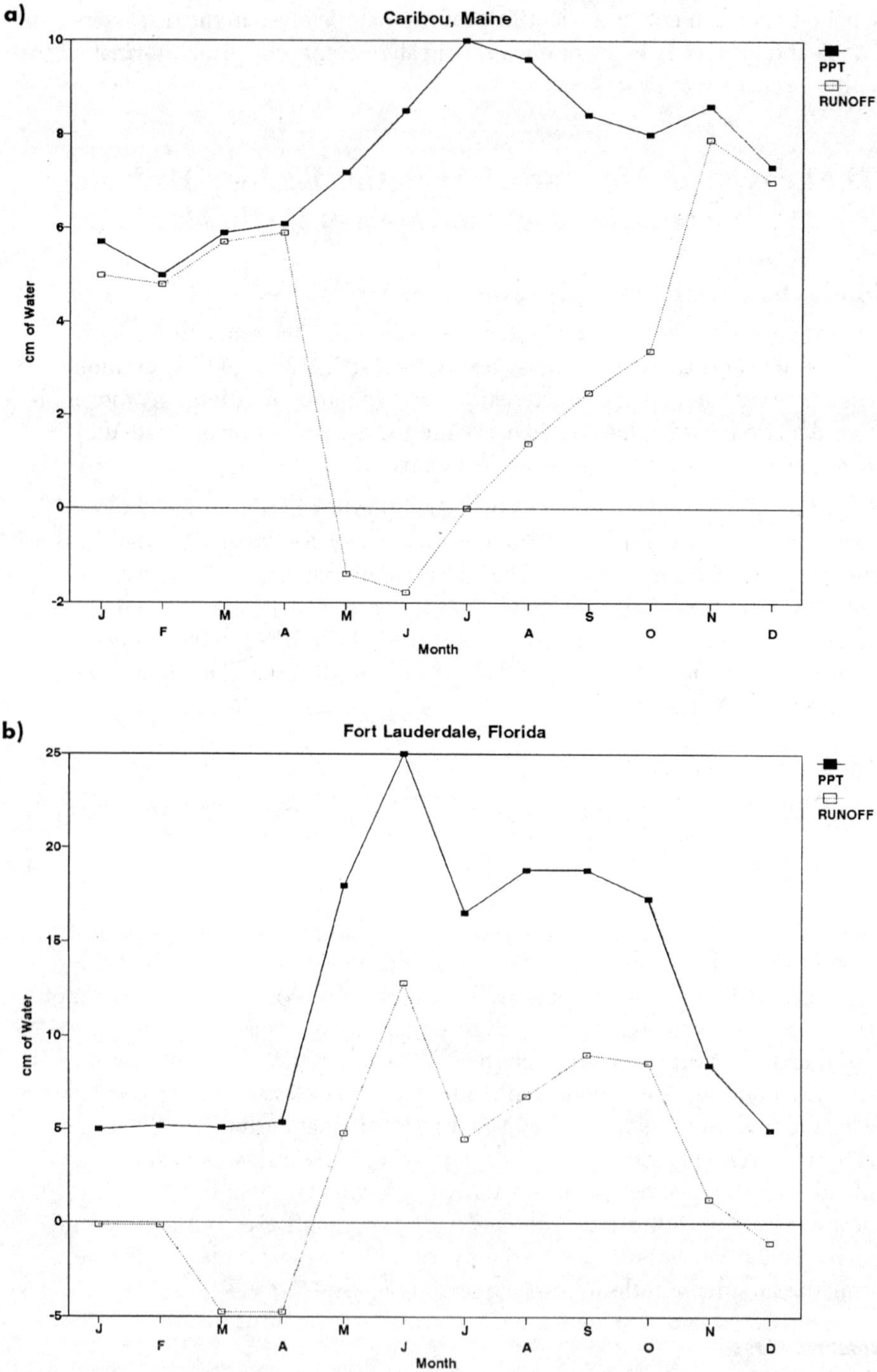

Figure 4-7 Relationship of total rainfall in cm to runoff in cm for a) Caribou, ME and b) Fort Lauderdale, FL

is generally linked to runoff and wetland positions. There are depressional, riverine, and fringe categories of geomorphologic settings.

Depressional wetlands include such landforms as kettles, potholes, vernal pools, and Carolina bays. They frequently occur high in drainage systems; thus, they typically depend heavily upon local precipitation when compared to other geomorphic settings. In climates where ET exceeds P, depressions such as vernal pools tend to be dry much of the time, or they depend upon ground water (Zelder 1987; Brinson 1993). In climatic regions where $R > 0$ for a significant portion of the year, depressions may accumulate sufficient peat to develop a domed topographic relief. These types of wetlands receive their water from precipitation, not from ground water or overbank flooding.

Extensive peatlands are usually the terminal condition of peat accumulation in depressions, followed by radiating paludification. When such conditions occur, they create domed landscapes where the highest elevation receives precipitation as the sole source of water. These are generally nutrient-poor environments. They may cover large areas of land such that the peat substrate dominates the movement and storage of water, the mineral nutrition of the plants, and the patterns of the landscape (Moore and Bellamy 1974). Extensive peat formations caused by paludification across the landscape may develop surface patterns that are independent of the underlying topography. As a consequence, there is a gradient from the headwater ombrotrophic wetlands with diffuse outlets to ones further downstream with fen-like characteristics (Siegel and Glaser 1987).

Riverine wetlands form as linear strips parallel to streams but are generally separated from the stream channel by natural levees. A riverine wetland may occupy most of the floodplain in large rivers (high-order streams) in the lower coastal plain but may be very small or nonexistent in low-order streams in the Piedmont regions of the South (Theriot 1988; Hook et al. 1994). Hydroperiods range from short and flashy in low-order streams to long and steady in higher-order streams. The slope of the stream channel determines whether a given section of the floodplain is predominately erosional or depositional.

Freshwater fringe wetlands are restricted to freshwater tidal zones associated with estuaries. These types of wetlands are generally riverine (alluvial), in nature but some may be headwaters (nonalluvial). The latter occur in small drainages that feed into rivers near estuaries.

Hydrodynamics

The source of water for freshwater wetlands may be precipitation, groundwater discharge, surface or near-surface inflows, or any combination of these. Many depressional wetlands receive their water from precipitation runoff. These types of wetlands occupy depressions in the landscape that are above the general water-table level (Figure 4-8a). They are generally separated from the water table by a layer of relatively impermeable soil that restricts the rate of water movement downward

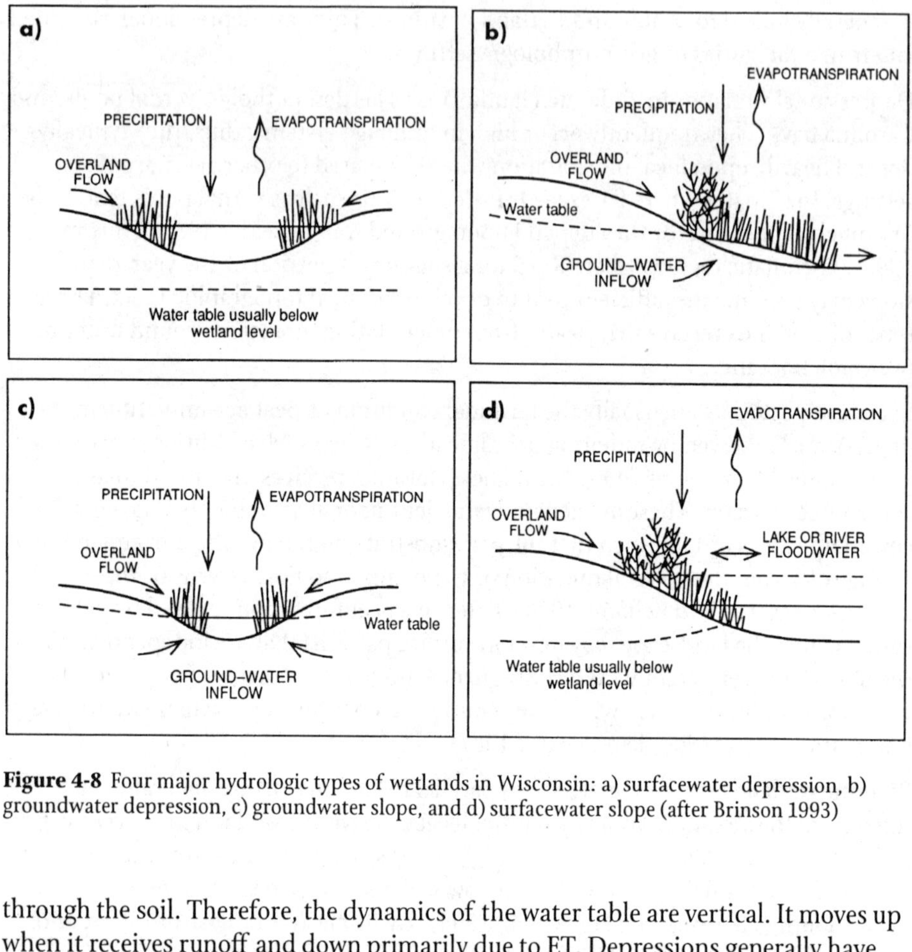

Figure 4-8 Four major hydrologic types of wetlands in Wisconsin: a) surfacewater depression, b) groundwater depression, c) groundwater slope, and d) surfacewater slope (after Brinson 1993)

through the soil. Therefore, the dynamics of the water table are vertical. It moves up when it receives runoff and down primarily due to ET. Depressions generally have no inlets or outlets, or, if they are present, they receive or drain water only during or after storm events. They tend to be disconnected hydrologically from the surrounding landscape and the substrate below the restrictive layer. However, during high-water events, some water may spill out of the depression beyond the restrictive layer and come into contact with the substrate below. Research in Florida has shown that the cypress domes may be more interconnected than originally thought (Riekerk 1993). Depending on size, geomorphology, and regional location, they may develop distinct zonational vegetation and structural patterns in relation to the time and duration of inundation and fluctuation of the water table. Nutrient input into these systems is primarily by precipitation. On a relative scale, they tend to have low productivity. However, productivity may vary with the geology, climatic conditions, and types of soils and vegetation that develop.

Some depressional wetlands receive ground water in addition to runoff from precipitation (Figures 4-8b, 4-8c, 4-8d). If the groundwater table intersects the slope at or within the depression, water enters from below as well as from runoff. Ground water may enter wetlands or create wetlands on slopes where the water table intersects the soil surface (Figure 4-9). Such areas can best be visualized as seeps or springs. However, relatively large wetlands can occur on slopes.

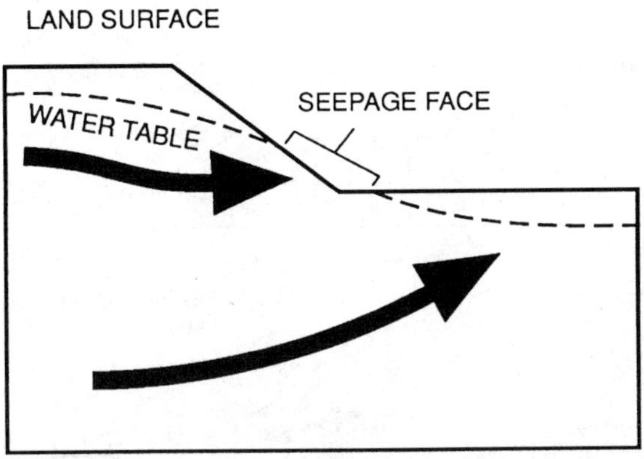

Figure 4-9 Relationship of land surface and water table to seepage face (after Brinson 1993)

If ground water enters a wetland, it has been in contact with the mineral content of an aquifer or soil. Depending on the time of contact and the composition of the lithology, such water normally has higher mineral content than water derived from precipitation. Consequently, plant communities in wetlands that receive groundwater discharge tend to be more productive than rainwater wetlands (depressions). Furthermore, the hydrodynamics of the system are apt to be more stable than in precipitation-driven wetlands (i.e., dry-downs may not be as severe and as rapid). The dynamics of the water table in these types of wetlands tend to be vertical in relation to water inputs and outputs (Figure 4-10a).

The source of water in riverine wetlands may be from overbank flooding, ground water, and precipitation. The dominant water source is not always evident even after extensive exploration. A study in the Piedmont of South Carolina showed that a fourth-order stream received periodic overbank flooding on average about 3 times/y during the dormant season. However, during the growing season, the wetland was driven entirely by precipitation (Hook et al. 1994). In contrast, in a fifth-order stream in coastal Georgia, water came from overbank flooding during the growing season as well as the dormant season, but between major rainfall events in the watershed, precipitation and ground water influenced the wetland to varying degrees depending on topographic relief. Pesiometric studies showed that micro topography had important influences on drainage patterns and sources of water between flood events (Saul 1995).

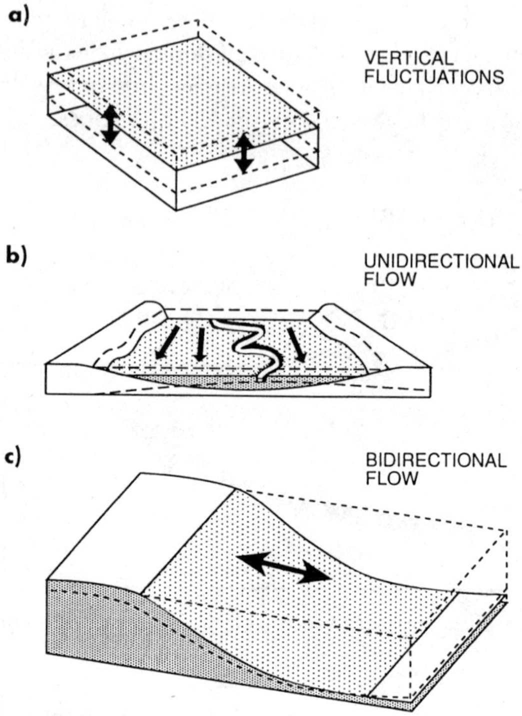

Figure 4-10 Categories of hydrodynamics based on dominant flow pattern: a) vertical fluctuations normally are caused by evapotranspiration and precipitation, b) unidirectional flows are horizontal surface and subsurface, and c) bidirectional flows are horizontal across the surface (after Brinson 1993)

The water in a floodplain tends to flow unidirectional down stream (Figure 4-10b), but depending on topography depressions in the floodplain, it may take on vertical dynamics when the river is not in flood stage. In the lower reaches of rivers influenced by tides, the fringe wetlands may be subjected to bidirectional flows similar to those in estuaries (Figure 4-10c). The variation in hydrodynamics among wetlands and within localities of a wetland must be carefully considered if contaminant studies are to successfully identify key transport and exposure pathways to biota.

Biogenic and fluvial deposition in wetlands tend to be causally related to water flow rate (energy; Figure 4-11a). Hydrologic energy, hydrodynamics, nutrient availability, temperature, salinity, fire frequency, and herbivory are also related in a general manner to wetland type and core factors (Figure 4-11b).

When a wetland has 2 or more water sources, it can be difficult to separate their relative contributions. For riverine systems, records of time, frequency, depth, and duration of overbank flooding are necessary to evaluate the extent of individual contributions, effects of overbank flooding on the wetland, and how contaminants may be delivered, retained, and transported. Some rivers have stream gauges

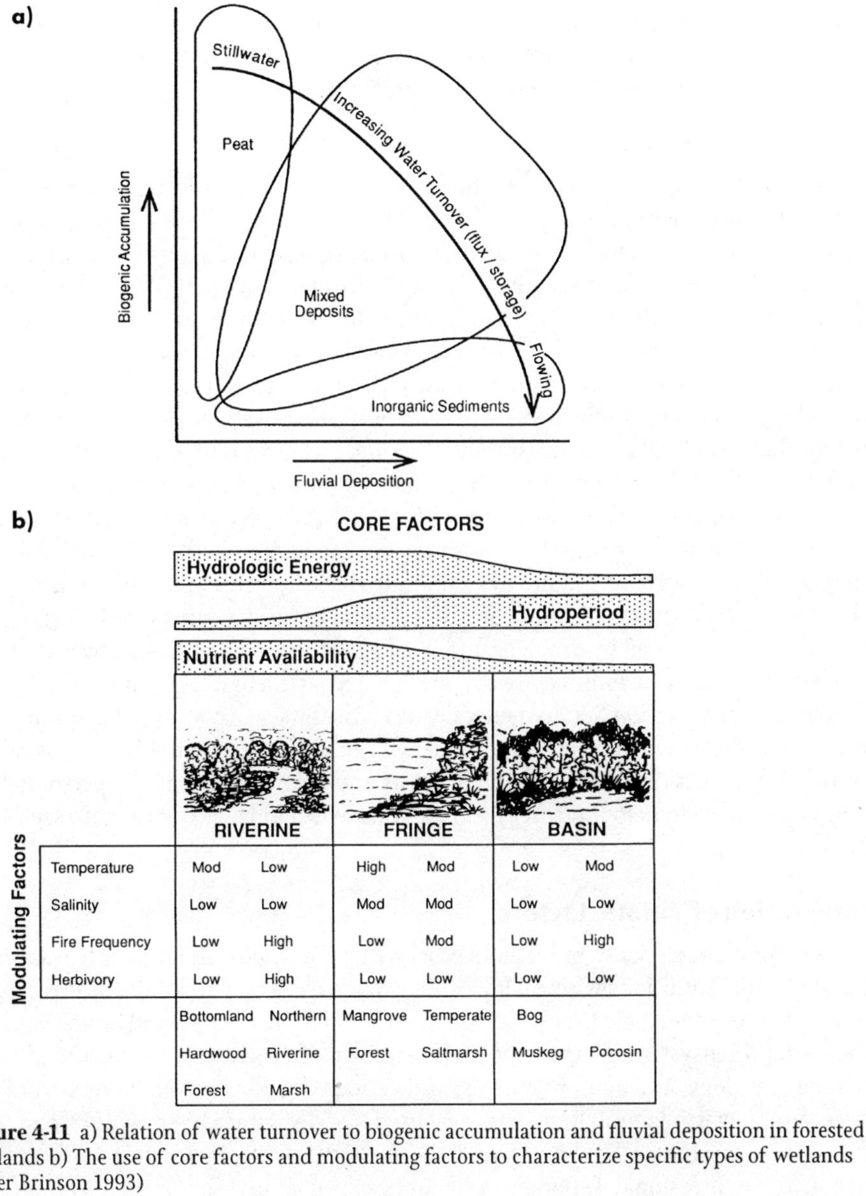

Figure 4-11 a) Relation of water turnover to biogenic accumulation and fluvial deposition in forested wetlands b) The use of core factors and modulating factors to characterize specific types of wetlands (after Brinson 1993)

maintained by the U. S. Geological Survey (USGS) for various durations. Such records are invaluable for ecological and toxicological studies and evaluation of various wetland functions. In the absence of such records, stream flow or pesiometric (soil saturation) studies are necessary to quantify many characteristics of a wetland. Problems arise in determining how long monitoring must have occurred to be useful. For example, a 38-y record for one wetland in eastern North Carolina demonstrated that, depending on which 3- or 5-y period was selected for measurement, the site could be classified either as a wetland or nonwetland using jurisdictional criteria (W. Skaggs, personal communication).

Use of soil surveys

Many, if not most, counties in the United States have surveys of the soils. The surveys contain more general traits that will help determine the potential characteristics of a specific wetland. They identify soils by series and drainage class and provide information on productivity, amount of organic matter (OM), general information on the degree of soil saturation or flooding, times of hydroperiods, and occasionally the duration of hydro events. In addition, if the wetland is forested, the data bank may include information on site index for various tree species. This provides another clue to the relative productivity of the wetland (site index is the height that a tree will reach at a specified age and has proven to be a very good measure of the productivity of the site). Again, these are general traits for a soil series, but they provide the researcher with a fairly extensive array of characteristics about the wetland site in question. It is necessary to verify whether the soil information is truly indicative of the site by examining the soil profile and other salient characteristics of the site. Is the vegetation natural or has it been altered? Has the hydrology been altered by drainage and blockage of drainages? Assistance with this process can usually be found close by. The U.S. Department of Agriculture Natural Resources Conservation Service generally has offices in each county, with trained personnel who can help interpret soil survey information and sometimes assist with actual field checks. In addition, county agents and university extension personnel may be available to help interpret the data or provide guidance on where to seek help.

Integration of abiotic factors

The salient characteristics of wetland ecosystems are embodied in the integration of local climatic conditions with geology and hydrodynamics. The results of this integration over geologic time are evident in the soils, vegetation, and biota. Thus, the wetland ecosystem is a result of the interaction of specific abiotic factors (climate, geology, and hydrodynamics) and various organisms over a long period of time. However, can abiotic traits alone be used to determine what processes and functions a specific wetland may have? The answer is—only in a general context. For instance, a depressional wetland would not be expected to be involved in carbon transport or to actively transport pollutants or nutrients out of the system. Furthermore, the system would not be expected to be highly productive, but caution is needed for the latter. If the depression has a groundwater source that is rich in nutrients, its productivity may be high; thus, it could act as an efficient buffer or transformer. Additionally, the amount of OM in the soil will influence its potential to support microorganisms for decomposition and other soil reactions.

Geomorphic settings and traits can be a practical starting point for identifying the basic type of wetland as well is its principal ecosystem functions and associated ecological significance (Table 4-5). Moreover, the relationship of abiotic factors to wetland characteristics is useful for identifying those generic functional traits that should be addressed in a wetland-specific risk assessment. The approach can be simplified to a protocol that incorporates 7 steps:

1) Determine the geomorphic setting. Is it a depression or basin, a riverine system, or a fringe wetland?
2) Determine the dominant source of water. Is it rain water, ground water, or overbank flooding?
3) Determine the dynamics of the hydrological mechanisms. Does the water table fluctuate vertically? Is it primarily unidirectional or bidirectional? Do the dynamics change with water-table level or season? Use the water balance equation and determine when R exceeds 0. This will identify the seasons or times that the water table is apt to be the highest or lowest.
4) Use all available resources, i.e., aerial photographs, maps, interviews with local people, field reconnaissance in and around the wetland, to determine if the hydrology has been significantly altered. If it has, try to determine how the alterations may have affected the hydroperiods, timing, frequency, and flow patterns that would be expected to be associated with the existing geomorphic setting.
5) Use soil surveys to determine soil series, texture, drainage class, vegetation, hydroperiods and hydrodynamics, and the relative productivity based on site index or other site productivity documentation in the survey.
6) Scout the entire area to determine the patterns of inundation, vegetation types, and vegetation densities to identify any zones or patterns that may affect how toxins may enter the wetland and how they could be influenced by open water, vegetation traits, and seasonality of hydrodynamics.
7) Determine where and how the wetland is positioned in the watershed and whether it may have been impacted by long-term chronic conditions (disturbance) of any type. Look for differences in vegetation. Does the regeneration match what is expected for the site? If not, is the regenerating vegetation more hydric or more mesophytic than is characteristic for the wetland type?

Analyzing these abiotic factors is the fist step in an ecosystem approach to wetland risk assessment. Although abiotic traits alone can provide valuable clues for targeting ecotoxicological investigations or other studies, one must also overlay information on the biology and ecology of the system in order to conclusively identify and evaluate the full range of potential issues or problems for a given assessment.

Knowledge of wetland science is necessary in order to effectively address the biotic components of wetland ecosystems in the context of risk assessment. A discussion of some of the key principles is given here to point out important factors that must

Table 4-5 Relationships between geomorphic setting and ecosystem attributes of freshwater wetlands

Geomorphic setting	Qualitative evidence	Quantitative evidence	Hydrologic functions	Ecological significance
No apparent inlet or outlet	Topographically isolated from other surface water	Drydowns frequent; water table frequently below the wetland	Retains inflow; losses mostly by infiltration or evapotranspiration (ET)	Inaccessible to aquatic life dependent on streams; endemics likely
Positioned on local topographic high; surface output only	Outlet may be defined by contours or intermittent streams	Drydowns frequent; water table frequently below the wetland	Temporary flood storage; outlet may overflow during high surface water or flow continuously during high ground water; outlet controls maximum depth	Wetland open to immigration and emigration of aquatic life; potential for recolonization if drydowns cause local extinctions
Located in marginally dry climate; variable inlets and outlets	Inlets and outlets may be defined by contours or intermittent streams	Water conductivity high = wetland is recharging underlying aquifer; if low = aquifer is supplying the wetland	Retains inflow; loss primarily by ET or infiltration; may be subject too wide for migrating fluctuations in water depth	Import and export detritus; critical habitat for migrating waterfowl; vulnerable to eutrophication and toxic accumulation due to long retention time
Both surface inlet and outlet; large catchment sustains marginal riverine features	Inlets and outlets may be defined by contours or intermittent streams	Water budget dominated by lateral surface flows or strong groundwater discharge	Temporary flood storage; drainage back to stream or continuously saturated	Import and export detritus; provides fish and wildlife habitat
Located on break in slope	Soil saturated most of the time	Chemically indicative of ground water; discharge from slope base or face	Inflow steady and continous; seasonal loss by ET; low surface storage capacity	Provides stable source of moisture; contributes to biodiversity
Ombrotrophic bog	Peat substrate saturated most of the time; plants indicate ombrotrophic bog; surface flows are negligible	Peat confirmed by organic content and thickness; ombrotrophy evident from low pH and ion content	Some storage of storm runoff; groundwater conservation when water table is below surface	Upland habitat scarce; species composition is unique to bog conditions
Rich fen	Peat substrate saturated most of the time; graminoid species indicative of groundwater supply	Peat confirmed by organic content and thickness; minerotrophy evident from circumneutral pH and high ion content	Subsurface water supply maintains saturation to surface and hydraulic gradient to maintain flow	Allows lateral movement of water without channelized flow; exhibits moderate level of primary productivity and detritus export

Table 4-5 (*continued*)

Geomorphic setting	Qualitative evidence	Quantitative evidence	Hydrologic functions	Ecological significance
Streamside zones of intermittent streams	Headwater position; first-order stream	Flows not continous; no headwater flooding or overbank flows	Interface of landscape where ground water and surface water change to fluvial environment	Riparian zone critical to maintain buffer between the stream and uplands
High-gradient downcutting portions	Bedrock-controlled channel	Substrate lacks alluvium; flow may be continuous but flashy	Downslope transport is dominant feature	Scour prevents extensive wetland development
High-gradient aggrading portions	Substrate controlled by fluvial processes	Stratigraphy shows imbedding of coarse particles within fines	Wetland on coarse substrate maintained by upslope groundwater source	Unstable substrate in a scour-prone environment colonized by pioneer species Allochthonous organic supply
Middle-gradient landform	Channelized flow; evidence of oxbows and meanders consistent with fluvial processes	Flow likely continous with moderate to high base flows	Channel process establishes variation in topography, hydroperiod, and habitat interspersion on a floodplain	Interspersion of plant communities increases biodiversity
Low-gradient alluvial; floodplain of bottomland hardwood	As above, but in low-gradient landform	Flow continuous with cool season flooding; high suspended sediments in stream	Flood storage; conserves groundwater discharge	Major habitat for wildlife; biogeochemial activity and nutrient
Shoreline of large lakes	Subject to seiches; lake level controls position	Year-to-year trends in zonation follow climatic cycles; wind-generated fluctuations possible	Lake is water supply for wetland and establishes hydroperiod gradient for wetland zonation	Stabilizes shoreline; transition habitat used by aquatic and terrestrial biota
Coastal sea-level location	Subject to tides; sea-level controlled	Elevation relative to tides and changing sea level	Wetland is responsive to tides and sea level	Barrier to saltwater encroachment; retains sediment; nursery habitat for estuarine organisms

be considered when identifying biological characteristics of a wetland. These characteristics may ultimately affect the direction of the risk assessment as well as the effectiveness of subsequent risk management.

Biological processes and ecosystem functioning

In addition to the complexity introduced by the myriad of interactions of external factors, differential biotic responses to these external factors also yield a complex set of interactions among the biota (organisms, species, populations, communities), the critical processes they perform (photosynthesis, microbial action, decomposition, etc.), and the way these organisms and their processes are expressed through ecosystem functions (production, biomass accumulation, biogeochemical processes, etc.). To a large extent, the complex structure and function of wetlands reflect the divergent properties of their biota. Most wetlands are dominated by a flora of vascular plants that are adapted to a greater or lesser extent to flooded conditions, but that are, in most respects, structurally and physiologically similar to their terrestrial ancestors. Yet, wetlands may also have features similar to deepwater aquatic ecosystems, including sediment biogeochemical and biotic processes mediated through predominantly anoxic conditions and aquatic food webs of algae, invertebrates, and vertebrates. Although wetlands show structural and functional overlap with terrestrial and aquatic systems, they often serve as the interface between these 2 systems. Wetland structure, internal critical processes, and ecosystem functions are sufficiently different from terrestrial and aquatic systems to require a knowledge base specific to wetlands. We provide here only a brief discussion of certain unique aspects of wetland ecosystems. The reader is encouraged to review relevant published literature for a more complete foundation in wetland ecology. Recommended readings include Ethrington (1983), Mitsch and Gosselink (1993), and NRC (1995).

Wetlands can best be viewed as complex temporal and spatial mosaics of habitats with distinct structural and functional characteristics. Variation in vegetation structure represents one of the most striking examples of spatial and temporal pattern in wetland habitat. Depending upon the type of wetland, the system may be dominated by emergent herbaceous or woody macrophytes, with open water relegated to relatively small areas among blades of emergent plants or to small open patches within the emergent stand. However, regardless of the dominant vegetation, horizontal zonation is a common feature of wetland ecosystems, and in most wetlands, relatively distinct, often concentric bands of vegetation develop in relation to water depth. Bottomland hardwood forests and prairie pothole wetlands provide excellent illustrations of zonation in 2 very divergent wetland types (Figures 4-12 and 4-13).

Wetlands may display dramatic temporal shifts in zonation patterns in response to changing hydrology. Entire systems may even shift, for example, between predominantly emergent and open water zones. In periods of little or no water, some

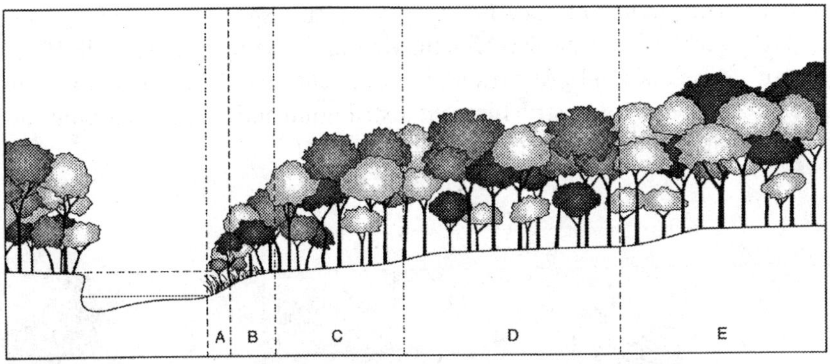

Figure 4-12 Vegetation zones along South Skunk River, IA (and similar-sized rivers in central hardwoods forest region). A–B) Deposition bank with A) herbaceous plants and tree seedlings grading to B) dominance by *Salix interior* and young *Salix nigra* and *Populus deltoides.* C) Floodplain with maturing *Salix nigra, Populus deltoides* and *Acer saccharinum*. D) First terrace dominated by *Celtis occidentalis, Junglans nigra*, and *Fraxinus pennsylvanica*. E) Second terrace dominated by *Quercus macrocarpa* and/or *Acer nigrum* depending on soil type and aspect. In larger river bottoms, area C is much expanded with relatively less of areas D and E.

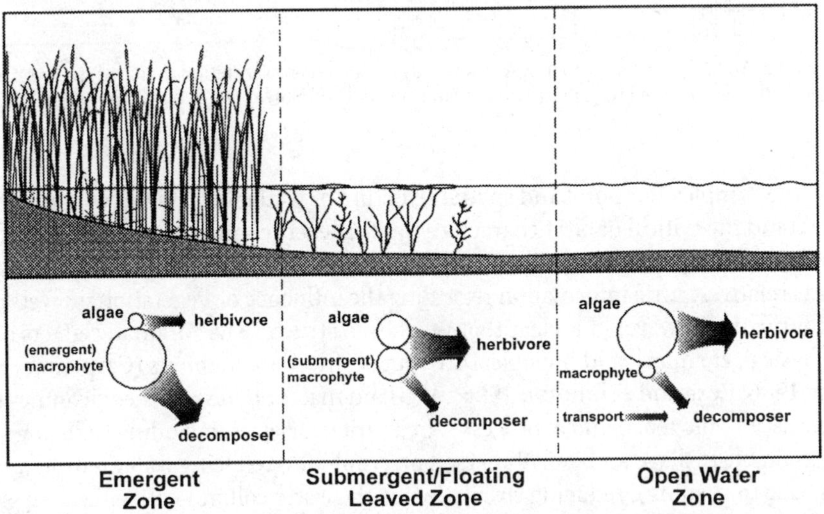

Figure 4-13 Spatial pattern in vegetation and energy flow in prairie pothole wetlands

wetlands may temporarily become almost terrestrial in form and function. Yet, the same system in other years or in other seasons of the same year may be flooded to the extent that the system becomes, in small or significant part, largely aquatic in nature. Temporal patterns are in fact important characteristics of many wetland types. Seasonal cycles are a major feature of floodplain forests, for example. These systems are flooded during winter and spring periods of high stream flow and bankfull discharge but are typically dry by mid to late summer due to drainage and ET. Longer-term cycles are a major feature of prairie pothole wetlands, which undergo dramatic, more or less cyclic changes in response to a variety of environmental factors including water-level fluctuations and grazing (van der Valk 1989; Mitsch and Gosselink 1993). As a result, these systems may exhibit major year-to-year variations in vegetation structure and distribution and in the relative importance of vegetated and open water zones (Figure 4-14).

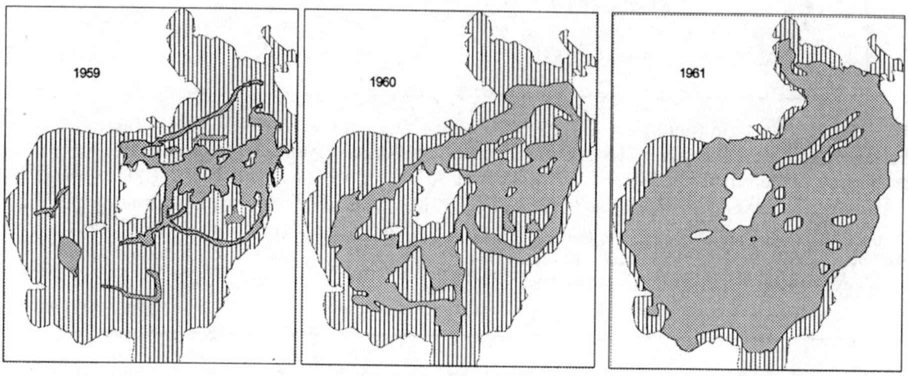

Figure 4-14 Annual changes in open water (shaded) and emergent vegetation (hatched) in a prairie pothole wetland (reprinted with permission from University of Notre Dame, Weller and Spatcher 1965)

Given the complex temporal and spatial structure of wetlands, it is important to understand the critical habitat characteristics that exert control over major aspects of wetland function. In comparison to our understanding of vegetation dynamics, there is relatively little information regarding the influence of vegetation on wetland environments. However, it is clear that vegetation structure has dramatic effects on the physical, chemical, and biological attributes of wetland habitats (Carpenter and Lodge 1986; Rose and Crumpton 1996). Wetland macrophytes affect environmental attributes and biogeochemical processes in a variety of ways, including reducing light available to algae and/or submersed macrophytes, reducing water temperatures (due to shading), reducing circulation of the water column with effects on gas exchange and material transport, increasing inputs of detrital carbon, enhancing transport of gases to and from the sediment (rhizosphere), and either reducing or enhancing mineral uptake and release. In addition to direct and indirect effects on biogeochemistry (see Chapter 3), vegetation structure is one of the most important factors affecting foodweb structure and bioenergetics in wetland ecosystems. Despite the obvious oversimplification, it is useful to distinguish 3 broad classes of primary producers in wetlands with regard to foodweb dynamics:

1) emergent macrophytes,
2) submergent and floating leaved macrophytes, and
3) planktonic and periphytic algae.

Emergent macrophytes are similar to terrestrial plants in that their biomass is high in structural components such as cellulose and lignin. Their leaves and stems have the low nutrient content and high carbon-to-nitrogen ratios typical of terrestrial plants of similar growth form, and their food value is relatively low. In general, herbivory on emergent macrophytes is very low, and most of their production is transferred to the detrital pool. Nonetheless, the impact of herbivore activity may be extensive at times. For example, the complete destruction of emergent vegetation by muskrats in freshwater marshes has been documented numerous times (van der Valk 1989). However, even during these events, muskrats prefer roots and shoot bases and rarely consume leaves and stems of emergent macrophytes. These tougher materials are instead discarded or used to build lodges, thus entering the detrital pool. Due to the prevalence of structural compounds such as cellulose and lignin, detritus derived from emergent macrophytes is relatively resistant to digestion or decomposition, especially under anaerobic conditions. Nutrient content is even lower and carbon-to-nitrogen ratios higher than in the living plants, and as a result, decomposition frequently requires nutrient subsidy from external sources such as chemical fertilizers.

In contrast to emergent macrophytes, submergent and floating leaved macrophytes have substantially less structural material. Their tissues generally have higher nutrient content and lower carbon-to-nitrogen ratios. Due to their higher nutrient content, the food value of submergent and floating leaved plants can be relatively high in comparison to emergent macrophytes. Herbivory on submergent and floating leaved macrophytes is highly variable, but in comparison to emergent macrophytes, a larger portion of their production may be consumed by herbivores rather than being transferred directly to the detrital pool. The principal herbivores consuming submergent and floating leaved macrophytes include waterfowl, macroinvertebrates, and fish. Due to the relative paucity of structural compounds, detritus derived from submergent and floating leaved macrophytes is relatively labile and relatively easily digested or decomposed.

Planktonic and periphytic algae, of course, have very little structural material. Their tissues have very high nutrient content and low carbon-to-nitrogen ratios. Algae have very high food value and are easily consumed and digested by a wide range of herbivores including microzooplankton, macroinvertebrates, and fish. Although grazing rates vary, much of the algae produced in wetlands is consumed by herbivores rather than being transferred directly to the detrital pool, significantly more than in the case of emergent or submergent macrophytes. Detritus derived from algae is very labile and easily digested or decomposed.

Most freshwater wetlands are assumed to be dominated to a lesser or greater extent by a food chain that is weblike and detritus-based (Mitsch and Gosselink 1993). However, based on the preceding discussion, it is clear that spatial heterogeneity in vegetation structure can result in a mixture of detritus-based and producer–herbivore-based food webs (Figure 4-13). For example, emergent macrophytes dominate production in the emergent zone of freshwater marshes. Most of this production could be expected to enter the detrital pool, with relatively little consumption by herbivores. In contrast, phytoplankton dominate production in the open water zone of freshwater marshes, and much of their production would probably be consumed directly by herbivores. In wetland zones dominated by submergent and floating leaved macrophytes, these macrophytes and their attached algae might both contribute significantly to total production. In either case, a significant proportion of the total production would probably be consumed directly by herbivores. Given these relationships, it is probably better to characterize the food webs of freshwater marshes and most other wetlands not as either detritus-based or producer-herbivore based, but rather as complex mosaics of habitats with distinct food webs. It is important to understand that seasonal as well as longer-term shifts in habitat mosaics and in their associated food webs and biogeochemistry are fundamental aspects of the character of many wetland ecosystems (Figure 4-14).

Applying the Ecological Factors to a Wetlands-specific Risk Assessment

As part of the data collection for the risk assessment, keep in mind that, as a general rule, ecotoxicological or other types of tests that might be applicable for coastal or marine wetlands may not be suitable for freshwater wetlands and vice versa (Kent et al. 1994). It is incumbent on those using any of the tests or undertaking the laboratory or field studies to fully understand their applicability, limitations, and interpretation.

The ecosystem approach given here was constructed to maximize flexibility in approaching the risk assessment, made necessary by the diversity of freshwater wetlands that may be encountered, in addition to the multitude of factors or stressors that may be at work in the particular wetland under study (Kusler and Kentula 1990; Zentner 1994). Figure 4-15 provides a simple hypothetical illustration of the stressors or factors at work in a wetlands at 2 different times to explain that the magnitude of these stressors is highly dynamic. This figure further emphasizes that all forms of stressors, biological, chemical, and physical, are integrated within the overall risk faced by ecological receptors, such as wetlands, and that the interlinkage of these stressors must be understood and recognized when conducting a risk assessment (Kentula et al. 1993).

An ecosystem approach stresses the key concept of interlinkage of the wetland components (NRC 1992, 1995). An additional overarching provision is that the approach to data collection and evaluation should be tiered (or phased) so that resources are focused effectively and there is ample opportunity for the risk assessor and risk manager to discuss the scientific and policy implications as the risk assessment proceeds (USEPA 1994a, 1997).

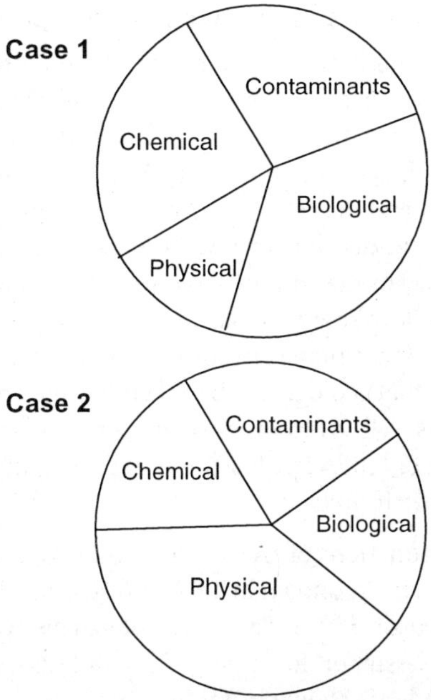

Figure 4-15 Main groups of stressors in the environment. Note that the relative proportions of the stressors to the whole stress are dynamic, both temporally and spatially, and not evenly divided.

Problem formulation

There are several main points to consider when beginning a wetland risk assessment. First is to gather and review previously developed information such as aerial photographs, historical maps, land use documents, previous biological or chemical studies, etc. Also important is to gain an understanding of the hydrology and geology driving the wetlands under study. For example, is the wetland riparian, a prairie pothole, or another type? As noted earlier, wetlands vary in their structure primarily due to hydrological and geological conditions, both of which will influence the focus of the risk assessment (NRC 1995) as well as the data collection process. Another key aspect is to determine or define the spatial extent of the area under study. For some wetlands, this will amount to only a few acres; for others, it may encompass an entire watershed of several thousand acres or more.

An early step in problem formulation, with respect to wetlands, is the use of wetland evaluation models (e.g., Brinson 1993; Bartoldus et al. 1994), which can help establish the important characteristics of the wetland under study. More importantly, however, these and other models can be useful when discussing assessment and measurement endpoints.

Development of assessment and measurement endpoints

One of the most important steps in the problem formulation phase is establishing clear assessment endpoints because they set the stage for all of the forthcoming effort. Assessment endpoints specific to freshwater wetlands can vary tremendously due to the diversity of potential wetland types that may be encountered and due to the myriad functions the wetland may serve. In a diversion from the general practice in ecological risk assessment, under the proposed USEPA framework (USEPA 1992) the assessment endpoints may or may not be biologically or ecologically based. For example, the hydrology, geomorphology, soils, and other aspects of the wetlands may be far more important a focus than some of the biological resources (Brinson 1993). This is not to suggest that ecologically based endpoints are not important, but that they entail abiotic as well as biotic considerations. In fact, directing the risk assessment at the ecosystem or landscape level requires recognition of the abiotic and biotic components and their linkage.

Some important values and functions of freshwater wetlands, from which assessment endpoints can be derived, are shown in Table 4-6 (see also Brinson 1993; Bartoldus et al. 1994; Richardson 1994). These are not exhaustive but can be used as starting points in the risk assessment. Examples of possible assessment endpoints specific to freshwater wetlands are shown in Table 4-7.

Table 4-6 Important values and functions of freshwater wetlands

Value or function	Mechanism or activity
Hydrological	
Flood protection	Water storage and control
Water quality	Sediment control; nutrient production or export
Ecological	
Habitat	Vegetative growth and maintenance
Human	
Recreation	Fishing, hunting, wildlife watching
Commercial	Fishing, timber harvesting

Table 4-7 Possible assessment endpoints for freshwater wetlands

Assessment endpoint	Significance
Hydrological	
Maintain natural supply of water to wetland	Key to maintaining proper level of hydration
Provide sediment control	Reduces turbidity and sediment loading to nearby waterbodies
Geomorphological	
Maintain bank stability	Reduces erosion of stream and river banks
Ecological	
Maintain level of primary productivity	Underpins food web stability

A hypothetical case helps illustrate the development of assessment endpoints and the shift in focus of the risk assessment. Assume that the freshwater wetland under study is one that is dependent on a constant supply of high-quality ground water. In this example, one assessment endpoint might be to protect the supply of high-quality ground water to the wetlands by preventing exposure of the ground water to nonchemical stressors (physical diversion of the ground water for other purposes). Albeit an oversimplification of an actual situation, this illustrates a shift from ecologically driven assessment endpoints to hydrologically driven endpoints. However, as stressed in the ecosystem approach given here, the ecology, hydrology, and geomorphology are inseparable and, in fact, define the ecosystem being protected. In this situation, protection is afforded against that which poses a risk to the sustainability of the wetland: loss of ground water, without which the wetland ceases to exist.

In one of the most extensive ecological risk assessments conducted in a wetland environment, the Clark Fork River (CFR) Superfund Site in Montana (Pascoe and DalSoglio 1994; Linder et al. 1994; see also Chapter 5), none of the assessment endpoints for the riparian wetlands or the river itself included protection of the water supply per se. This does not imply that the risk assessment was done incorrectly, but that the primary focus was to protect ecological resources (primarily plants and animals) versus the one key component responsible for the wetlands themselves: water. Further, this does not mean that there were no important biologically driven assessment endpoints, but that the assessment endpoints for wetlands should include other parameters that are crucial to the long-term sustainability of the wetland itself.

Under the hypothetical case described above, another important consideration could be ensuring that the ground water is meeting a minimum "quality" standard. Quality could be defined as a particular range of pH, turbidity, or specific conductance, or as an absence of chemical stressors at some threshold concentration (e.g., dissolved Se concentrations below 5 g/L. Regardless of the situation, it is important to establish the assessment endpoints clearly in the context of what is vital to sustaining or improving the health of the freshwater wetland, recognizing the inseparability of the ecological, hydrological, and geomorphological components.

Likewise, measurement endpoints may or may not have a biological or ecological basis. Nevertheless, they must be relevant to and linked directly with the assessment endpoints. In the hypothetical case, measurement endpoints may be analytical determinations of contaminant concentrations in the water supplying the wetlands, the specific conductance or suspended solids levels in the water, the flow of water to the wetlands, and others. Implicit, too, is the understanding that biologically driven assessment and measurement endpoints may be included as well.

Numerous endpoints can be used to assess impacts to biological functions. Following is a synopsis of some key biological measurement endpoints for wetland risk assessment (Table 4-8).

Table 4-8 Important hydrogeomorphic, biogeochemical, ecological, and compound-specific parameters for assessing exposure in freshwater wetlands (field and/or laboratory measurements)

Hydrogeomorphic information	Biogeochemical information	Ecological information	Compound-specific information
Type of water input (capillary, precipitation, etc.)	Soil-sediment origin and characterization	Plant communities	Volatility
Type of water flow (surface, subsurface, etc.)	Microbial activity	Aquatic and benthic community structure	Hydrophobicity
Type of water outputs (percolation, evaporation)	Oxidation/reduction conditions	Wildlife survey	Water solubility
Suspended-sediment load and characterization	OM content of sediments		Octanol/water partition coefficient
Sedimentation rate			Hydrolysis Photolysis Biodegredation

Methods and endpoints for wetlands

While numerous field and laboratory methods are available for evaluating aquatic habitats and sediments within wetlands, relatively few are available for testing wetland soils. Sources of information regarding aquatic and sediment contamination evaluation are listed below, and only more recently developed soil test methods will be summarized here for use in wetlands risk assessment.

Whether qualitative and reliant on published information or quantitative and implemented as part of a designed study, aquatic field surveys and biological tests for evaluating wetland risks can be achieved by evaluating biological effects associated with chemical, physical, or biological stressors. Frequently, these tools are used in the measurement or monitoring of wetland populations and community structure through structural endpoints such as relative abundance, species richness, community organization (diversity, evenness, similarity, guild structure, and presence or absence of indicator species), and biomass. Functional endpoints, such as cellular metabolism, individual or population growth rates, and rates of material or nutrient transfer (e.g., primary production, organic decomposition, or nutrient cycling) are less commonly measured. While functional measurements are important in interpreting the significance of an observed change in population or community structure, functional measures are difficult to interpret in the absence of structural information, have not been standardized, and require considerable understanding of the system and processes involved.

Species richness and relative abundance

Species richness (the number of species in a community) and relative abundances (the number of individuals in any given species compared to the total number of individuals in the community) are structural endpoints commonly measured in field surveys of periphyton, plankton, macroinvertebrates, and fish regardless of whether the habitat is a wetland or flowing surfacewater feature. Estimates of relative abundance or species richness can yield readily interpretable information on the degree of contamination of wetland habitat (Pascoe et al. 1994). Loss of a particular species can be critical when that species plays an important role in a community or ecosystem (Karr et al. 1986).

Biomass

Biomass measurements, defined as the mass of tissue present in an individual, population, or community at a given time, are another potential structural endpoint critical to wetland risk assessment. As summarized by LaPoint and Fairchild (1989), biomass can be directly measured gravimetrically on wet or dry tissue. For example, biomass may be estimated gravimetrically by using pooled samples of individuals or by an indirect method, e.g., invertebrate or fish biomass can be indirectly estimated by using empirical or published length:weight regressions. Biomass of periphyton communities is also commonly measured. Measurements of phytoplankton or periphyton biomass can be estimated on the basis of ash-free dry mass (AFDM) or chlorophyll *a* content (APHA 1992). Chlorophyll measurements are performed by solvent extraction, followed by spectrophotometry or fluorometry (APHA 1992).

Indicator species

The presence or absence of indicator species is commonly used to assess adverse effects to ecological communities (Karr et al. 1986; Hilsenhoff 1988; Plafkin et al. 1988). While originally derived from the saprobian system in which certain species and groups were found to generally characterize stream and river reaches subject to organic wastewaters (Kolkwitz and Marsson 1902; Gaufin 1958; Sheehan 1984), the application of indicator species to wetlands is clearly practiced, e.g., within the delineation process. History has shown that the indicator species concept lacks broad applicability to all types of contaminant stress, however. Furthermore, species selection may occur in aquatic habitats that are chronically polluted with low levels of contaminants over sufficiently long periods. In some wetlands, as well as flowing surface water, the IBI may be pertinent to the risk assessment process.

Indices

Biological indices in wetland risk assessments, as in other ecological risk assessment applications, can be used to mathematically reduce taxonomic information to a single number, or index, to simplify data for interpretation or presentation. Indices can be classified among several types:

1) evenness (measuring how equitably individuals in a community are distributed among the taxa present),
2) diversity (calculating the abundance of individuals in 1 taxon relative to the total abundance of individuals in all other taxa),
3) similarity (comparing likeness of community composition between 2 sites), and
4) biotic indices (examining the environmental tolerances or requirements of individual species or groups).

Although indices may aid in data reduction, they should never be divorced from the actual data on species richness and abundance. Relying on a single index such as the Shannon-Weiner may be misleading for any system at risk, including wetlands. For example, a few individuals evenly distributed among several species could give a relatively high index of diversity, even though a habitat is grossly polluted. In addition, statistical assumptions of independence, normality, and homogeneity of variance are frequently invalid for these derived, proportional measures. Hence, when indices are used, statistical transformations (e.g., arc sine) or rank-order statistics are recommended (Siegel 1956; Green 1979; Hoaglin et al. 1985).

Guild structure

For wetland communities, data generated at the species level can be analyzed according to guild structure. Guilds, or functional feeding groups, are classifications based on the manner in which organisms obtain their food and energy. Invertebrates can be classified among such functional groups as collector-gatherers, piercers, predators, scrapers, and shredders (Merritt and Cummins 1984; Cummins and Wilzbach 1985); and fish can be classified as omnivores, insectivores, and piscivores (Fausch et al. 1984; Karr et al. 1986). Avian communities in wetlands are increasingly being analyzed within the context of guild structure (Adamus 1993a, 1993b). Shifts in community guild structure may reflect changes in the trophic-dynamic status of a wetland. For example, contaminant impacts on a wetland may eliminate or reduce periphyton and thus concomitantly reduce the relative abundance of scrapers (herbivores) in relation to other invertebrate guilds such as collector-gatherers. Effects must be fairly strong to assess changes in guild structure. For contaminant studies in wetlands, community and guild analysis should also be supported by physical habitat and chemical information, since these may alter production and dynamics of biological populations and, consequently, confound the interpretation of wetland community data. Needless to say, the selection of appropriate reference locations is critical to wetland assessments that incorporate community and guild analysis.

Plankton

Many devices are available for sampling plankton for their enumeration and analysis. Sampling techniques for phytoplankton and zooplankton are similar in various surfacewater habitats. The choice of an individual sampling technique, sample size, and sample numbers, whether for zooplankton or phytoplankton, will depend upon the characteristics of the aquatic habitat (in terms of depth, density of organisms, and spatial variation).

Macroinvertebrates

Benthic invertebrates are the most common fauna used in ecological assessments of contaminants, whether sediments are in wetlands or other surfacewater habitats. Numerous excellent references deal with the collection, identification, and analysis of benthic invertebrate populations (e.g., Southwood 1978; APHA 1992). Typical measurement endpoints include relative abundance and species (or taxon) richness. Trophic guild structure can be determined from taxonomic identifications to species (Merritt and Cummins 1984; Cummins and Wilzbach 1985). Indices of diversity, evenness, and community similarity can also be calculated. In any given contaminant effects study, careful consideration must be given to the comparability of samples among stations.

Fish

In biological monitoring and evaluation, as well as in wetland risk assessment, fish may be recommended for use because

1) regulators and the public can easily understand the implications of the effects of pollution on fish;
2) fisheries have economic, recreational, and aesthetic values;
3) the identification of fishes is relatively easy (compared to that of micro- and macroinvertebrates);
4) the environmental requirements of fish are well known; and
5) fish are perceived as "integrators" of effects at lower trophic levels (Hendricks et al. 1980).

However, the size, distribution, and response of freshwater fishes are sometimes difficult to quantify because variations in spatial distribution and year classes are large (Lagler 1978). Additional difficulties in the quantification of fish populations are caused by the selectivity and efficiency of the sampling gears used (Hendricks et al. 1980). However, consideration of these factors can allow unbiased comparisons of different wetland habitats that support their being considered as part of the wetland risk assessment process.

The types of analyses performed on data from the collected fish include relative abundance, species richness, and size structure. One method for fish community assessment is the IBI (Karr 1981; Karr et al. 1986), where IBI is weighted on the basis of individual species tolerances for water quality and habitat conditions. The IBI was developed to determine the effects of decreased habitat quality on fish communities of midwestern streams, but for some wetlands it may be quite applicable to the risk-assessment process. The index is composed of 12 individual metrics divided into the fields of species composition and richness, trophic composition, abundance, and condition. Scores of each metric are classified as "best," "average," or "worst" (each class having a numerical weighting) in relation to reference data (Fausch et al. 1984).

Sediment and soil methods and endpoints for wetlands risk assessment

While not as readily available as aquatic or sediment toxicity test methods (e.g., Peltier and Weber 1985; Weber et al. 1988), methods have been identified for testing soil biota (e.g., USEPA 1989). For wetlands, the application of biological tests should provide a comparative toxicity database upon which wetland-specific soil evaluations can be completed. Screening (unamended wetland soils yielding percent effect) and definitive tests (amended soils potentially yielding median effective concentrations) may be completed with standardized test species to evaluate toxicity within a biological assessment. Additionally, to assure adequate information for ecological evaluations of soil contamination, species having site-specific relevance may also be tested (Parkhurst et al. 1989). When performed in parallel with standard test methods, these site-specific tests (e.g., using resident plant species) may be diagnostic and indicate biological responses (e.g., development of metal resistance) that are associated with soil exposures. Presently, the application of laboratory bioassays to wetland risk assessment is increasing, particularly in developing biological databases that contribute to the ecological risk assessment process. To enhance the ecological relevance of site-specific biological tests and to reduce the potential extrapolation error associated with interspecific comparisons, use of standard and site-specific test species in ecological assessment should be considered in soil testing (see Linder et al. 1993).

Plant test methods

Plants associated with wetlands have been used extensively to assess water and sediment quality. The wide variety of tests developed has targeted the effects of both water column and sediment-borne toxic materials. The types of aquatic vegetation used for these purposes range from microscopic unicellular algae to relatively large flowering plants. The 3 most commonly applied test methods include chlorophyll *a* concentration, growth, and contaminant uptake.

Growth measurements (biomass accumulation per unit of time) have been widely applied as an assessment method for a variety of freshwater estuarine and marine species. Much of the testing has been conducted on sediments in the laboratory, using unicellular phytoplankton such as *Selenastrum capricornutum* (freshwater) and *Skeletonema costatum* (marine) (e.g., Thomas et al. 1990; Ankley et al. 1993). Until recently, use of rooted wetland macrophyte growth has been limited. Growth is perhaps the least specific measurement endpoint. A response such as reduced growth rate is not tied to specific sites within the plant where reactions or processes are altered by specific chemicals. This is especially true for rooted macrophytes. The advantage of measuring growth is that it is an integrator of all effects of toxicants on plants, it is relatively easy to measure, there is a wide range of past use, and it can be done with acceptable precision in both the field and laboratory.

The physiology of chlorophyll production and maintenance is quite well known. Chlorophyll occurs in virtually all plants and is the primary pigment involved in the important ecological process of photosynthesis. The correlation between chlorophyll concentration and photosynthetic rate commonly is strong. Chlorophyll concentration relative to contamination of water or soils has been measured in unicellular algae, macrophytes, and periphyton communities (e.g., Bassi et al. 1990). Chlorophyll concentration generally reflects the mass of plant material present, as well as being an indication of the health of the material. Toxicants can affect the chlorophyll molecule directly or through the process of energy transfer during photosynthesis. A method recently applied for determining the effects of toxicants on chlorophyll (and photosynthesis) involves the measurement of delayed fluorescence. The technique appears to be highly sensitive and relatively easy to conduct.

Contaminant uptake by plants has been applied primarily to rooted macrophytes. It is assumed that most of the uptake occurs through the roots and that the concentration of the contaminant compounds in leaf tissues is directly related to the concentration in the soil or sediment. Uptake has received wide application in fresh and marine systems and has been carried out under both laboratory and field conditions (e.g., Kovacs 1978; Lee et al. 1981). Uptake of contaminants relies on several assumptions that must be taken into account for interpretation of results. Chemicals may be modified to form nontoxic compounds by the plant. Certain chemicals are not concentrated, while others are, which may bias the interpretation of what chemicals are present in the test medium. However, these uptake measurements are more relevant for evaluating risks to herbivores (and bioavailability of chemicals in sediment) than for deciding what is there per se. Finally, uptake rates may be inhibited by the toxicity of other materials in the medium, and the test organism may be inhibited in its ability to accumulate the contaminants.

While measurements of plant growth, chlorophyll content, and contaminant uptake are the most commonly used methods, several other are in various stages of development and implementation. These methods include measurements of photosynthetic rate, chloroplast morphology, peroxidase activity, root growth, seed germination, seedling growth, and reproduction.

The strongest approach to the assessment of wetland subsystems may be to use a combination of several methods to evaluate contamination of water and sediments. This combination would indicate both ecological and physiological responses of the plants to the media and would increase the power of the analysis through verification of responses using several endpoints.

Seed germination and root elongation

Techniques modified from methods originally developed in the plant and weed science disciplines have yielded short-term tests that assess toxic chemical effects on plants. The seed germination and root elongation bioassays are laboratory toxicity tests that directly and indirectly assess toxicity of soils and evaluate toxicity endpoints (seed germination and root elongation) pertinent to ecological assessments for terrestrial and wetland habitats. Seed germination tests measure toxicity associated with soils directly, while root elongation tests consider the indirect effects of water-soluble constituents which may be present in site samples. These methods have been used extensively in soil contamination evaluation, including a comprehensive wetlands risk assessment (Linder et al. 1994; Pascoe and DalSoglio 1994; Pascoe et al. 1994).

Rooted aquatic plants

Wetland soils frequently complicate standard methods for phytotoxicity assessment, owing to the saturated character of their soils. Wetland soils may resemble sediments in many respects, particularly when seasonal or ephemeral climatic conditions alter soil water-holding capacity, which may confound interpretations of germination and growth responses in standard plant testing species (e.g., buttercrunch lettuce, *Lactuca sativa*). Standardized rooted aquatic plant toxicity tests, however, have been developed and should be considered on a site-specific basis for hydric soils and freshwater or estuarine sediment evaluations. The most well-developed method uses *Hydrilla verticillata*, but additional test methods using sago pondweed (*Potamogeton pectinatus*) may also be valuable in evaluating wetland soils or sediments (Byl and Klaine 1991; Fleming et al. 1992).

Laboratory evaluations with wetland and upland plants

Freshwater marsh plants may be used to evaluate sediments or hydric wetland soils as outlined by Walsh et al. (1991). The method was originally designed to test single toxicants or defined chemical mixtures in defined media, but it can be modified to test field-collected sediments or wetland soils that may be appropriate to wetland risk assessment. In general, the method utilizes rooted marsh plants and evaluates the effects of contaminated soils and sediments on early seedling growth and survival. For example, *Echinochloa crusgalli* is one species of marsh plant specifically identified in the test procedure, but alternative marsh plants (e.g., *Spartina alterniflora*) may be identified on a site-specific basis and tested, provided the selected plants are amenable to the test format outlined.

Primarily in response to the assessment needs associated with land disposal of dredging materials, the U.S. Army Corps of Engineers Waterways Experiment Station (WES) has developed a test method for evaluating phytotoxicity and bioaccumulation potential in a freshwater plant, the yellow nutsedge (*Cyperus esculentus*). The method is applicable to wetland risk assessments and can be used in either flooded wetland or upland habitats. From an ecological perspective, the test evaluates toxicity endpoints (e.g., growth) that may directly relate to field observations regarding plant cover or vegetative vigor (WES 1989; Folsom and Price 1992). It is also useful for evaluating bioaccumulation of contaminants in the diet of herbivores.

Alternative test species in seed germination, root elongation, and early seedling survival and vegetative vigor tests

In these tests, measurement endpoints are frequently similar (e.g., growth, germination), but the species being tested differ. In part, these differences reflect soil matrix characteristics that might limit the success of any given test system, especially in wetland soils. For example, lettuce seed is frequently used in seed germination tests, but some soils may not be amenable to testing with a domesticated species selected for optimal growth in a particular soil matrix. Contaminant effects and matrix effects may potentially be confounded when the life history characteristics of a test species preclude or potentially limit its usefulness in any given phytotoxicity test method. Additionally, for interpretation of wetland-specific ecological effects, the support of a comparative toxicity database may be insufficient within a risk assessment context. Thus, more relevant test species may be beneficial to evaluate ecological effects with a wetlands risk assessment, and measurement endpoints (e.g., survival and growth) used to evaluate relationships between ecological indicators and soil toxicity may be considered using methods modified for tests with alternative species. For example, methods to evaluate seed germination using various species of plant seeds (agricultural crops, vegetables and herbs, flowers, and trees and shrubs) are briefly summarized by the Association of Official Seed Analysts (AOSA) in their Rules for Testing Seeds (1990). Here, exposure conditions specific to various species are tabulated, including suggested substrates and optimum incubation temperatures for germination testing as well as test duration specifications. Furthermore, special pretreatment of native seeds, e.g., prechilling or scarification, is also specified, and methods for distinguishing between nongerminated seeds and nonviable seeds are identified (e.g., tetrazolium and embryo excision tests). On a wetland-specific basis, these alternative test species may be more conducive to ecological interpretation, especially when soil matrix effects unique to wetlands can potentially confound contaminant effects on seed germination and emergence.

Soil biota biomass and diversity

Without question, wetlands are complex biological systems, and wetland soils are critical components in the characterization process. A thorough consideration of the methods applicable to wetland soils characterization with a risk assessment setting is beyond our present scope. However, wetlands functions and processes are clearly dependent upon a healthy soil. For example, nutrient cycling would not occur without organisms to perform the majority of the critical processes. Soil organisms perform many wetland processes, and in unimpacted soil, there usually (but not always) are several organism groups that perform any particular process. For example, the dependency of vegetation on the presence of mycorrhizal fungi and on a functional soil–organism nutrient cycling system may be quantified within a wetlands risk assessment, and evidence is accumulating that at least some plants are dependent on symbiotic organisms for establishment or survival (Reeves 1985; Janos 1987). Clearly, other measurement endpoints could be identified (Linder et al. 1992), and while not exhaustive, methods are available to evaluate these within the context of wetland risk assessment:

1) bacterial biomass and community structure,
2) fungal biomass and community structure,
3) protozoan diversity, and
4) nematode diversity and community structure.

Solid-phase and aqueous-phase Microtox

While aqueous-phase testing with Microtox has been readily available for 10 to 15 years, solid-phase testing has only recently been commercially available (Microbics 1992). As previously summarized (Warren-Hicks et al. 1989), Microtox relies upon measurements of bioluminescence for an evaluation of a sample's toxicity. The test, whether aqueous- or solid-phase, utilizes freeze-dried cultures of the marine bacterium *Photobacterium phosphoreum* and is based on the inhibition of bioluminescence by toxicants (Bulich 1979, 1982, 1986). The results of several studies of pure compounds and complex chemical mixtures suggest that aqueous-phase testing with Microtox generally agrees with standard fish and invertebrate toxicity tests (Curtis et al. 1982). Solid-phase testing with Microtox, however, does not have a comparable database established for developing statements regarding its correspondence with standard soil tests using, for example, earthworms.

Earthworms tests

While not applicable to all wetland soils, earthworms have become a primary test organism for soil contamination evaluations. From an ecological perspective, earthworms are significant in improving soil aeration, drainage, and fertility (Edwards and Lofty 1972), although the comparative database does not unequivocally suggest that earthworm toxicity measurements are reflective of soil health. To enhance the ecological relevance of site-specific biological tests and to reduce the potential extrapolation error associated with interspecies comparisons, testing with site-specific species should be considered in soil evaluations. The earthworm bioassay most frequently used is a modification of a method described by Goats and Edwards (1982) and Edwards (1984) and uses lumbricoid earthworms as the test species. *Eisenia foetida* may be used in these tests because it is easily cultured in the laboratory and reaches maturity in 7 to 8 weeks at 25 °C. *E. foetida* is responsive to a wide range of toxicants, and the comparative database suggests that similar toxicity responses can be anticipated regardless of the subspecies being tested (Neuhauser et al. 1986).

Nematodes tests

Soil-inhabiting nematodes represent one of the most readily available soil invertebrates that should be studied during soil contamination evaluations within an ecological effects assessment for a wetland. Owing to their usually high numbers, their role in soil decomposition processes, and their significant contribution to soil nutrient dynamics (e.g., dispersion and grazing on microflora, potential stimulation of bacterial activity, and promotion of nutrient mineralization), soil nematodes directly as well as indirectly reflect the health of the wetland soil. *Panagrellus redivivus* has a relatively well-developed literature in aquatic toxicity testing (Samoiloff et al. 1980) and has been used for evaluating single chemicals and complex chemical mixtures (Samoiloff et al. 1983), including applications to sediment evaluations. Most frequently, *P. redivivus* has been used in conjunction with other biological assessments (e.g., *Daphnia magna* or *Ceriodaphnia dubia* testing) for evaluations of water quality, but the test system has also been applied to sediment toxicity testing (Samoiloff et al. 1983). Work with *P. redivivus* has been well described in the comparative toxicity literature, but another, more recently developed nematode test using *Caenorhabditis elegans* (e.g., van Kessel et al. 1989; Williams and Dusenbery 1990) may be applicable for ecological effects assessments. *P. redivivus* and *C. elegans* tests measure acute—lethal—and subacute or sublethal effects related to growth, reproduction, and mutagenicity. Both methods are short-term tests and generally require less than 4 to 5 d for completion, although long-term tests that measure reproductive effects (e.g., number of offspring) may require 7-d exposures.

Unlike *P. redivivus*, *C. elegans* is a native soil-dwelling nematode (Briggs 1946 as cited by van Kessel et al. 1989), and tests with this nematode may more closely reflect soil contaminant effects in terrestrial habitats. Williams and Dusenbery (1990) studied the toxic effects of metals in aqueous solutions using *Caenorhabditis elegans*, and in their comparative analysis, *C. elegans* acute toxicities (LC50s) for single-compound metal exposures complemented and were consistent with acute toxicity results from *Daphnia magna* and sediment macroinvertebrates. As suggested by various authors (e.g., Popham and Webster 1979; Haight et al. 1982; Doelman et al. 1984; van Kessel et al. 1989), for some toxicants like heavy metals, the existing toxicity database for nematodes was developed, and extending these methods to soils should be considered within ecological effects assessments. For example, while the testing with either *P. redivius* or *C. elegans* was originally developed for testing surface water or sediment pore waters, nematode tests are directly applicable to evaluating soil extracts or interstitial waters.

Arthropods (insects) tests

Various methods have been developed for evaluating chemical effects on terrestrial insects, especially pesticide effects on nontarget species (e.g., USEPA 1982), and these methods are directly applicable to wetlands risk assessment. As ecological indicators of soil contamination, terrestrial insects, and soil arthropods in general, are potentially critical targets within an ecological effects assessment. Within ecological contexts, terrestrial invertebrates play a role in communities and ecosystems that involves integrated functions such as decomposition, grazing, predation, and pollination (Croft 1990). While methods that evaluate adverse biological effects in terrestrial invertebrates exposed to soil contaminants are not widely considered in the ecological effects assessment process at present, their contributions have increased and should continue to increase in the near future, especially for wetlands risk assessment. Through strategies similar to those used with aquatic invertebrates (e.g., Plafkin et al. 1989; Klemm et al. 1990), terrestrial insects would be amenable to soil contaminant evaluations for wetlands, particularly given field survey information regarding insect community structure and population numbers in wetlands at risk. For example, to evaluate soil microarthropods quantitatively and qualitatively, techniques are readily available to extract, enumerate, and identify these organisms in reference and impacted soil samples. Soil microarthropods are easily extracted from the soil using Tulgren high-efficiency extractors (e.g., Seastedt and Crossley 1980; Anderson 1988). The extracted organisms can then be counted using dissecting microscopes and identified to genus, or form-group. Recent innovations in computer-assisted identification (Hypercard) have also reduced the time required to identify these organisms (Moldenke et al. 1991).

Terrestrial arthropod (non-insect) and isopod tests

Outside of North America, terrestrial arthropods other than insects have been considered from the perspective of accidental or coincidental exposure to potentially harmful chemicals (Croft 1990). While not exclusively focused on wetlands, these methods are directly applicable to the risk assessment process for wetlands. For example, to evaluate effects of agrichemical pesticides or biological control agents on nontarget invertebrates, laboratory methods have been standardized for evaluating chemical effects on mites (e.g., Sewell and Lighthart 1988). While terrestrial arthropod tests methods are few and present a limited history in ecological effects assessments for wetlands, their role in the environment (Croft 1990) requires that these organisms should receive consideration as ecological receptors during the risk assessment process. The methods developed for pesticide evaluations could be directly applied to wetland soils contamination evaluation. Alternatively, soil-derived eluates could be used in the testing process, if the study design indicated that indirect routes of exposure were likely to occur, e.g., nonpoint source runoff into wetlands from agricultural lands. While a variety of test species have been used in the standard tests developed in Europe and the United States (Hassan 1985; Hassan et al. 1987; Croft 1990), the laboratory test methods using non-insect arthropods are relatively straightforward and easily could be modified to directly meet the requirements of a soil contaminant evaluation for wetlands.

Similarly, biological assessments using terrestrial isopods have historically been considered in soil contamination evaluations, although standardization, e.g., through the American Society for Testing and Materials (ASTM) or the Organization for Economic Cooperation and Development (OECD), is lacking. As field indicators of contaminant exposure, the isopod literature suggests that whole-body and organ-specific contaminant bioaccumulation may be monitored with these animals, particularly for some environmental chemicals, e.g., metals (Beyer et al. 1984; Beyer and Anderson 1985; Hopkin 1986, 1990).

Mollusk tests

Wetlands are habitats that are frequently impacted by hazardous waste disposal sites, and mollusks are often regarded as representative invertebrates characteristic of these habitats (Pennak 1978). Coincident with these habitat-related questions, some families of freshwater mussels (Unionidae) have been identified as critical species for ecological risk assessments for some environmental chemicals (agri-chemicals) (USDOI 1989). Accordingly, methods potentially amenable to ecological effects assessments at Superfund sites have been developed to evaluate chemical effects and acute toxicity for sensitive life stages in various mollusk species (Johnson 1990). In contrast to concerns regarding habitat loss and contaminant effects on freshwater mollusks, efforts to develop effective molluscides have also yielded test methods (e.g., Getzin and Cole 1964; Crowell 1979) that may be applicable to the ecological assessment needs for wetlands. Historically, marine and estuarine mollusks have been used in toxicity and ecological effects assessments within the Office of Pesticides Program (USEPA 1995), and these methods could be equally applicable to contaminant-related questions for wetlands risk assessments. Analogous tests with freshwater mollusks have recently been developed. For example, the Unionidae mollusks are characteristic freshwater mussels, and numerous species could be considered within a toxicity assessment setting. In developing a freshwater mussel test, *Anodonta imbecilis* was initially selected as a representative unionid mollusk; however, the techniques described by Johnson (1990) should be applicable for testing mussels with similar reproductive strategies. Most frequently, the tests involve the early developmental stages of the mussel, or glochidia, and juvenile mussels, depending upon endpoints being measured. Guidance for developing the test with freshwater mussels followed ASTM E729 (1997b), and while not widely used at this time, toxicity assessments with freshwater mussels should be considered within an ecological effects assessment for wetlands.

In contrast to the freshwater mussel test that was primarily developed in response to ecological risk assessment questions related to agrichemical use, test methods that evaluate terrestrial snails and slugs were developed as efficacy tests for evaluating molluscides (e.g., Getzin and Cole 1964; Crowell 1979). These methods, however, are readily adapted for wetland risk assessment.

Amphibian test methods

Wetlands are habitats that are frequently impacted by hazardous waste sites, and evaluating and monitoring these transition zones between upland and surfacewater areas will require a variety of field and laboratory techniques (Tiner 1984; Adamus and Brandt 1990). Amphibians—frogs and salamanders—may be representative of the fauna potentially critical to ecological effects assessments for wetlands. Amphibian test systems are standardized through ASTM (T29 1997b, E1439 1997c). Early embryos of the African clawed-frog (*Xenopus laevis*) are used in the standardized test; however, much work has been completed with alternative test species and should be considered on a site-specific basis (e.g., Linder et al. 1990; ASTM E1439 1997c; Linder, Wyant et al. 1991).

Interplay of risk management and risk assessment

Important to all risk assessments, whether for wetlands or terrestrial environments, are the early discussions held between the risk assessor and the risk manager. These should define the scope, timing, level of effort, and constraints involved with the risk assessment. There will need to be resolution of issues specific to freshwater wetlands, and the particular type of wetland, between the risk manager and risk assessor before any work is begun.

This discussion may have several important outcomes. First is agreement on the spatial extent or magnitude of the wetland. Small, easily managed wetlands may require a reduced or screening-level assessment to satisfy the requirements of the risk manager. On the other hand, wetlands that are tens or hundreds of acres, that reside in the midst of major industrial activities, or that are complex in terms of their hydrology, soils, geomorphology, etc. may require a much greater level of effort on the part of the risk assessor. In this latter situation, landscape and ecosystem issues arise and can readily complicate the effort. For example, some wetlands may be dependent on source water outside of the study area, or for that matter, in another state, region, or watershed. Like a number of stressed wetlands in North America, the wetland may be vitally important in controlling floods in a particular area but may not represent a highly valuable habitat (e.g., a *Phragmites* sp.-dominated wetlands) (Bartoldus et al. 1994).

It is also important for the risk manager and the risk assessor to decide on the important stressors and receptors that will be the focus of the assessment. As data are collected and evaluated, additional stressors and receptors may become evident and may justify a realignment of the focus. A confounding issue that often arises at this time is whether the risk assessment will take a multi-stressor or single-stressor approach. It is rare that only a single stressor will be present, yet to approach the risk assessment using multiple stressors requires advancement beyond current science. Today there is inadequate understanding of how to deal with multiple stressors only qualitatively because there is no recognized, validated method for integrating impacts from multiple stressors. Thus, without a clear understanding of what is driving the risk management decision and of the regulatory and jurisdictional issues, the risk assessor may be left with insufficient or at least unclear guidance.

Exposure assessment

Inputs of chemical and nonchemical stresses to freshwater wetlands occur through geological, biological, and hydrological pathways typical of other ecosystems (Mitsch and Gosselink 1993). Geological input from weathering of parent rock, although poorly understood, may be an important source of exposure in some wetlands. Biological inputs include photosynthetic uptake of C, N fixation, and biotic transport of materials by animals. Except for gaseous exchanges such as C and N fixation or aerial deposition, however, inputs to wetlands are generally dominated by hydrology. Hydrologic transport to freshwater wetlands may occur through precipitation, surfacewater flow, or groundwater flow. The hydrologic exposure pathways of freshwater wetlands are determined by their flooding regime or by the balance between precipitation and evapotranspiration.

Hydrodynamics will affect exposure levels in both the aquatic and soil-sediment compartment of a wetland, as it will to a large extent determine the soil-sediment chemistry by producing anaerobic conditions, importing and removing OM, and replenishing nutrients. Exposure can occur in transition zones between the wetland and surrounding upland areas. It is important to consider this area as well when examining potential exposure scenarios.

Ideally, exposure in the wetland ecosystem is assessed based on representative monitoring data. In the absence of measured data, exposure can be predicted in the context of a wetland-specific hydrogeomorphic, biogeochemical, and ecological setting. In the case of a chemical exposure assessment, information on the inherent properties of substances should be used in combination with the wetland characteristics in order to derive exposure concentrations or levels. Describing the level and distribution of a stressor in the wetland environment and its changes with time (e.g., in concentration or chemical form) is a complex process and needs to include a rigorous evaluation of what drives exposure. In order to ensure that predicted aquatic and sediment exposures are realistic, all available knowledge of the wetland ecosystem should be integrated in the exposure evaluation of a chemical stressor. Some measurements or parameters that can be important when evaluating or predicting exposure of chemical and/or nonchemical stressors in freshwater wetlands are listed in Table 4-8.

Compound-specific information and biogeochemical processes affecting exposure in the different compartments are usually derived and extrapolated from standard laboratory tests or literature data. Applicability of literature data and data from standard tests to freshwater wetland ecosystems requires review and, ideally, field verification.

Biological assessment

Defined earlier, biological assessments are primarily ecotoxicological tests performed in either a field or laboratory setting. While there are many issues related to the conduct and application of ecotoxicological tests (Levin et al. 1989), they represent one of the main sources of effects information available to the risk assessor. It is beyond the scope of this section to detail the methods or protocols for these tests. However, the publications cited in Table 4-4 include standard testing protocols as well as those developed through the auspices of the OECD.

Once the key stressors and receptors have been identified, the biological assessment should consider toxicity to wetland organisms or plants in the overlying water as well in the sediments, provided the stressor is likely to enter and persist in the sediments. In addition, the assessment may need to extend to the transition zones surrounding the wetlands because some stressors will impact adjacent terrestrial environments. These areas should be evaluated only if there are clear, potential pathways for exposure of receptors. Because the primary focus of the biological assessment should be at higher levels of organization, the risk assessor should be cognizant of which tests or series of tests are designed to measure population-, community-, or ecosystem-level effects. Furthermore, the endpoints of the test, whether lethality, reproductive impairment, growth, etc., should be understood and their linkage to the assessment endpoints clearly defined before any work is begun.

Depending on their scope, biological assessments in the aquatic environment could include representative, and ideally sensitive, species of

1) primary producers,
2) primary consumers,
3) microbial community,
4) saprophages or detrivores, and
5) carnivores.

Potential tests for the primary producers could include tests with algae and vascular plants, both submerged and emergent forms. Effects on primary consumers could be evaluated by testing representative species of protozoa, invertebrates, insects, and amphibia. Inhibition of microbial activity, important in wetland's nutrient recycling and transport, could be evaluated by studying the effect on aerobic and/or anaerobic respiration. Toxicity tests with crustacea and insects can be used to assess effects on the saphrophages/detrivores community. Finally, standard acute and chronic tests are available to assess effects on fish.

Biological assessments of the benthic communities should take into account pathways of exposure. In addition, observed effects will be strongly influenced by sediment-soil biogeochemical conditions such as organic carbon content, particle size distribution, sulfide content, redox potential (RP), and time period allowed for equilibration to occur between dissolved and sorbed fractions of chemical stressors (USEPA 1990). Available test methods concern detrivores or mixed detrivores/ herbivores/carnivores and include insect, annelida, and crustacea species with both acute and chronic endpoints (USEPA 1990).

Recently, the OECD reviewed aquatic testing methods for pesticides and industrial chemicals (OECD 1995). The review included both pelagic and benthic test methods. An overview of the recommended test methods—applied to freshwater wetlands—is shown in a foodweb frame in Figure 4-16.

It was recommended by OECD that the guidelines and tests take the form of a framework for taxonomic groups rather than for single species, whenever possible. This should make it possible to test representatives from different wetland compartments and facilitate extrapolation of obtained test results to the wetland of interest. Furthermore, the guidelines and tests should include both acute and subchronic or chronic toxicity endpoints, depending on the assessment endpoints.

Most of the impacts on freshwater wetlands will occur in the aquatic environment, i.e., the sediment and overlying water. Even so, the terrestrial environment surrounding or transitioning to the freshwater wetland may also be at risk, depending on the type of stressor and the exposure. Species that are dependent on the wetland structure and function (e.g., insects, amphibians, reptiles, small mammals, and birds, and transition-zone plants, trees, and shrubs) should be considered when potential effects are evaluated. Standardized toxicity tests are currently available for many insects, some amphibians, and numerous small mammals and birds, but few have been adapted for the species most often associated with freshwater wetlands. Acute and chronic bioassays with rodents and lagomorphs have been used for many years to determine the toxicity of chemicals and other materials that may also pose a risk to humans. Similarly, standard acute and chronic tests with species of waterfowl and upland birds have been widely used in the field of environmental toxicology.

There are, however, few tests that have been developed for nonfood plants, although the tests currently used in regulatory programs for pesticides and herbicides may be useful. For example, tests for root elongation and shoot development, seed germination, and other methods are known and may be useful in evaluating toxicity of soils in the transition zone. Other soil tests, some using earthworms, might be useful in this context. Keep in mind that the primary focus of the assessment is the wetland itself, and it is there that the effort should begin.

Unfortunately, few tests lend themselves easily to determining the potential toxic effects on trees and shrubs that may inhabit the transition zones. In those situations, it may be more plausible to determine impacts in situ on those trees and shrubs located adjacent to the wetlands of concern. Methods developed by forestry scientists (e.g., measuring growth rate, stand composition, and overall vigor) can be utilized for this.

Using standardized toxicity tests brings up several important considerations, some of which are mentioned in Chapter 9. One of these concerns data interpretation and is driven primarily by the fact that most easily maintained species used in testing are not the same species generally found in freshwater wetlands. Thus, the uncertainty of extrapolating from one species to another within the same genus could be as large

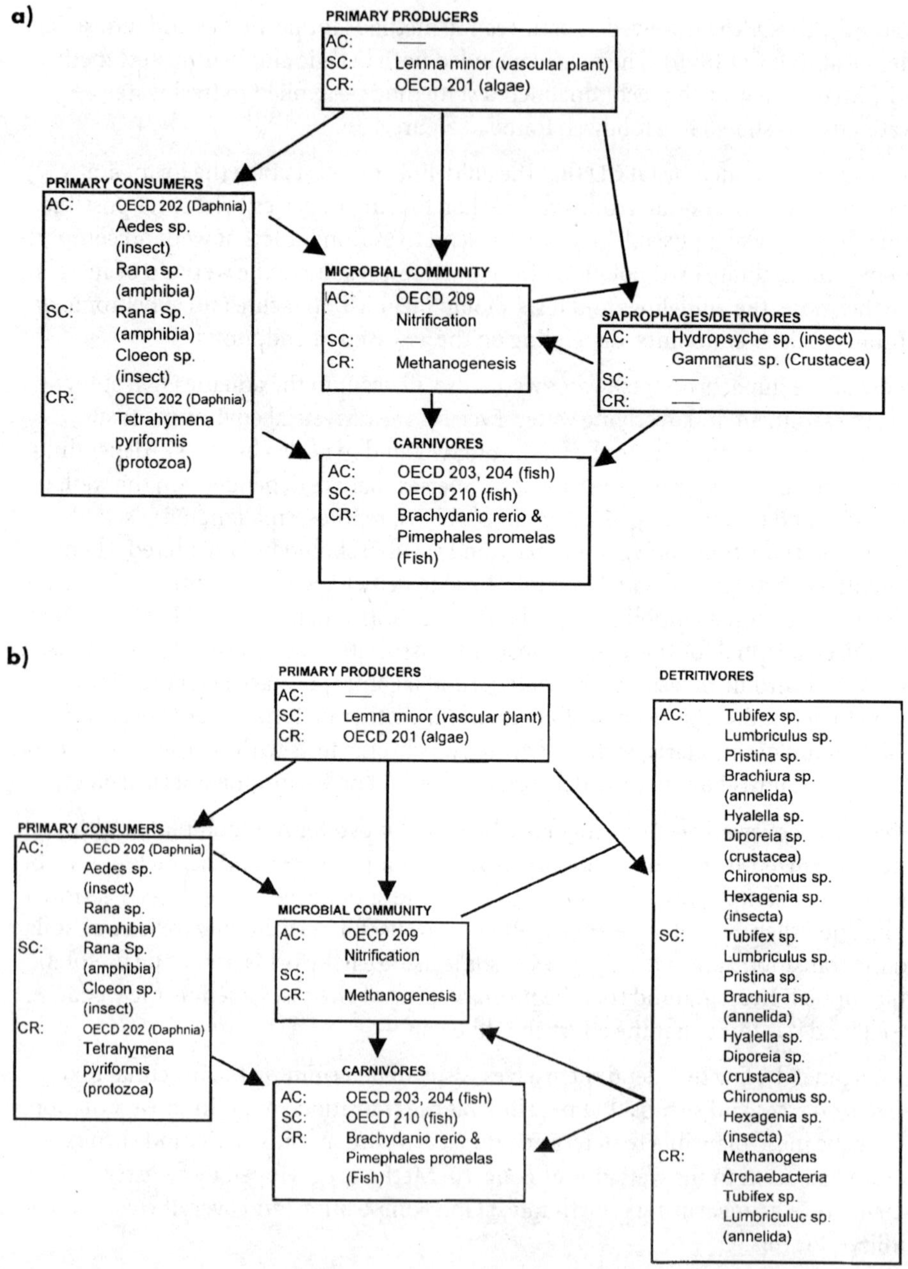

Figure 4-16 Taxonomic grouping of test organisms recommended for freshwater wetland risk assessment by the OECD (1995): a) Primary producer-herbivore-carnivore food web, b) Detritus-based food web. AC= acute tests, SC= subchronic tests, CR= chronic tests

as extrapolating from rodents to humans. Therefore, it is important to understand the limitations of surrogate species testing and its application to risk assessment. Other uncertainties arise when acute exposure test data are extrapolated to chronic exposure situations, high concentration-response studies to low-concentration exposures, laboratory to field results, and others. All of the results from the biological assessment should be taken in context with other data that will be developed as part of the risk assessment.

Selection of biological tests for wetland ecotoxicity evaluation should be driven by the exposure assessments affected by the hydrogeomorphic and biogeochemical characteristics of the wetland of interest.

Ecological assessment

Ecological assessment primarily determines the impacts of stressors at the population, community, or ecosystem level. In general, standardized ecotoxicology tests do not lend themselves to this type of assessment, and few provide useful ecosystem-level information (Kelly and Harwell 1989; Cairns and Niederlehner 1992). In addition, there are significant temporal and spatial issues that come into play. Measuring a significant change in an ecosystem or at the landscape level may require years or decades of study, yet the risk assessor and risk manager are faced with a much more compressed time line. Just as important, it is difficult to isolate easily studied areas of the wetlands from the surrounding ecosystem that supports it, which may require the risk assessor to include caveats and large uncertainties in the risk assessment.

Given this situation, most ecological assessments are field studies that measure structural components of the ecosystem, including the size and make-up of the habitat, the biomass or standing crop of important plants and animals, and the abundance and diversity of plants and animals. There are, however, functional measurements (Bartoldus et al. 1994; Richardson 1994) that might be useful in understanding the ecological integrity of the wetland. For example, wetlands are extremely important to biogeochemical processing and nutrient cycling (e.g., N and P) (NRC 1995; Chapter 3, this volume) as well as in primary productivity and C, N, P export (Chapter 2, this volume). These functional aspects of wetlands, often considered to be indicative of ecosystem-level processes, depend heavily on microbial communities, water flow, benthic macroorganisms, and other parameters (Brinson 1993). As a result, these functions may be important areas for the risk assessor to consider when designing and conducting the ecological assessment, especially when the assessment focuses on effects at the ecosystem level. Similarly, population- or community-based measures may be useful, provided they have a direct relationship to the assessment endpoints and have been validated scientifically.

Net primary productivity and carbon or energy flow also offer wetland processes that may be measured to assess ecosystem-level effects, provided the measures are integrated across the entire wetland. In this situation, the measure is made of a wetland's net product, resulting from an integrated, interconnected process.

Often, results of the biological and ecological assessments can become inputs to various trophic-level or foodweb models. Such models can give the risk assessor a useful tool to develop a refined conceptual model of how stressors could impact the various processes in the wetlands. The problem with some of the trophic-level or foodweb models is that they require a substantial amount of data, preferably site-specific in nature, lest the uncertainty remain high. Given that fact, the risk assessor and risk manager should decide early on whether the size of the wetland or the complexity of the problem warrants such data-intensive assessments.

Evaluation of Case Studies using the Ecosystem Framework

In retrospect: Would ecosystem-based wetland planning have altered the outcome of the Kesterson episode?

Kesterson Reservoir (see Chapter 6) provides a case history that can be used to assess how well the ecosystem approach performs in evaluating risks associated with proposed wetlands. Limited availability of water was the key issue driving the development of Kesterson's wetlands. Since the 1890s, diversion of water for agricultural use had taken a tremendous toll on the quantity of wetlands remaining in the San Joaquin Valley of California. By the 1970s, when Kesterson was developed, the view generally held by wetland managers in the valley was that any water was better than no water. Viewed in hindsight, the rationale for this thinking is clearly flawed because of water quality issues such as selenium contamination, but at the time, there was no equivalent wetland from which to draw information. However, had an environmental planner been present using the ecosystem approach, would the resultant risk assessment have effectively identified and predicted the problems that eventually occurred?

In order to answer this question, we must look at the basic components of the ecological framework (Figure 4-2). A key factor indicated in the assessment process for Kesterson would have been to thoroughly characterize the water sources and hydrologic regime, i.e., quantity and quality of irrigation drainage, in the context of the arid climate present at the site. Had this step been performed adequately, several key pieces of information should have emerged to guide the decision process. First, it should have been apparent that the evaporative nature of the climate would maximize the likelihood that salts and chemical contaminants in the water source could become concentrated in the wetlands. Second, knowing that the intended water source was subsurface irrigation drainage and not fresh water, adequate chemical characterization would have been indicated. A water quality analysis would have revealed the presence of elevated concentrations of Se, B, and, in some instances, As or other elements. Even though much of the toxicity database that now exists for these trace elements would not have been available then, it should still have been clear that the water source contained an atypical concentration of salts and trace elements. This, in turn, would have signaled a risk factor that required further investigation. The ecological framework would have indicated to the planner that thorough biological effects testing was necessary to determine whether the water source was acceptable for developing the wetland to meet its primary goal, i.e., as habitat for migratory waterfowl and shorebirds. Carrying out these effects studies would have quickly revealed the toxic hazards from trace elements and indicated that irrigation drain water should not be used to develop Kesterson.

The critical failure in the Kesterson episode was lack of recognition that water quality is a primary consideration in wetland development. Kesterson also illustrates the difficulty of using 1 wetland to achieve 2 objectives. In the case of Kesterson, these were wildlife habitat and disposal of irrigation drainage. Clearly, these were not compatible objectives from the standpoint of water quality. The ecological framework to risk assessment could have identified this problem early in the planning stage and recommended steps to avoid the wildlife toxicity problems that eventually developed.

Current evaluation: Application of the ecosystem framework to risk assessment at Milltown Reservoir Wetlands

The work at Milltown Reservoir Wetlands (MRW) (see Chapter 5) illustrates the strengths and limitations of an integrated ecosystem-based approach to ecological risk assessment. This work at MRW also illustrates how the approach, when applied within a risk assessment context, provides resource managers with tools that would enhance their decision-making process and minimize or at least clearly identify sources of uncertainty. At MRW, the ecosystem approach outlined in this chapter clearly provided a framework for minimizing the heavy-metal–related problems that have developed and are being evaluated throughout the MRW-CFR watershed today. For example, at MRW, land-use and water-use planning was poorly implemented in the up-front siting of the construction project for the hydroelectric facility located at the confluence of the Blackfoot and Clark Fork Rivers of western Montana. This historic, and in many instances current, practice of pursuing widespread land-use and water-use practices with only limited forethought for the interconnectedness within ecological systems is a serious flaw that quickly becomes apparent when the ecosystem-based approach is applied. Whether these resource-use practices are mining, agriculture, forestry, or recreation oriented, various environmental problems have arisen throughout the western U.S. in the absence of an ecosystem-based approach to risk assessment.

Using MRW as our example, the initial decision to site a hydroelectric facility at the Hellsgate of the Clark Fork just east of Missoula, MT might have been reconsidered, especially if the watershed had been more fully characterized and appreciated. For example, the relationships between the upstream source areas near Anaconda and

Butte were clearly not understood at the turn of the century when the hydroelectric facility was constructed at Milltown. If an analysis of the hydrology (surface and subsurface) as well as the geomorphology had been completed as part of the current problem formulation phase of the risk assessment process, the facility might have been constructed at an alternative location, or other measures to reduce sedimentation behind the dam would have been considered.

The current problems from metals and arsenic associated with the soils and sediments are a direct consequence of an incomplete analysis of the surface and subsurface hydrology within the CFR watershed. While this criticism is retrospective, the history of the MRW nonetheless reinforces the value that the ecological risk assessment framework offers to resource managers today. Again, using MRW as it looks today, the available risk analysis for the wetland clearly indicates that the present and near-term risks are low relative to metal- and As-related questions in the wetland, and the focus of attention upstream from the reservoir is well deserved from a management perspective. Here again the ecosystem-based approach has served decision-makers well, and while more subtle issues remain regarding incompletely answered questions (e.g., regarding rhizosphere exposures in the wetland), within a risk assessment context, sufficient information was available to address the current and near-term issues related to the wetland. More importantly, the uncertainty associated with these decisions was more clearly understood and characterized in the ecological risk assessment for the wetlands at Milltown Reservoir, primarily because of the risk analysis activities indicated by the framework. Even in the comprehensive ecological risk assessment for MRW that is currently available, incomplete knowledge is apparent. However, when pursued within an ecosystem context, the uncertainties associated with those data gaps were manageable within the near-term and long-term plans for the wetland and the CFR watershed.

As the work at MRW illustrates, environmental contaminant problems in wetlands often are not a simple problem of chemicals alone, but instead are a complex set of interconnected issues that involve a large noncontaminant component. More often than not, habitat alteration has provided an equal, if not greater, contribution to a multiple stressor setting for resources at risk like those at MRW. Within the ecosystem-based approach, the ability to distinguish between and among various stressors will be required more frequently in resource management decisions that are focused on low-concentration exposures to environmental contaminants and the potential subacute effects that may result. While our present state-of-the-science achieves varying degrees of completeness for any particular risk assessment, the ecosystem approach clearly supports a decision-making process that will minimize uncertainty and potentially yield resource management decisions that are dynamic and achievable in the near and distant future.

In the future: Will the Everglades restoration be successful? A challenge of hydrological, chemical, and biological linkages

Restoration of the Everglades involves several policy, partnership, and technical challenges. The policy and partnership issues are beyond the scope of this chapter, but the technical issues that will influence policy decisions are clearly on-point here. Successful Everglades restoration will hinge on the ability of scientists to integrate the concepts discussed in this chapter and provide consensus advice to decision-makers. If this integrative approach is not used, the end result will be a lack of environmentally sound management policies, i.e., an even bigger disruption of the natural wetland ecology than now exists.

From the time the earliest explorers came to south Florida, the challenge was how to drain the region so that productive use could be made of the land. These efforts began in earnest during the 1880s with the work of Hamilton Disston and his projects to connect Lake Okeechobee to the Caloosahatchee River. By the mid-20s, the state had completed the main north–south canals from the lake to the coast, and agriculture became an important part of the region's economy. By 1970, the USACOE completed the major components of its Central and Southern Florida Project, which linked all the drainage canals and water management structures into a comprehensive water management system. The project has been completely successful in meeting its major objectives of flood control, agricultural water supply, and protection of urban well fields from saltwater intrusion.

However, the project, and the 5 million people now able to live in the region, is producing unexpected side effects. The wading-bird population of south Florida has diminished to less than 10% its level of 50 years ago. Florida Bay is experiencing vast algal blooms, which are killing sponge and seagrass beds vital to shrimp and fish populations living there. Nutrient runoff from dairy, citrus, and sugar farms around Lake Okeechobee is transforming the river of sawgrass to large cattail communities. Citizens and government are looking for ways to restore much of the lost biological function in the Everglades.

For the past 20 years, scientists and technical managers have examined the problem from within their areas of expertise. The water managers worked on the water management problems. The land-use managers worked the land-use problems. The chemists and toxicologists studied the effects of the various chemicals and nutrients, using their established protocols and approaches. The biologists studied various biological problems, but usually in a very narrow context rather than with an ecosystem perspective. The only clear agreement from all of these investigations is that the altered (drained) system is causing a series of effects that no one understands very well.

The progress that is needed will depend on linking the analysis in ways suggested in the section entitled "The ecosystem approach: integrating ecology, hydrology, geomorphology, and soils of wetlands." For example, the analysis of nutrient effects on sawgrass cannot be complete without an appropriate analysis of different hydrological alternatives. The source of elevated mercury levels in the food chain is a vexing dilemma. Altered hydrology is cited as one of many possible causes, with a restored hydrology proposed as the solution. However, the changes in water quality parameters other than Hg, as well as shifts in plant and animal life that would likely accompany these hydrological modifications, must also be considered. The soils in the region vary greatly, and engineers routinely design water-control structures based on their compatibility with the soil conditions. However, less studied and understood are the possible influences of changing water regimes on biology and groundwater hydrology. Most importantly, land-use assumptions and decisions will continue to have a decisive impact on all of these analyses and outcomes.

The critical challenges in south Florida will be to develop an ecosystem approach and a landscape view to our science. Both of these areas represent critical gaps in our knowledge, but both are the focus of current initiatives to adjust our approach. Without an ecosystem approach, the information is incomplete and consensus is impossible. Without a landscape view, the issues become intractable and solutions impossible. The ecological framework to risk assessment allows scientists to examine the issues in a context that can provide the consensus necessary for success.

Research Needs and Recommendations

Previous ways of assessing wetlands have been expanded into the ecosystem approach outlined in this chapter. This approach integrates ecology, hydrology, geomorphology, and soils of wetlands for the evaluation of impacts and risks from chemical, biological, and physical stressors. When the ecosystem method to wetlands-specific risk assessment was applied, it became apparent that there is a need to establish and implement a consistent operational framework in order to make full use of this approach. Several concerns are evident. The effect of multiple stressors (chemical, physical, and biological, of anthropogenic or natural origin) must be an integral component of the assessment process. Standardization of reliable acute, subchronic, and chronic tests is necessary. Alternative exposure–effects scenarios must be evaluated. Understanding fate and transport of chemicals and their interaction with physical, chemical, and biological toxicity-modifying factors is critical. The parameters that must be measured on-site to determine potential pathways and fate of toxins need to be better quantified. There are also specific information needs for organismic, population and community, and ecosystem levels of organization.

Organismic

The levels of uncertainty resulting from presently used, standardized toxicity tests have not been carefully scrutinized in the context of freshwater wetland ecosystems. For example, plant toxicity data are generally based on one green alga *(Selenastrum capricornutum, Scenedesmus* sp. or *Chlorella* sp.) and one vascular aquatic plant (duckweed species, *Lemna minor* or *Lemna gibba*), but there may be a need to represent different groups of photosynthetic and nonphotosynthetic wetland organisms. Using a species battery approach could lessen the potential errors associated with interspecies extrapolation. This is also true for micro- and macroinvertebrates. Laboratory-to-field extrapolations of single-species tests may therefore be improved by using ecologically relevant species batteries with subsequent field validation.

Population and community

As with interspecies comparisons, errors and uncertainty associated with inter-organizational extrapolation need to be evaluated. This would include scaling issues associated with transitions between different levels of biological organization.

Ecosystem

The ecosystem approach proposed here uses HGM characterization together with wetland functions as the criteria for establishing transport, fate, and effects of both chemical and nonchemical stressors. Coupled with toxicity assessments at 3 organizational levels—organismic, population and community, and ecosystem—this approach may be used to describe exposure and effects of stressors in freshwater wetlands, both as a predictive tool and to describe existing conditions. Practical application of the approach will provide a better understanding of how physical, chemical, and biological factors modify the intensity of the stressors. Tools for integrating and analyzing these complex ecosystem interactions need to be refined or, in some cases, still need to be developed. Approaches for evaluating the influence of seasonal and spatial variability are especially necessary.

Toxicity assessments involve tests of varying complexity (single-species, mesocosm, ecosystem assessments, etc.). As a rule of thumb, costs escalate with increasing complexity and single-species laboratory bioassays being the least expensive. From a cost-benefit perspective, the least complex test that can adequately predict ecosystem effects should be the method of choice, providing proper validation has been carried out. The ecosystem approach may reduce the overall cost of risk assessment by identifying key biological, chemical, and physical parameters that must be evaluated early in the assessment process.

References

Adamus PR, Brandt K. 1990. Impacts on quality of inland wetlands of the United States: a survey of indicators, techniques, and applications of community level biomonitoring data. Corvallis OR: U.S. Environmental Protection Agency, Environmental Research Laboratory. USEPA/600/3-90/073

Adamus PR, Stockwell LT. 1983. A method of wetland functional assessment: Volumes I and II. Washington DC: Offices of Research and Development, Federal Highway Administration, U.S. Department of Transportation. Report No. FHWA-1P-82-23.

Adamus PR, Clairain EJ, Smith RD, Young RE. 1987. Wetland evaluation technique (WET). Volume II: Methodology. Vicksburg MS: U.S. Army Corps of Engineers, Waterways Experiment Station. Operational Draft Technical Report Y-87-TR.

Adamus PR. 1993a. Users manual: Avian richness evaluation method (AREM) for lowland wetlands of the Colorado Plateau. Corvallis OR: U.S. Environmental Protection Agency, Environmental Research Laboratory. EPA/600/R-93/240.

Adamus PR. 1993b. Computer program: Avian richness evaluation method (AREM) for lowland wetlands of the Colorado plateau. Corvallis OR: U.S. Environmental Protection Agency, Environmental Research Laboratory.

Anderson JM. 1988. Spatiotemporal effects of invertebrates on soil processes. *Biol Fertil Soils* 6:216–227.

[AOSA] Association of Official Seed Analysts. 1990. Rules for testing seeds. *J Seed Technol* 12:1–122.

[APHA] American Public Health Association. 1992. Standard methods for chemical analysis of water and wastewater, 18th edition. Washington DC: APHA.

[ASTM] American Society for Testing and Materials. 1997a. Annual book of ASTM standards. Volume 11.05, Biological effects and environmental fate; biotechnology, pesticides. West Conshohocken PA: ASTM.

[ASTM] American Society for Testing and Materials. 1997b. Standard guide for conducting acute toxicity tests with fishes, macroinvertebrates, and amphibians. Annual Book of Standards. Philadelphia PA: ASTM. E729.

[ASTM] American Society for Testing and Materials. 1997c. Standard guide for conducting the frog embryo teratogenicity test: Xenopus. Annual Book of Standards. Philadelphia PA: ASTM. E1439.

Ankley GT, Mattson VR, Leonard EN, West CW, Bennett JL. 1993. Predicting the acture toxicity of copper in freshwater sediments: evaluation of the role of acid-volatile sulfide. *Environ Toxicol Chem* 12:315–320.

Bailey RG, Avers PE, King T, McNab WH, editors. 1994. Ecoregions and subregions of the United States. Washington DC: U.S. Forest Service.

Bailey RG. 1994. Ecoregions of the United States (colored map, scale 1:7,500,000). Revised edition. Washington DC: U.S. Forest Service.

Bartoldus CC, Garbisch EW, Kraus ML. 1994. Evaluation for planned wetlands (EPW). A procedure for assessing wetland functions and a guide to functional design. St. Michaels MD: Environmental Concern. 306 p.

Bassi M, Corradi MG, Favali MA. 1990. Effects of chromium in freshwater algae and macrophytes. In: Wang W, Gorsuch JW, Lower WR, editors. Plants for toxicity assessment. Philadelphia PA: ASTM. ASTM STP 1090. p 204–224.

Beyer WN, Anderson A. 1985. Toxicity to woodlice of zinc and lead oxides added to soil litter. *Ambio* 14:173–174.

Beyer WN, Miller GW, Cromartie EJ. 1984. Contamination of the O_2 soil horizon by zinc smelting and it effect of woodlouse survival. *J Environ Qual* 13:247–251.

Brinson MM. 1993. A hydrogeomorphic classification for wetlands. Vicksburg MS: U.S. Army Corps of Engineers, Waterways Experiment Station. Technical Report WRP-DE-4.

Bulich AA. 1979. Use of luminescent bacteria for determining toxicity in aquatic environments. In: Markings LL, Kimerle RA, editors. Aquatic toxicology. Philadelphia PA: ASTM. p 221–237

Bulich AA. 1982. A practical and reliable method for monitoring the toxicity of aquatic samples. *Process Biochem* 17:45–47.

Bulich AA. 1986. Bioluminescence assays. In: Dutka BJ, Bitton G editors. Toxicity testing using microorganisms. Vol 1. Boca Raton FL: CRC Pr. p 57–74.

Byl TD, Klaine SJ. 1992. Peroxidase activity as an indicator of sublethal stress in the aquatic plant *Hydrilla verticillata* (Royle). In: Gorsuch JW, Lower WR, Wang W, and Lewis MA, editors. Plants for toxicity assessment. Volume 2. Philadelphia PA: ASTM. STP 1115. p 101–106.

Cairns J, Niederlehner BR. 1992. Predicting ecosystem risk: genesis and future needs. In Cairns J, Niederlehner BR, Orvos DR, editors. Predicting ecosystem risk. Princeton NJ: Princeton Scientific. p 327–343.

Carpenter SR, DM Lodge. 1986. Effects of submerged macrophytes on ecosystem processes. *Aquat Bot* 26:341–370.

Chapman GA, Denton DL, Lazorchak JM. 1995. Short-term methods for estimating the chronic toxicity of effluents and receiving waters to west coast marine and estuarine organisms. Cincinnati OH: National Exposure Research Laboratory. EPA/600/R-95/136. 661 p.

Croft BA. 1990. Arthropod biological control agents and pesticides. New York NY: Wiley. 723 p.

Crowell H. 1979. Chemical control of terrestrial slugs and snails. Corvallis OR: Agricultural Experiment Station, Oregon State Univ. Station Bulletin 628.

Culotta E. 1995. Bringing back the Everglades. *Science* 268:1688–1689.

Cummins KW, Wilzbach MA. 1985. Field procedures for analysis of functional feeding groups of stream macroinvertebrates. Contribution 1611 to Appalachian Environmental Research Laboratory. Frostburg MD: Univ of Maryland. 21 p.

Curtis C, Lima A, Lazano SJ, Veith GD. 1982. Evaluation of a bacterial bioluminescence bioassay as a method for predicting acute toxicity of organic chemicals to fish. In: Person JG, Foster RB, Bishop WE, editors. Aquatic toxicology and hazard assessment. Philadelphia PA: ASTM. ASTM STP 766. p 170–178.

Doelman P, Nieborer G, Schrooten J, Visser M. 1984. Antagonistic and synergistic toxic effects of Pb and Cd in a simple foodchain: nematodes feeding on bacteria and fungi. *Bull Environ Contam Toxicol* 32:717–723.

Edwards CA. 1984. Report of the second stage in development of a standardized laboratory method for assessing the toxicity of chemical substances to earthworms. Brussels, Belgium: Commission of the European Communities. EUR 9360 EN. 98 p.

Edwards CA, Lofty JR. 1972. Biology of earthworms. London UK: Chapman and Hall. 415 p.

Ethrington JR. 1983. Wetland ecology. London UK: Edward Arnold. 67 p.

Fausch KD, Karr JR, Yant PR. 1984. Regional application of an index of biotic integrity based on stream fish communities. *Trans Am Fish Soc* 113:39–55.

[FEMA] Federal Emergency Management Agency. 1992. National comprehensive plan for incident response and management. Washington DC: FEMA.

Federal Register. 1995. Natural resource damage assessments. Proposed rule. *Federal Register* 60(149):39803–39834.

[FICWD] Federal Interagency Committee for Wetland Delineation. 1989. Federal manual for identifying and delineating wetlands. Cooperative technical publication. Washington DC: U.S. Army Corps of Engineers, U.S. Environmental Protection Agency, U.S. Fish and Wildlife Service, and U.S. Department of Agriculture/Soil Conservation Service.

Fleming WJ, Ailstock MS, Momot JJ, Norman CM. 1992. Response of sago pondweed, a submerged aquatic macrophyte, to herbicides in 3 laboratory culture systems. In: Gorsuch JW, Lower WR, Wang W, Lewis MA, editors. Plants for toxicity assessment. Volume 2. Philadelphia PA: ASTM. ASTM STP 1115. p 267–275.

Folsom Jr BL, Price RA. 1992. A plant bioassay for assessing plant uptake of contaminants from freshwater soils or dredged material. In: Gorsuch JW, Lower WR, Wang W, Lewis MA, editors. Plants for toxicology assessment. Volume 2. Philadelphia PA: ASTM. ASTM STP 1115. p 172–177.

Frayer WE, Peters DD, Pywell HR. 1989. Wetlands of the California central valley: status and trends—1939 to mid-1980's. Portland OR: U.S. Fish and Wildlife Service. 29 p.

Gaufin AR. 1958. The effects of pollution on a mid-western stream. *Ohio Journal of Science* 58:197–208.

Getzin S, Cole S. 1964. Evaluation of potential mulloscides for slug control. Station Bulletin 658. Pullman WA: Washington Agricultural Experiment Station.

Goats G, Edwards CA. 1982. Testing the toxicity of industrial chemicals to earthworms. Harpenden UK: Rothamsted Experimental Station. p 104–105.

Green RH. 1979. Sampling design and statistical methods for environmental biologists. New York NY: Wiley. 257 p.

Haight M, Mundry T, Pasternak J. 1982. Toxicity of seven heavy metals on *Panagrellus silusiae*: the efficacy of the free-living nematode as an in vivo toxicology assay. *Nematologica* 28:1–11.

Hammer DA. 1990. Constructed wetlands for wastewater treatment. Boca Raton FL: Lewis. 856 p.

Hassan SA. 1985. Standard methods to test the side effects of pesticides on natural enemies of insects and mites developed by the IOBC/WPRS work group "Pesticides and beneficial organisms." *Bull OEPP/EPPO* 15:214–255.

Hassan SA, Albert R, Bigler F, Blaisinger P, Bogenschütz H, Boller E, Brun J, Chiverton P, Edwards P, Engloert WD, Huang P, Inglesfield C, Naton E, Oomen PA, Overmeer WPJ, Rieckmann LO, Samsoe-Petersen L, Staubli A, Tuset JJ, Viggiani G, Vanwetswinkel G. 1987. Results of the third joint insecticide testing programme by the IOBC/WPRS working group "Pesticides and beneficial organisms." *J Appl Ent* 103:92–107.

Hendricks ML, Hocutt CH, Stauffer Jr JR. 1980. Monitoring of fish in lotic habitats. In: Hocutt CH, Stauffer Jr JR, editors. Biological monitoring of fish. Lexington KY: Lexington Books. p 205–233.

Hilsenhoff WL. 1988. Rapid field assessment of organic pollution with a family biotic index. *J North Am Bentholog Soc* 7:65–68.

Hoaglin DC, Mosteller F, Tukey JW. 1985. Exploring data tables, trends and shapes. New York NY: Wiley. 527 p.

Hook DD. 1993. Wetlands: history, current status, and future. *Environ Toxicol Chem* 12:2157–2166.

Hook DD, McKee Jr WH, Williams TM, Jones S, Van Blaricom D, Parsons J. 1994. Hydrologic and wetland characteristics of a Piedmont bottom in South Carolina. *Water Air Soil Poll* 77:293–320.

Hopkin SP. 1986. The woodlouse *Porcellio scaber* as a "biological indicator" of zinc, cadmium, lead, and copper pollution. *Environ Pollut* (Series B) 11:271–290.

Hopkin SP. 1990. Species specific differences in the net assimilation of zinc, cadmium, lead, copper, and iron by the terrestrial isopods *Oniscus asellus* and *Porcellio scaber*. *J Appl Ecol* 27:460–474.

Janos DP. 1987. VA mycorrhizas in humid tropical ecosystems. In: Safir GR, editor. Ecophysiology of VA mycorrihizal plants. Boca Raton FL: CRC Pr. p 107–134.

Johnson I. 1990. Proposed guide for conducting acute toxicity tests with the early life stages of freshwater mussels. Report to Ecological Effects Branch, Office of Pesticide Programs under USEPA Contract Number 68-02-4278, 87018 4-EEB-08. Gainesville FL: KBN Engineering and Applied Sciences Inc.

Karr JR. 1981. Assessment of biotic integrity using fish communities. *Fisheries* 6:21–27.

Karr JR, Fausch KD, Angermeier PL, Yant PR, Schlosser IJ. 1986. Assessing biological integrity in running waters: a method and its rationale. Champaign IL: Illinois Natural History Survey. Special Publication No. 5. 28 p.

Kelly JR, Harwell MA. 1989. Indicators of ecosystem response and recovery. In: Levin SA, Harwell MA, Kelly JR, Kimball KD, editors. Ecotoxicology: problems and approaches. New York NY: Springer-Verlag. p 9–39.

Kent DJ, Jenkins KD, Hobson JF. 1994. Ecological risk assessment of wetlands. In: Kent DM, editor. Applied wetlands science and technology. Boca Raton FL: Lewis. p 79–103.

Kentula ME, Brooks RP, Gwin SE, Holland CC, Sherman AD, Sifneos JC, Hairston AJ, editors. 1992. An approach to improving decision making in wetland restoration and creation. Corvallis OR: Wetlands Research Program, U.S. Environmental Protection Agency, Environmental Research Laboratory. EPA-600/R-92/150.

Kentula ME, Brooks RP, Gwin SE, Holland CC, Sherman AD, Sifneos JC. 1993. An approach to improving decision making in wetland restoration and creation. Boca Raton FL: CRC Pr. 151 p.

Klemm DJ, Lewis PA, Fulk F, Lazorchak JM. 1990. Macroinvertebrate field and laboratory methods for evaluating the biological integrity of surface waters. Cincinnati OH: United States Environmental Protection Agency, Environmental Monitoring Systems Laboratory. EPA/600-4-90/030.

Klemm DJ, Morrison GE, Norberg-King TJ, Peltier WH, Heber MA. 1994. Short-term methods for estimating the chronic toxicity of effluents and receiving waters to marine and estuarine organisms. Cincinnati OH: Environmental Monitoring Systems Laboratory. EPA/600/4-91/003. 483 p.

Kolkwitz R, Marsson M. 1902. Grundsatz für die bilogische Beunteilung des Wassers nach seiner Flora und Fauna. Mitt. PrufAnst. WassVersorg. *Abwasserbeseit Berlin* 1:33–72.

Kovacs M. 1978. Element accumulation in submerged aquatic plant species in Lake Balaton, Hungary. *Acta Bot Aca Sci Hung* 24(3–4):139–284.

Kusler JA, Kentula ME. 1990. Wetland creation and restoration: the status of the science. Washington DC: Island Pr. 594 p.

Lagler KF. 1978. Capture, sampling, and examination of fishes. In: Bagenal T, editor. Fish production in fresh waters. IBP Handbook No. 3. London UK: Blackwell Scientific.

LaPoint T, Fairchild J. 1989. Aquatic surveys. In: Warren-Hicks W, Parkhurst B, Baker Jr S, editors. Ecological assessment of hazardous waste sites. Corvallis OR: U.S. Environmental Protection Agency, Environmental Research Laboratory. EPA/600/3-89/013.

Lee CR, Sturgis TC, Landin MC. 1981. Heavy metal uptake by marsh plants in hydroponic solution cultures. *J Plant Nutrition* 3(1–4):139–151.

Leibowitz SG, Abbruzzese B, Adamus PA, Hughes LE, Irish JT. 1992. A synoptic approach to cumulative impact assessment: a proposed methodology. Corvallis OR: U.S. Environmental Protection Agency, Environmental Research Laboratory. EPA/600/R-92/167.

Lemly AD. 1994. Irrigated agriculture and freshwater wetlands: a struggle for coexistence in the western United States. *Wetlands Ecol Manage* 3:3–15.

Levin SA, Harwell MA, Kelly JR, Kimball KD. 1989. Ecotoxicology: problems and approaches. New York NY: Springer-Verlag. 547 p.

Linder G, Barbitta J, Kwaiser T. 1990. Short-term amphibian toxicity tests and paraquat toxicity assessment. In: Aquatic toxicity and risk assessment, thirteenth symposium, ASTM STP 1096. Philadelphia PA: American Society for Testing and Materials. p 189–198.

Linder G, Bollman M, Wilborn D, Nwosu J, Baune W, Smith S, Ott S, Callahan C. 1991. Final technical report for the preliminary field survey and on-site, in situ and laboratory Evaluations Completed at Milltown Reservoir. Prepared for U.S. Environmental Protection Agency, Region 8, Helena, Montana by ManTech Environmental Technology, Inc. Corvallis OR.

Linder G, Wyant J, Meganck R, Williams B. 1991. Evaluating amphibian responses in wetlands impacted by mining activities in the western United States. In: Comer RD, Davis PR, Foster SQ, Grant CV, Rush S, Thorne O, Todd J, editors. Issues and technology in the management of impacted wildlife. Boulder CO: Thorne Ecological Institute. p 17–25.

Linder G, Ingham E, Henderson G, Brandt CJ. 1993. Evaluation of terrestrial indicators for use in ecological assessments at hazardous waste sites. Corvallis OR: U.S. Environmental Protection Agency, Environmental Research Laboratory. EPA-600/R-92-183.

Linder G, Hazelwood R, Palawski D, Bollman M, Wilborn D, Malloy J, DuBois K, Ott S, Pascoe G, DalSoglio J. 1994. Ecological assessment for the wetlands at Milltown Reservoir, Missoula, Montana: characterization of emergent and upland habitats. *Environ Toxicol Chem* 13:1957–1970.

Linder G, Ingham E, Brandt J, Henderson G. 1992. Evaluation of terrestrial indicators for use in ecological assessments at hazardous waste sites. Corvallis OR: USEPA Environmental Research Laboratory. EPA/600/R-92/183.

Lowrance RR, Todd RL, Fail J, Hendrickson O, Leonard R, Asmussen L. 1984. Riparian forests as nutrient filters in agricultural watersheds. *Bioscience* 34: 374–377.

Merritt RW, Cummins KW, editors. 1984. An introduction to the aquatic insects of North America. Dubuque IA: Kendall/Hunt. 441 p.

Microbics. 1992. Microtox™ manual. Carlsbad CA: Microbics Corporation.

Mitsch WJ, Gosselink JG. 1993. Wetlands. 2nd ed. New York NY: Van Nostrand Reinhold. 539 p.

Moldenke A, Shaw C, Boyle JR. 1991. Computer-driven image-based soil fauna taxonomy. *Agr Ecostst Environ* 34:177–185.

Moore PD, Bellamy DJ. 1974. Peatlands. New York NY: Springer-Verlag. 476 p.

Moore SB, Winckel J, Detwiler SJ, Klasing SA, Gaul PA, Kanim AR, Kesser BE, Debevac AB, Beardsley A, Puckett LA. 1990. Fish and wildlife resources and agricultural irrigation drainage in the San Joaquin Valley, California. Sacramento CA: San Joaquin Valley Drainage Program. 974 p.

Mount DI, Brungs WA. 1967. A simplified dosing apparatus for fish toxicology studies. *Water Res* 1:21–29.

Mount DI, Stephan CE. 1967. A method for establishing acceptable limits for fish—malathion and the butoxyethanol ester of 2,4-D. *Trans Am Fish Soc* 96:185–193.

[NRC] National Research Council. 1992. Restoration of aquatic ecosystems: science, technology and public policy. Washington DC: National Academy Pr. 552 p.

[NRC] National Research Council. 1995. Wetlands: characteristics and boundaries. Washington, DC: National Academy Pr.

Neuhauser EF, Durkin PR, Milligan MR, Anatra M. 1986. Comparative toxicity of ten organic chemicals to four earthworm species. *Comp Biochem Physiol* 83C(1):197–200.

[OECD] Organization for Economic Cooperation and Development. 1995. Review and evaluation of aquatic test methods for pesticides and industrial chemicals. Paris, France: OECD.

Omernik J. 1987. Ecoregions of the coterminous United States. *Annals of the Association of American Geographers* 77:118–125.

Parkhurst B, Linder G, McBee K, Bitton G, Dutka B, Hendricks C. 1989. Toxicity tests. In: Warren-Hicks W, Parkhurst B, and Baker, Jr S, editors. Ecological assessment of hazardous waste sites. Corvallis OR: U.S. Environmental Protection Agency, Environmental Research Laboratory. EPA/600/3-89/013.

Pascoe GA. 1993. Wetland risk assessment. *Environ Toxicol Chem* 12:2293–2307.

Pascoe GA, DalSoglio JA. 1994. Planning and implementation of a comprehensive ecological risk assessment at the Milltown Reservoir-Clark Fork River Superfund Site, Montana. *Environ Toxicol Chem* 13:1943–1956.

Pascoe GA, Blanchet RJ, Linder G, Palawski D, Brumbaugh WG, Canfield TJ, Kemble NE, Ingersoll CG, Farag A, DalSoglio JA. 1994. Characterization of ecological risks at the Milltown Reservoir-Clark Fork River Sediments Superfund Site, Montana. *Environ Toxicol Chem* 13:2043–2058.

Peltier WH, Weber CI. 1985. Methods for measuring the acute toxicity of effluents to freshwater and marine organisms. 3rd ed. Cincinnati OH: U.S. Environmental Protection Agency, Environmental Monitoring and Support Laboratory. EPA/600/4-85/013.

Pennak R. 1978. Pelecypoda. In: Freshwater invertebrates of the United States. 2nd ed. New York NY: Wiley. p 736–768.

Philips JD. 1989. Nonpoint source pollution control effectiveness of riparian forests along a coastal plain river. *Journal of Hydrology* 110:221–237.

Plafkin JL, Barbour MT, Porter KD, Gross SK. 1988. Rapid bioassessment protocols for use in streams and rivers: benthic macroinvertebrates and fish. Draft Report RTI82A. EA Engineering, Science and Technology, Inc., to the U.S. Environmental Protection Agency, Monitoring, and Data Support Division, Washington DC.

Plafkin JL, Barbour MT, Porter KD, Gross SK, Hughes RM. 1989. Rapid bioassessment protocols for use in streams and rivers: benthic macroinvertebrates and fish. Washington DC: USEPA Office of Research and Development. EPA/444/4-89/001.

Popham JD, Webster JM. 1979. Cadmium toxicity in the free-living nematode, *Caenorhabditis elegans*. *Environ Res* 20:183–191.

Reeves FB. 1985. Survival of VA mycorrhizal fungi: interactions of secondary succession, mycorrhizal dependency in plants and resource competition. *N Amer Conf on Mycorrhizae* 6:110–113.

Richardson CJ. 1994. Ecological functions and human values in wetlands: A framework for assessing forestry impacts. *Wetlands* 14:1–9.

Riekerk H. 1993. Groundwater flow in pine-cypress flatwoods. In: General Technical Report SO-93, Proceedings of the Seventh Biennial Southern Silvicultural Research Conference. USDA, Forest Service, Southern Forest Experiment Station, New Orleans LA. 65 p.

Rose C, Crumpton WG. 1996. Effects of emergent macrophytes on dissolved oxygen dynamics in a prairie pothole wetland. *Wetlands* 16:495–502.

Roth E, Olsen R, Snow P, Sumner R. 1993. Oregon freshwater wetland assessment methodology. McCannell SG, editor. Salem OR: Oregon Division of State Lands.

Samoiloff M, Bell J, Birkholz D, Webster G, Arnott E, Pulak R, Madrid A. 1983. Combined bioassay-chemical fractionation scheme for the determination and ranking of toxic chemicals in sediment. *Environ Sci Technol* 17:329–333.

Samoiloff M, Schulz S, Jordan Y, Denich K, Arnott E. 1980. A rapid simple long-term toxicity assay for aquatic contaminants using the nematode *Panagrellus redivius*. *Can J Fish Aquat Sci* 37:1167–1174.

Saul B. 1995. Nutrient exchange between floodwater and groundwater in a forested riparian zone in the southeastern coastal plain. [Master's thesis]. Clemson SC: Clemson University, Department of Forest Resources.

Seastedt TR, Crossley Jr DA. 1980. Effects of microarthropods on the seasonal dynamics of nutrients in forest litter. *Soil Biol Biochem* 12:337–342.

Sewell DK, Lighthart B. 1988. Standard practice for conducting fungal pathogenicity tests on the predatory mite *Metaseiulu occidentalis* (Acari: Phytoseiidae). 600/3-89/046. U.S. Environmental Protection Agency, Environmental Research Laboratory, Corvallis, OR.

Sheehan PJ. 1984. Effects on community and ecosystem structure and dynamics. In: Sheehan PJ, Miller DR, Butler GC, Bourdeau P, editors. Effects of pollutants at the ecosystem level. New York NY: Wiley. p 51–99.

Siegel JR, Glaser PH. 1987. Groundwater flow in a bog-fen complex, Lost River Peatland, northern Minnesota. *Journal of Ecology* 75: 743–754.

Siegel S. 1956. Nonparametric statistics for the behavioral sciences. New York NY: McGraw-Hill. 312 p.

Southwood TRE. 1978. Ecological methods. New York NY: John Wiley and Sons. 524 p.

Suter GW. 1991. Endpoints for regional ecological risk assessments. *Environ Manage* 14:19–23.

Swanson SM, Rickard CP, Freemark KE, MacQuarrie P. 1991. Testing for pesticide toxicity to aquatic plants: recommendations for test species. In: Gorsuch JW, Lower WR, Wang W, Lewis MA, editors. Plants for toxicity assessment. Volume 2. Philadelphia PA: American Society for Testing and Materials. ASTM STP 1115. p 77–97.

Theriot R. 1988. Relationship of bottomland hardwood species to natural water regimes. In: The ecology and management of wetlands. Volume 1. Ecology. London UK: Croom-Helm. p 344–351.

Thomas MW, Judy BM, Lower WR, Krause GF, Sutton WW. 1990. Time-dependent toxicity assessment of herbicide contaminated soil using the green alga *Selenastrum capricornutum*. In: Wang W, Gorsuch JW, Lower WR, editors. Plants for toxicity assessment. Philadelphia PA: American Society for Testing and Material. ASTM STP 1091. p 235–254.

Thompson SP, Merritt KL. 1988. Western Nevada wetlands—history and current status. *Nevada Public Affairs Review* 1:40–45.

Tiner Jr RW. 1984. Wetlands of the United States: current status and recent trends. Washington DC: Department of the Interior, U.S. Fish and Wildlife Service, National Wetlands Inventory.

[USACOE] U.S. Army Corps of Engineers. 1982. Guidelines for delineating physical boundaries of wetlands. 40 CFR 23.4 *Federal Register*.

[USACOE] U.S. Army Corps of Engineers. 1987. Beneficial uses of dredged material: proceedings of the First Interagency Workshop, 7–9 October 1986, Pensacola, FL. Vicksburg MS: USACOE Waterways Experiment Station. Technical Report D-87-1. 271 p.

[USDOI] U.S. Department of the Interior, Fish and Wildlife Service. 1980. Habitat evaluation procedures (HEP). Washington DC: U.S. Department of the Interior, Fish and Wildlife Service. ESM 121.

[USDOI] U.S. Department of Interior. 1989. Endangered and threatened wildlife and plants. 50 CFR 17.11 and 17.12.

[USEPA] U.S. Environmental Protection Agency. 1973. Biological field and laboratory methods for measuring the quality of surface waters and effluents. Cincinnati OH: National Environmental Research Center, USEPA. EPA/670/4-73/001.

[USEPA] U.S. Environmental Protection Agency. 1982. Sampling protocols for collecting surface water, bed sediment, bivalves, and fish for priority pollutant analysis. Washington DC: Office of Water, Regulations, and Standards, USEPA.

[USEPA] U.S. Environmental Protection Agency. 1986. Hazard evaluation division standard evaluation procedure. Ecological risk assessment. Washington DC: USEPA Office of Pesticide Programs. EPA 450/9-85-001.

[USEPA] U.S. Environmental Protection Agency. 1987. A compendium of Superfund field operations methods. Washington DC: Office of Emergency and Remedial Response, USEPA. EPA/540/p-87/001.

[USEPA] U.S. Environmental Protection Agency. 1989. Protocols for short term toxicity screening of hazardous waste sites. Corvallis OR: USEPA, Environmental Research Laboratory. EPA/600/3-88/029.

[USEPA] U.S. Environmental Protection Agency. 1990. Macroinvertebrate field and laboratory methods for evaluating the biological integrity of surface waters. Washington DC: USEPA Office of Research and Development. EPA/600/4-90/030.

[USEPA] U.S. Environmental Protection Agency. 1991a. Ecological assessment of Superfund sites: an overview. In ECO Update, Vol. 1, Number 2. Washington DC: USEPA, Office of Solid Waste and Emergency Response, Office of Emergency and Remedial Response, Hazardous Site Evaluation Division (OS-230). Publication 9345.0-05I.

[USEPA] U.S. Environmental Protection Agency. 1991b. Technical support document for water quality-based toxics control. Washington DC: USEPA. EPA/505/2-90-001.

[USEPA] U.S. Environmental Protection Agency. 1992. Framework for ecological risk assessment. Washington DC: Risk Assessment Forum. EPA/630/R-92/001.

[USEPA] Environmental Protection Agency. 1994a. Managing ecological risks at EPA: issues and recommendations for progress. Washington DC: USEPA. EPA/600/R-94/183.

[USEPA] U.S. Environmental Protection Agency. 1994b. Methods for measuring the toxicity and bioaccumulation of sediment-associated contaminants with freshwater invertebrates. Duluth MN: Office of Research and Development, Environmental Research Laboratory. 140 p.

[USEPA] U.S. Environmental Protection Agency. 1994c. Considering wetlands at CERCLA sites. Washington DC: USEPA. EPA/540/R-94/019.

[USEPA] U.S. Environmental Protection Agency. 1995. Methods for estimating the chronic toxicity of effluents and receiving waters to west coast marine and estuarine organisms. Washington DC: USEPA. EPA/600/R-95-136.

[USEPA] U.S. Environmental Protection Agency. 1997. Ecological risk assessment guidance for Superfund. Washington DC: USEPA. EPA/540/R-97/006.

[USEPA] U.S. Environmental Protection Agency. 1998. Guidelines for ecological risk assessment. Washington DC: USEPA. EPA/630/R-95/002F.

[USFWS] U.S. Fish and Wildlife Service. 1992. Draft documentation guidelines for natural resource damage assessment. Washington DC: USFWS Division of Environmental Contaminants.

van der Valk AG. 1989. Northern prairie wetlands. Ames IA: Iowa State Univ Pr. 533 p.

van Kessel W, Brocades-Zaalberg R, Seinen W. 1989. Testing environmental pollutants on soil organisms: a simple assay to investigate the toxicity of environmental pollutants on soil organisms, using $CdCl_2$ and nematodes. *Ecotoxicol Environ Safe* 18:181–190.

Walsh GE, Weber DE, Simon TL, Brashers LK. 1991. Toxicity tests of effluents with marsh plants in water and sediment. In: Gorsuch JW, Lower WR, Wang W, Lewis MA, editors. Plants for toxicity assessment. Volume 2. Philadelphia PA: American Society for Testing and Materials. ASTM STP 1115. p 517–525.

Wang W. 1991. Higher plants (common duckweed, lettuce, and rice) for effluent toxicity assessment. In: Gorsuch JW, Lower WR, Wang W, Lewis MA, editors. Plants for toxicity assessment. Volume 2. Philadelphia PA: American Society for Testing and Materials. ASTM STP 1115. p 68–76.

Warren-Hicks W, Parkhurst B, Baker Jr S. 1989. Ecological assessment of hazardous waste sites. Corvallis OR: USEPA Environmental Research Laboratory. EPA/600/3-89/013.

Weber CI, editor. 1993. Methods for measuring the acute toxicity of effluents and receiving waters to freshwater and marine organisms. 4th ed. Cincinnati OH: USEPA, Environmental Systems Monitoring Laboratory. EPA/600/4-90/027F. 293 p.

Weber CI, Horning WB, Klemm DJ, Neiheisel TW, Lewis PA, Robinson EL, Menkedick J, Kessler F. 1988. Short-term methods for estimating the chronic toxicity of effluents and receiving waters to marine and estuarine organisms. Cincinnati OH: USEPA, Environmental Monitoring and Support Laboratory. EPA 600/4-87/028.

Weller DM, Spatcher AT. 1965. Long-term changes in vegetation zones and open water in a prairie pothole wetland. *Am Midland Natural* 7:105–119.

[WES] U.S. Army Corps of Engineers Waterways Experiment Station. 1989. A plant bioassay for assessing plant uptake of heavy metals from contaminated freshwater dredged material. Vicksburg MS: U.S. Army Corps of Engineers Waterways Experiment Station. Technical Note EEDP-04-11.

Williams PL, Dusenbery BD. 1990. Aquatic toxicity testing using the nematode, *Caenorhabditis elegans*. *Environ Toxicol Chem* 9:1285–1290

Zelder P. 1987. The ecology of southern California vernal pools: A community profile. Biological Report 85(7.11). Washington DC: U.S. Fish and Wildlife Service.

Zentner J. 1994. Enhancement, restoration and creation of freshwater wetlands. In: Kent DM, editor. Applied wetlands science and technology. Boca Raton FL: Lewis. p 127–166.

Chapter 5

Case Study: An Ecological Risk Assessment for the Wetlands at Milltown Reservoir, Missoula, Montana

Greg Linder, Gary A. Pascoe, Julie A. DalSoglio

The ecological risk assessment for the wetlands at Milltown Reservoir near Missoula, MT illustrates the implementation of a comprehensive evaluation of risks for a wetlands that had long been impacted by anthropogenic activities. From a regulatory perspective, the Milltown Reservoir Wetlands (MRW)–Clark Fork River (CFR) area is a Superfund site that consists of approximately 160 km along the upper CFR from Milltown Dam to Warm Springs, MT (Figure 5-1). The ecological risk assessment for the MRW and the upper CFR was extensively reported in a series of papers that appeared in *Environmental Toxicology and Chemistry* in 1994 (Volume 13, No. 12) and addressed risk assessment activities for 2 sample units: MRW and the reach of the CFR from just down river of Warm Springs Ponds to the upriver boundary of Milltown Reservoir. Our present focus, however, lies with the operable unit that contains the wetlands associated with the hydroelectric facility and reservoir.

Chapter Preview

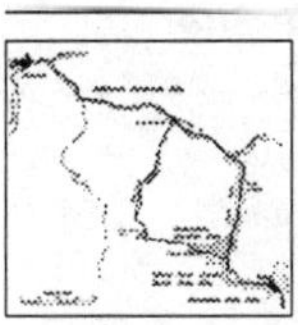

Ecotoxicology and Risk Assessment for Wetlands. Michael A. Lewis et al., editors.

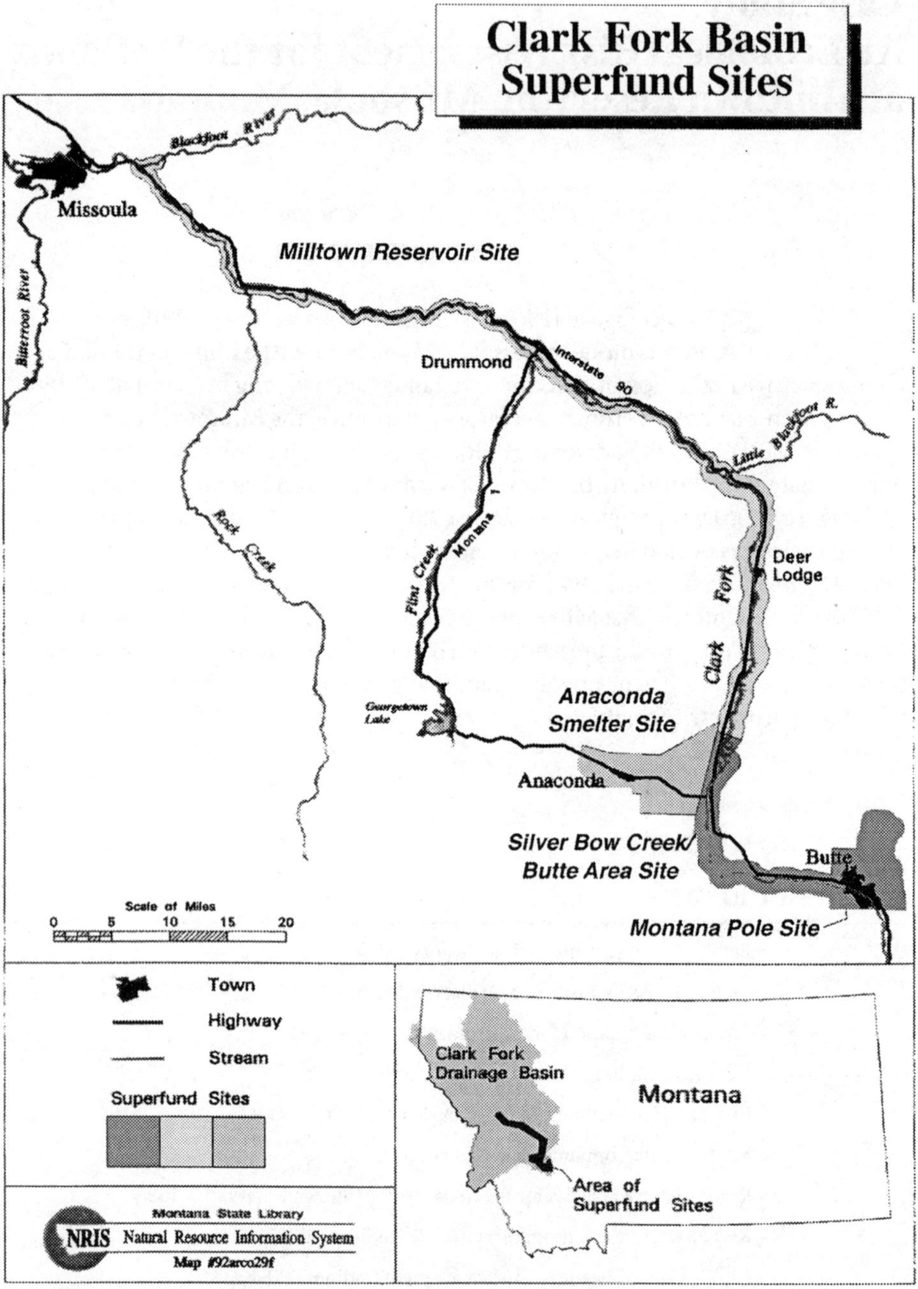

Figure 5-1 MRW-CFR Superfund site in western Montana, which follows the Clark Fork River and extends from Butte and Anaconda, MT to Missoula, MT

Environmental Setting and Site History

Milltown Reservoir is on the CFR in western Montana, 6 miles east of Missoula (Figure 5-2). Within regulatory contexts, the reservoir operable unit extends from Milltown Dam to the maximum pool elevation (995 m), which extends about 2 miles upstream beyond an unused railroad right-of-way. Milltown Dam is a hydroelectric project owned and operated by Montana Power Company. The reservoir was formed in 1907 following the construction of a hydroelectric facility located on the CFR immediately downstream from its confluence with the Blackfoot River.

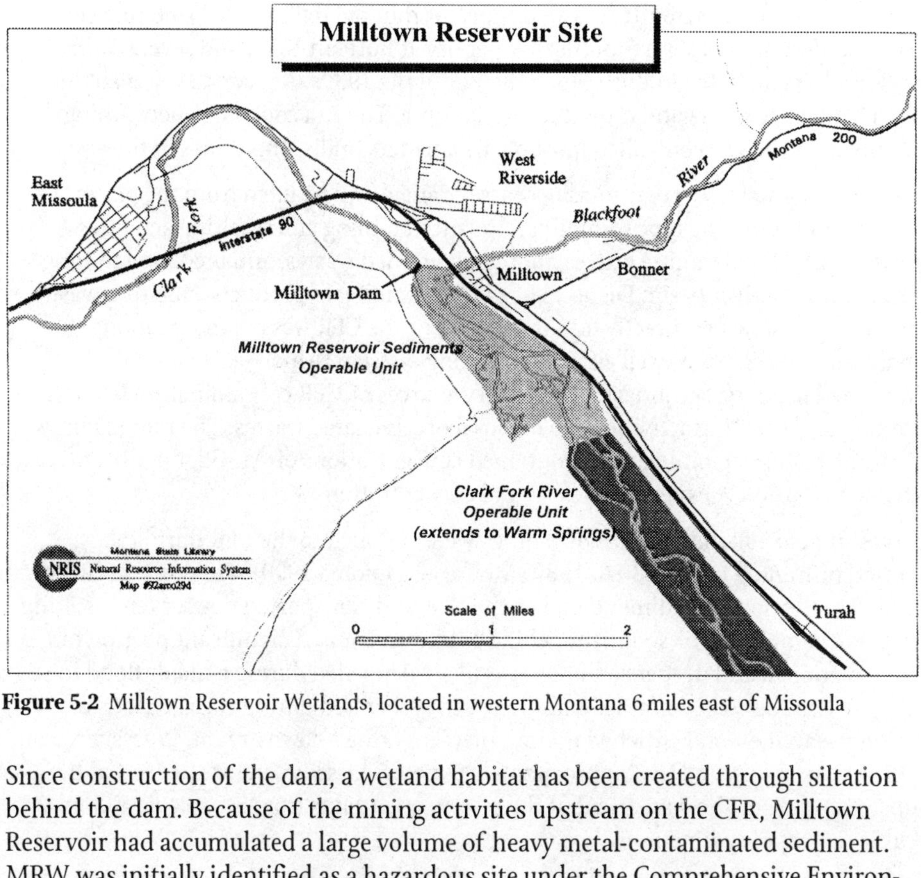

Figure 5-2 Milltown Reservoir Wetlands, located in western Montana 6 miles east of Missoula

Since construction of the dam, a wetland habitat has been created through siltation behind the dam. Because of the mining activities upstream on the CFR, Milltown Reservoir had accumulated a large volume of heavy metal-contaminated sediment. MRW was initially identified as a hazardous site under the Comprehensive Environmental Response, Compensation, and Liability Act (CERCLA, or Superfund) in 1981 after local community well-water samples were found to have arsenic levels that ranged from 0.22 to 0.51 mg/L; the U.S. Environmental Protection Agency (USEPA) recommendation for potable water supplies suggested that arsenic not exceed 0.05 mg/L. Within an ecological context, the impact of the contaminated sediments on the wetlands had not been well characterized, and as part of the baseline risk assessment activities for the MRW/CFR site, the wetlands at Milltown Reservoir were evaluated for the extent of contaminant and its impact on the indigenous wildlife and vegetation characteristic of the site. Contaminant sources were characterized by metals- and arsenic-enriched sediments, the presence of metals and arsenic in local surface water and ground water, and dispersed and subsequently exposed sediments and wetland soils above the reservoir banks that potentially contribute to ecological impacts on the wetlands at Milltown Reservoir.

The contamination at MRW is directly related to historical activities in the upstream areas of Butte and Anaconda, MT. As early as 1864, when gold was discovered at Butte, the CFR watershed had been the setting for mining and smelting-related activities, and by 1881 Butte was an important mining, milling, and smelting center. At least 25 companies were mining copper ore at Butte in 1885, and several mills and smelters operated in Butte from 1885 until the 1930s. Anaconda was also the site of major smelters and mills during that time. The Anaconda Copper Mining Company owned or controlled most of the smelters, mills, and mines in the area.

Early mining wastes were primarily coarse-grained and resulted from the placer mining and stamping type of milling. Advanced mining and smelting activities resulted in refined mining wastes, more fine-grained wastes, and increased mining impacts to the river basin. Disposal of tailings, milling byproducts, smelting wastes, and mine wastewater directly into tributaries of the CFR was common among the main mining centers as well as smaller mining districts. Moore and Luoma (1990) identified primary, secondary, and tertiary sources of CFR contamination from the mining and smelting activities and disposal of associated wastes. The mine tailings near the historical mining areas contained concentrations of As, Cd, Cu, Pb, and Zn that are 10 to 100× expected background concentrations.

An estimated 100 million tons of tailings were supplied to the CFR during the period of mining from 1880 to 1982 (Moore and Luoma 1990). These wastes were added to the normal sediment load of the CFR and transported downriver, resulting in the accumulation of sediment behind Milltown Dam. A significant portion of coarse-grained and deeper sediment was likely deposited during a major flood in 1908, when the coarse-grained mining wastes generated during early periods of mining activities, and enriched in trace metals, washed downstream. Woessner et al. (1984) have estimated that approximately 9 meters of sediment are present at the upstream face of the dam and that the reservoir contains from 3.5 to 4.6 million cubic meters of sediment.

Wetlands Risk Assessment at Milltown Reservoir

An ecological risk assessment may be considered an integrated evaluation of ecological effects and exposure, as detailed by USEPA (1992), Suter (1993) and others (see Figure 5-3). Within an ecological risk assessment for a wetlands like that at Milltown Reservoir, soil, sediment, surfacewater, and groundwater contamination evaluations must consider chemical and biological interactions associated with

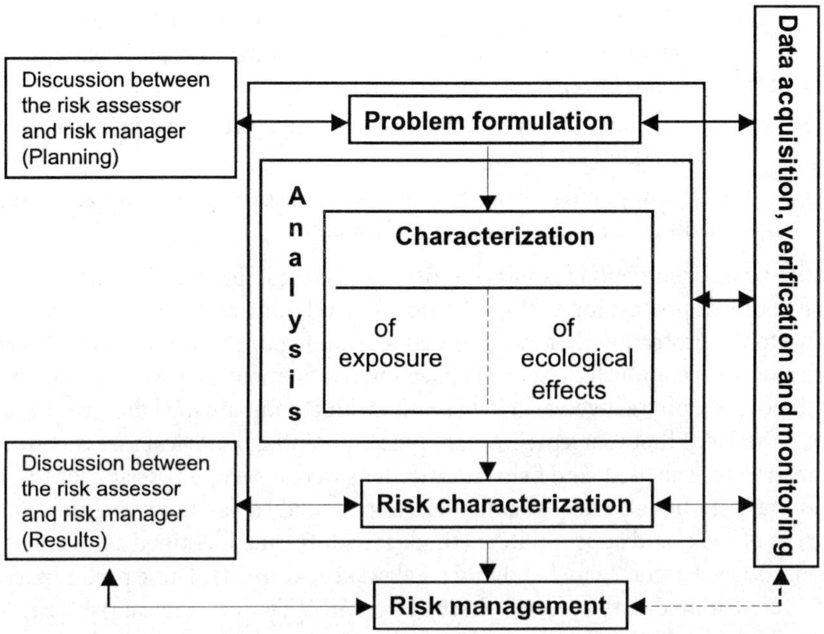

Figure 5-3 Ecological risk assessment process as developed in the framework document (USEPA 1992)

contaminant exposures that occurred in the wetland habitat. For the risk assessment at MRW, metal and arsenic contamination of the wetland could have been evaluated according to various assessment strategies. For example, both chemical-based and toxicity-based approaches have made significant contributions to ecological assessments for hazardous waste sites. From an ecological perspective, however, the strengths of each strategy were combined to evaluate ecological effects and exposure within a risk assessment setting. At MRW, ecological effects and exposure assessments were regarded as interrelated functions that yielded estimates of risks associated with environmental contaminants in various matrices sampled at a site.

Problem Formulation for the Ecological Risk Assessment at MRW

Early in problem formulation (Figure 5-3), plans were developed to address the site-specific requirements for an ecological risk assessment at MRW. Issues reflected in these assessment endpoints include the following:

1) Metals and arsenic may be elevated in wetland soils to concentrations that impact terrestrial invertebrates and vegetation.
2) Elevated metals concentrations in sediments may impact benthic ecology.

3) Primary consumers and higher-trophic-level organisms such as deer, waterfowl, and predatory birds may be exposed to elevated metals in water, soils, sediments, and lower-trophic-level food sources.
4) Muskrats and beaver may be exposed to elevated metals in aquatic vegetation and other wetland food sources.
5) Rainbow trout populations may be impacted by exposure to contaminated water, sediment, and invertebrate food sources.

Identifying environmental resources at risk was a critical first step in the ecological risk assessment process for MRW, as well as in developing cleanup alternatives relative to the protection that was afforded to wildlife populations on and adjacent to the site. To accomplish these data collection requirements, 2 phases of work were identified. Each phase involved a field season with accompanying laboratory work. During the Tier I first year's preliminary phase, potential biological assessment methods were evaluated, and field study designs were developed. Results of the preliminary studies also helped guide selection of study areas and refine the selection of tasks and appropriate methods for addressing identified assessment endpoints (see Pascoe, Blanchet, Linder, Palawski et al. 1994). These preliminary studies contributed to the second phase of the MRW Tier I ecological risk assessment, which involved definitive field and laboratory studies and the ecological characterization of the study area. Tier II studies were also proposed to answer information needs that might arise from the results of Tier I studies. These Tier II studies included multi-seasonal sampling and additional toxicity studies, particularly during early spring snowmelt, but they were not planned in detail as part of the baseline ecological risk assessment for MRW.

Preliminary studies of the terrestrial and wetland habitat consisted of ecological characterization tasks and limited field and laboratory studies. Results of the ecological characterization (e.g., a wetland delineation study was used to select emergent zone and upland sampling stations) helped identify wetland and upland sample and testing locations and supported the selection of test methods used in the risk analysis phase of the project, e.g., the utility of a plant rooting zone study (Linder, Bollman et al. 1991). The wetlands delineation also provided information on vegetation ecology of the terrestrial habitat (USFWS 1991a). Similarly, a wildlife survey (USFWS 1991b) provided semiquantitative ecological information on waterfowl, other birds, and small mammals. Results of these preliminary wetland and upland characterization studies helped focus the definitive year's studies on soil contamination and were used to establish locations of terrestrial sampling units shown in Figure 5-4.

While beyond the scope of the present overview of ecological risk assessment for wetlands, an extensive evaluation for aquatic habitats (including sediment-associated and flowing-water habitats) was also pursued as part of the MRW–CFR baseline risk assessment. The activities related to sediment and aquatic toxicity evaluations were coordinated with those for the wetlands risk assessment. From a

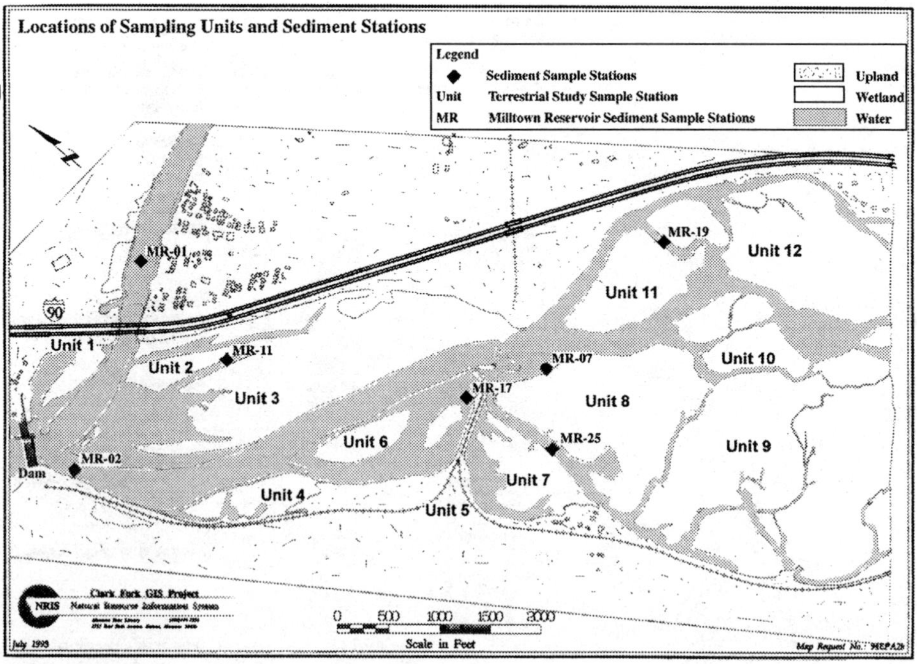

Figure 5-4 Sampling and testing units at MRW

study design perspective, results of the preliminary year's efforts helped identify sampling stations for the wetland and sediment evaluations, fish and sediment toxicity studies, and aquatic and terrestrial plant evaluations. The final sampling and testing locations covered a wide range of metals concentrations, water depths, and habitat characteristics in the upper CFR and at the MRW.

Based on the assessment endpoints developed from a review of existing information on MRW and on the results of the preliminary studies, a conceptual model of the ecological risk assessment was developed (Figure 5-5). The model identified the sources of contamination, the populations and communities potentially at risk, and the environmental pathways from the sources to these receptors. Selection of ecological receptors was based on a number of factors, including residence of the species, knowledge of species ecology and habitat uses, sensitivity of the wetland and its food webs to changes in species composition and populations, and responsiveness to the effects of multiple chemicals of concern at the site. The final component of the conceptual plan identified the specific study tasks: evaluate exposures to the receptors, identify ecological effects, and evaluate exposure–response relationships.

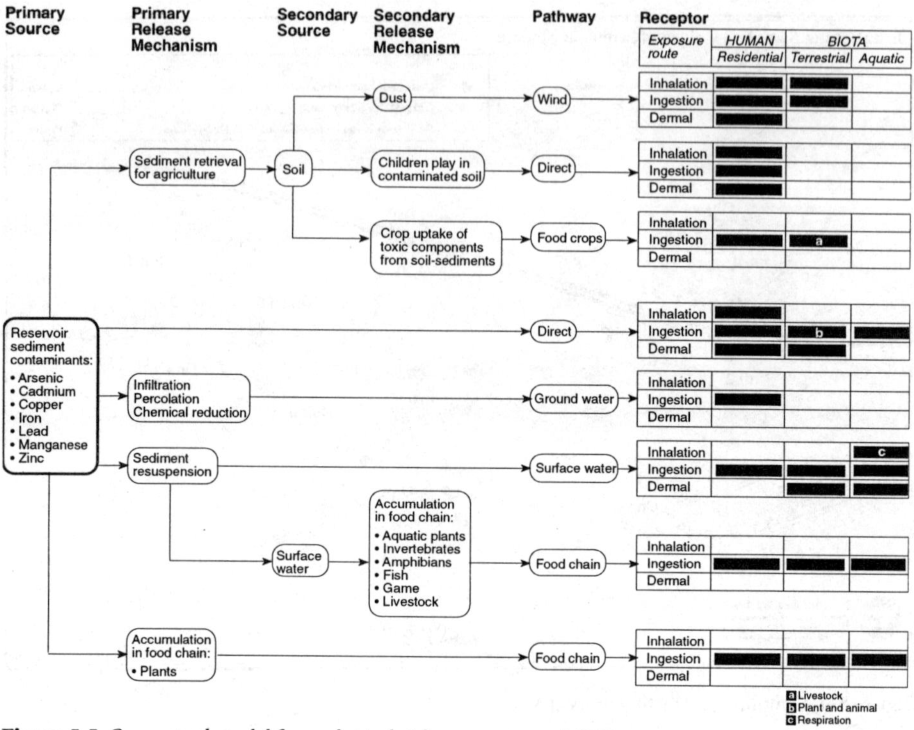

Figure 5-5 Conceptual model for ecological risk assessment at MRW

Definitive Studies for the Risk Analysis at MRW

Exposure assessment and ecological effects assessment

The ecological risk assessment for MRW was based on a triad of ecological risk assessment information (Pascoe 1993). In general, the triad consists of

1) chemical analyses to establish the presence, concentrations, and variabilities of specific chemicals of concern;
2) ecological surveys to establish whether adverse ecological effects have occurred; and
3) toxicity tests to establish a link between the adverse ecological effects and the chemistry of the wastes.

As described in USEPA guidance for conducting ecological assessments at hazardous waste sites (Warren-Hicks et al. 1989; USEPA 1997) and in Suter (1993), this triad of information may help establish cause–effect relationships between chemicals of concern and ecological effects.

For MRW, the ecological risk assessment was implemented through a tiered approach similar to those strategies previously developed in the hazard evaluation process (USEPA 1986, 1992). As indicated above, preliminary studies (as defined by Suter and Loar 1992) had screened and identified critical questions requiring further study and had helped define initial data requirements for a complete sampling and analysis plan for the definitive year's studies included in Tier I activities.

Potential reference environments for Milltown Reservoir were evaluated within the regulatory setting of CERCLA, and both the Blackfoot River and Thompson Falls Reservoir downstream on the CFR were considered as potential reference areas based on a set of reference area criteria (Pascoe and DalSoglio 1994). Sampling of Thompson Falls Reservoir was not performed within the scope of the field activities; although preliminary studies suggested that there might be unacceptable contamination within its reach, the Blackfoot River arm of the reservoir was selected as a reference area. Local wildlife refuges with wetland habitats (e.g., Lee Metcalf Wildlife Refuge near the Bitterroot River south of Missoula, MT) were also found to be only marginally suitable as reference areas for MRW, owing to physical habitat differences observed during preliminary sampling and field observations (Linder et al. 1994). In view of these questions regarding suitable reference environments, the integrated field and laboratory studies for the wetlands at Milltown Reservoir were designed to characterize trends in contaminant levels and biological effects within MRW itself.

The final selection of specific studies for preliminary and definitive years' studies for the MRW–CFR ecological risk assessment are listed in Table 5-1 and are briefly discussed in the following sections.

Biological tests and field activities

As part of the preliminary studies for the wetland, candidate biological test methods were evaluated, and soil and chemical analytical methods were identified. Biological test methods for the preliminary study included seed germination tests in laboratory and field (Linder et al. 1994), laboratory root elongation tests on soil eluates (Linder et al. 1994), earthworm tests in laboratory and field (Linder et al. 1994; Wilborn et al. 1997), amphibian tests in laboratory and field (Pascoe and DalSoglio 1994), and laboratory Microtox on soil eluates (Pascoe and DalSoglio 1994). As suggested above, these biological assessments completed during the preliminary year's activities were critical in the ecological assessment for MRW and helped identify tasks to be incorporated into the definitive year's work for Tier I studies. Also, in conjunction with the U.S. Fish and Wildlife Service, a small mammal trapping study was completed during the preliminary year, and provided site-specific information regarding metal burdens in resident small mammals for a food-chain contamination evaluation (see Linder et al. 1994).

Following the work completed during the preliminary year's studies, the definitive year's Tier I work was clearly defined and relied upon the sampling design established during the first field season. Methods in the definitive year's studies included vegetation surveys, earthworm tests in laboratory and field, root elongation tests on

Table 5-1 Field and laboratory methods applied to the baseline ecological risk assessment for MRW

Assessment task for Tier I studies	Laboratory test or field method	Reference
Conduct wetland delineaton, terrestrial vegetation assessment, and preliminary wildlife survey	Floristic survey[1,2]	FICWD 1989; Warren-Hicks et al. 1989; Kapustka 1989; Linder et al. 1992
	Wetland delineation[1]	FICWD 1989
	Wildlife survey[1,2]	SCS 1951; Gysel and Lyon 1980; McBee 1989; Warren-Hicks et al. 1989; Linder et al. 1992
	Screening-level microbial tests[1]	Warren-Hicks et al. 1989; Linder et al. 1992
	Seed germination and root elongation tests[1]	Warren-Hicks et al. 1989
	Early seedling growth[2]	Linder, Wyant et al. 1991
Evaluate rhizosphere exposures to contaminated ground water	Root elongation tests[2]	Warren-Hicks et al. 1989
Collect surface soil samples in areas of concern for metals analysis	Chemical analysis for metals in soil[1,2]	USEPA 1986
Complete soil quality characterization	Soil matrix characterization (soil texture analysis, cation exchange capacity, organic content, and pH)[1,2]	SCS 1951; Page et al. 1982
Determine food source contamination for site-specific receptors, and collect pertinent site samples for preliminary food-chain contamination survey	Small mammal trapping[1]	Warren-Hicks et al. 1989; Linder et al. 1992
	Chemical analysis for metals in herbivorous small mammals and food items[1,2]	USEPA 1986
Evaluate emergent zone habitats using amphibians	Screening-level amphibian tests[1]	Linder, Wyant et al. 1991
Collect composite samples of terrestrial invertebrates	Chemical analysis for metal bioaccumulation evaluation[1,2]	USEPA 1986
Collect sediment samples for preliminary evaluation of extent of contamination	Chemical analysis for metals in sediment[1]	USEPA 1986
Collect composite aquatic biota samples	Chemical analysis for metal bioaccumulation evaluation[1,2]	USEPA 1986

[1] Preliminary phase work
[2] Definitive phase work

groundwater samples, soil quality characterizations, and chemical analysis for metals in biological materials and soils. For Tier I activities, biological and chemical methods used during the preliminary year and the definitive year are listed in Table 5-1. Within the ecological triad approach, these risk analysis tasks were incorporated into the Tier I activities for both the MRW and the CFR baseline ecological risk assessment.

Ecological characterization

Studies of the wetland ecology of the Milltown Reservoir operable unit were planned to characterize MRW and to assist in location of sampling and testing stations. Ecological characterization consisted of a wetlands jurisdictional delineation (including a vegetation survey) (USFWS 1991a) and a semiquantitative wildlife survey (USFWS 1991b). Benthic communities in the wetland and CFR operable units were characterized by community structure analysis as part of the sediment quality triad approach to sediment evaluation (Canfield et al. 1994). Fish population and recruitment studies in the upper CFR have been and continue to be performed by Montana Department of Fish, Wildlife, and Parks (Lipton 1993) and Montana Power Company (1992).

Chemical analyses

Measurements of contaminant concentrations were planned for soils (Linder et al. 1994), sediments (Brumbaugh et al. 1994), surface waters (Linder et al. 1994), and terrestrial and aquatic biota (Linder, Bollman et al. 1991; Ingersoll et al. 1994). Chemical analyses were designed to provide information on potential exposures of ecological receptors and for an analysis of potential transfer of contaminants to higher trophic-level organisms in terrestrial and aquatic food chains.

Terrestrial invertebrate evaluation

Toxicity tests consisting of earthworm exposures to wetland soils in the laboratory and on site were planned as the primary terrestrial soil evaluation (Linder et al. 1994). The earthworm field test was one of the in situ toxicity studies developed for the Superfund program (Linder et al. 1992). Earthworm exposures also serve as a valuable measure of a contaminated food source to higher-level trophic animals.

Terrestrial vegetation evaluation

Toxicity tests of rooted macrophytes for the aquatic habitat (Linder et al. 1994) and a variety of terrestrial plant species, using measures of seed germination (Linder et al. 1994) and root elongation (Linder et al. 1994), were planned as measurements of potential impacts to wetland and terrestrial vegetation at the site. A greenhouse study (Linder, Bollman et al. 1991) was designed to provide additional information on early seedling survival and uptake of soil metals by plants; this information would later be used in the trophic transfer study.

Surfacewater evaluation

Metals contamination of surface waters arises primarily from upstream sources rather than from on-site sediment contamination. Thus, limited tests were planned for amphibian and bacterial exposures to surface water (Pascoe and DalSoglio 1994). Amphibians were representative of wetland exposures and were important sources of food for higher trophic-level organisms. The Frog Embryo Teratogenesis Assay *Xenopus* (FETAX) was planned for preliminary studies in depositional areas of the wetland, with possible expansion in Tier II studies. Microtox was planned as a rapid, inexpensive screening measurement of microbial function in surface waters and sediment pore waters, as well as in soil eluates.

Benthic invertebrate evaluation

The sediment quality triad approach was planned for evaluation of potential benthic impacts in wetland sediments (Canfield et al. 1994). The approach was designed to integrate site-specific information on sediment chemistry (Brumbaugh et al. 1994), toxicity to sediment invertebrates and trout (Kemble et al. 1994), sediment benthic community structure (Canfield et al. 1995), and bioaccumulation of sediment metals (Ingersoll et al. 1994). These studies were performed in conjunction with fish exposures to CFR sediments (Woodward, Brumbaugh et al. 1994; Woodward, Farag et al. 1994).

Fish evaluation

While not exclusively a wetlands issue, impacts to fish in the upper CFR were recognized as possibly related to the combined exposures of surface water, sediments, and food sources to contaminant metals (Woodward, Brumbaugh et al. 1994; Woodward, Farag et al. 1994). Toxicity studies on early life stages of rainbow and brown trout were planned to measure the impacts of exposures to metals in overlying water and diets comprised of contaminated invertebrates from the upper CFR. Traditional toxicity endpoints of survival and growth were supplemented with autopsies of exposed fish, measurements of ion regulation to assess potential interference with Ca and Na regulation, measures of lipid peroxidation as an indicator of oxidative stress induced by copper redox alterations, and determination of copper inclusions in macrophages as an indication of immune response stress (Farag et al. 1994). Fish population studies in the reservoir involved habitat evaluations and population estimates performed by Montana Department of Fish, Wildlife, and Parks (Lipton 1993) and Montana Power Company (1992).

Trophic transfer study

Ecological risk assessments performed under CERCLA traditionally have been based on a foodweb or linear food-chain analysis, consisting of modeling chemical uptake from contaminated sources to higher trophic levels, frequently in the absence of ecological studies. However, at each trophic level in MRW, field collections of soils, sediments, and biological materials (e.g., aboveground and below-ground plant samples, soil invertebrates, small mammals) were compared with appropriate criteria or literature toxicity information, as well as being used in a food-chain modeling approach. For the baseline risk assessment, a food-chain analysis was planned to complement the extensive site-specific information gathered on biological and toxicological parameters of lower trophic-level organisms (Pascoe et al. 1996). The food-chain analysis considered the potential for transfer of metals from sediments, soils, water, plants, and invertebrates to primary consumers and higher organisms such as fish, predatory birds, waterfowl, small mammals, and deer. Tissue residue analyses of various aquatic and terrestrial plant and animal specimens collected at the site, and the organisms evaluated in in-situ toxicity tests, supplemented the environmental media data for this study. Data on metals and arsenic concentrations in environmental media and field-collected specimens were also used to estimate contaminant bioavailability to terrestrial small mammals at the site (Pascoe, Blanchet, and Linder 1994).

Risk Analysis: Methods for Assessing Exposure and Ecological Effects

Exposure and ecological effects assessment study design

During the preliminary year's field activities, a stratified sampling design was developed, based largely upon the existing topography of the CFR. As indicated in Figure 5-4, MRW was stratified into 12 sample units. On the basis of the preliminary year's work, Sample Units 1 and 5 were excluded from subsequent definitive testing and evaluation. Sample Unit 1 was a recently vacated residential area and was characterized as disturbed prior to any potential impacts associated with heavy metals in soils and sediments, and Sample Unit 5 was a capped dredge-spoils disposal area considered only for groundwater monitoring. Within each sample unit, transects were established. To locate these transects initially, a randomly determined bearing to the first sampling station on each transect was taken in the field, then another random number yielded the distance in meters along that vector to that sampling station. Once this starting point was determined, sampling stations were systematically identified at 10-m intervals along the line. On larger sample units, transects formed grids with 10-m spacing to ensure sufficient sampling and testing locations. While more potential sampling stations were identified than were evaluated, sampling and testing consistently reflected an "equal-effort per sample unit basis" and generally involved work at a subset of 2 to 4 randomly selected sampling stations per sample unit. By stratifying MRW along the existing topographic bounds, sample units were segregated along depositional zones that had developed over the reservoir's 85-year history. Topographic delineation also indicated that these sample units would coincide with the emergent and upland features identified in the wetland delineation.

Field sampling

Within each sample unit, the locations of sample transect reference points were surveyed, then fixed using global positioning systems (Trimble Navigation/GPS Pathfinder); these reference points were later incorporated into the geographic information system database for the CFR (Natural Resource Information System, Montana State Library, Helena MT).

Samples collected at MRW during both preliminary and definitive phases of the Tier I risk assessment included soil, sediment, surfacewater, groundwater, and biological samples. Within each sampling unit, soils or groundwater samples were collected within a 1-m radius of each sampling station using stainless steel or carbon steel shovels, trowels, soil augers, mixing bowls, and well points, as appropriate. All nondisposable equipment was initially washed with site water, rinsed with 10% HCl, then rinsed with distilled or reverse osmosis water. For laboratory tests, soil samples were shipped at 4 °C by overnight carrier. Soil eluates were then prepared in the laboratory following USEPA methods (1989).

Wetland Soils Contamination Evaluation

Biological test methods

As previously noted, Table 5-1 lists the methods used in Tier I activities in both preliminary and definitive testing and survey work. Brief summaries of field and laboratory methods used for the biological assessment during the definitive studies at MRW are listed in the subsections that follow, but references cited in Table 5-1 should be consulted for detail.

Laboratory earthworm test method

In the laboratory, the earthworm (*Eisenia foetida*) test method directly evaluated biological effects associated with exposure to soils (ASTM 1997). Laboratory earthworm evaluations were terminated after 14 d. Upon termination, mortality data were collected for each replicate as well as behavioral observations and sublethal indicators of exposure. Percent effect values were calculated for the 14-d counts. All worms were then submitted for metals analysis; worms were not purged of gut contents prior to analysis.

On-site earthworm tests

In parallel with laboratory earthworm tests, on-site tests were conducted in order to address potential questions associated with laboratory-to-field extrapolation errors in the risk characterization (Wilborn et al. 1997). For on-site tests, 6 holes, 6 to 8 inches in diameter, were dug at each sampling station the day prior to test initiation; the excavated soil was saved for loading the exposure chambers. Following excavation, exposure chambers were placed in the holes. Exposure chambers were constructed from 4-inch, Schedule 40 polyvinyl chloride (PVC) pipe. The exposure chambers were 8 inches long; when the chambers were placed in the field, 7 inches of the pipe were placed into the soil, leaving a 1-inch rim above the soil's surface. Five of the PVC pipes were filled with excavated soil; hydrated artificial soil was placed in the sixth pipe for the control. The remaining excavated soil was then packed around all 6 PVC pipes to secure them in their respective positions at the sampling station. Two exposure chambers were used to monitor soil moisture (with an irrometer) and soil temperature (with a thermistor) at the sampling station being tested. The artificial soil-containing chamber was used to evaluate test organism health, independent of potential metal exposures in site soil.

To initiate the test, irrometers at each testing location were read. Then, based upon these soil moisture readings, exposure chambers were hydrated to 45% soil moisture on a dry weight basis. After each exposure chamber was readied, 10 worms were placed into each of the 3 soil replicates as well as the artificial soil control; screens were then tightly fitted over the artificial and site soil-containing exposure chambers. No top cover or screen was placed over chambers housing the irrometer or thermometer.

At test termination, final temperature and irrometer readings were recorded at the end of day 14, and each exposure chamber had its contents emptied onto a plastic bag. Earthworms were separated from the soil, then counted (survivorship) and evaluated for sublethal effects (e.g., dermopathology).

Laboratory root elongation test method

Root elongation evaluations estimated the adverse biological effects of groundwater and soil eluates on standard test species, e.g., lettuce seedlings (*Lactuca sativa*) in a 120-h test (USEPA 1989). Screening evaluations were completed using undiluted groundwater and soil eluates; if dilution tests followed these preliminary screens, the groundwater and soil eluates were diluted with reverse-osmosis (RO) water. Root elongation results were reported as percent reduction in root lengths in treatments relative to RO controls.

Soil analysis

Soil samples collected at MRW were analyzed for physical (e.g., soil texture and morphology) and chemical properties (e.g., cation exchange capacity [CEC] and total organic material). In addition, diethylenetriaminepentaacetic acid (DTPA) extractions were completed on all soil samples as an estimate of metal bioavailability (especially, Cu, Cd, and Zn). For soil characterization, all methods followed standard procedures detailed in Klute (1986) or Page et al. (1982).

Groundwater sampling

Groundwater sampling locations for the rooting zone study were identical to those terrestrial stations where on-site earthworm tests were completed. Soil samples from these same locations were also collected for laboratory earthworm tests and for preparation of soil eluates.

For sampling groundwater, well points (Redhead) were hand-driven into soils until the top of the screened portion of the well point was immediately below the water table (approximately 24 inches below the surface of the water table). Once groundwater was reached, 3 volumes of ground water (~ 500 ml each) were purged through Tygon tubing attached to a 1500-mL syringe before the sample was taken. For groundwater collection, samples were aspirated into a brown Nalgene high-density polyethylene (HDPE) sample bottle placed in-line to the sampling apparatus and filled to overflowing (Stollar 1990). After sample containers were filled, the lid was tightly secured, and the sample was then placed in an ice chest and held in complete darkness until the samples could be frozen. The samples were held frozen, shipped to the testing laboratory, and stored at 4 °C until test initiation. Immediately prior to root elongation testing, samples were warmed to ambient temperature, then filtered using a 0.45-m Millipore filter.

Metals analysis

Sample preparation for soils, sediments, and biological matrices followed USEPA methods (USEPA 1986); groundwater or surfacewater samples were digested with nitric acid prior to analysis (USEPA 1986). Once prepared, all samples were analyzed by flame (FAA) or graphite furnace atomic absorption (GFAA) spectrophotometry. For GFAA, a Perkin-Elmer (PE) Zeeman/3030 atomic absorption spectrophotometer with PE HGA-600 graphite furnace and AS-60 autosampler were used to measure As (193.7 nm), Pb (283.3 nm), and Cd (228.8 nm) on electrodeless discharge lamps (slit width, 0.7 nm). Predetermination temperature was set at 1300 °C, followed by a charring step at 2000 °C. Cu (324.7 nm) and Zn (213.9 nm) were determined by air/acetylene FAA on a PE 403 with HGA-2000 controller. Calibration curves bracketed all analytes and were within the linear range of element concentrations in samples. Data reduction and calculations for each sample were accomplished by linear regression based on least squares analysis.

Statistical methods

All laboratory and field data were tested for normality using the Kolmogorov-Smirnov tests, and variance homogeneity was evaluated using the Hartley test (Zar 1986). Any datasets that did not pass tests for normality and variance homogeneity were transformed (logarithmic or arcsin), then retested for normality and homogeneity. If transformed datasets did not satisfy normality or homogeneity assumptions for using parametric methods, then the nonparametric Friedman test (2-way and multiple comparison test methods) (Sprent 1989) was used. Additionally, Spearman's and Kendall's rank correlation procedures (Zar 1986) were performed on the metal subacute exposures versus subacute effects conducted with earthworms in the field.

Results of Risk Analysis for the Wetlands at Milltown Reservoir

Study area and ecological characterization

Upper Clark Fork River watershed

The CFR system (see Figure 5-1) drains over 57,000 km^2 and terminates after 550 km at Lake Pend Oreille in northern Idaho. The upper Clark Fork subbasin generally includes the headwaters of the CFR downstream to Milltown Dam, about 200 km (Moore and Luoma 1990).

Historically, the CFR was a major corridor and spawning ground for trout migrating out of Lake Pend Oreille. Migrations ceased with construction of the downstream dams (e.g., Cabinet Gorge Dam, Milltown Dam). The upper river currently supports high-quality game fish in certain river segments. The basin is also known for its big game, upland bird, and waterfowl hunting. These resources of the basin have created a large recreational and tourism industry.

Milltown Reservoir is the first major impoundment on the CFR. It is about 2 km in length and is generally shallow except for the 2 channels of the Clark Fork and Blackfoot Rivers (see Figure 5-2). Sediment accumulation in the impoundment behind Milltown Dam has created a 216-hectare wetland.

Wetland habitat classification

Milltown Reservoir is located in Missoula County, MT (T13 N; R18 S; Sections 20, 21, 27, and 28), approximately 10 km east of the city of Missoula. The study area was based upon jurisdictional wetland boundaries that were identified using the criteria of the Federal Interagency Committee for Wetland Delineation (FICWD 1989; USFWS 1991a). Wetland habitat types were classified using a hierarchical system described by Cowardin et al. (1979). The study area extended upstream beyond the full pool elevation of the reservoir to include the braided channel of the Clark Fork River and its associated wetlands as far upstream as the Harris Marsh and was bounded by Highway I-90 on the north, Milltown Dam to the west (Figure 5-2), and the abandoned railroad right-of-way to the south. The area west of the abandoned railroad bridge was characterized by slow-moving water with few islands. The area east of the abandoned bridge was characterized by faster-moving water and a highly braided river channel with many islands. Total jurisdictional wetland area comprised 186 hectares or approximately 86% of the total study area. Wetlands were classified into riverine (10%), palustrine (56%), or lacustrine (20%) systems and represented a highly diverse mosaic of habitats within the study area. The riverine system included moving-water areas contained within the river channel above the influence of Milltown Dam. Classes within the riverine system at Milltown Reservoir were not quantified but included rock bottom, unconsolidated bottom, aquatic bed, and unconsolidated shore. Approximately 21 hectares of riverine habitat occurred within the Milltown Reservoir study area.

The water pool created and influenced by Milltown Reservoir was classified as lacustrine. The lacustrine system was divided into limnetic (water depth greater than 2 meters) and littoral (water depth less than 2 meters) subsystems at Milltown Reservoir. The lacustrine system comprised approximately 43 hectares and included 18 hectares of limnetic habitat and 25 hectares of littoral habitat. Classes within the lacustrine system at Milltown were not mapped but included unconsolidated bottom, unconsolidated shore, and aquatic bed.

Most of the islands in the braided section of the river fell into the palustrine category, as did Harris Marsh and other water areas not influenced by either the river or Milltown Dam. Palustrine system wetlands at Milltown were divided into emergent wetland, aquatic bed, and scrub-shrub wetland classes. Emergent wetlands were mainly dominated by common cattail (*Typha latifolia*) and hardstem bulrush (*Scirpus acutus*). Aquatic beds were dominated by pondweed (*Potamogeton* sp.) and small duckweed (*Lemna minor*). Scrub-shrub wetlands were dominated by willow (*Salix amygdaloides*, *S. bebbiana*, and *S. exigua*), water birch (*Betula occidentalis*), and mountain alder (*Alnus incana*). Common understory plants included redtop bentgrass (*Agrostis stolonifera*), beaked sedge (*Carex rostrata*), Baltic rush (*Juncus balticus*), common tansy (*Tanacetum vulgare*), and field horsetail (*Equisetum arvense*). Balsam poplar (*Populus balsamifera*) trees occurred in scattered groves in the upper portion of the study area. The palustrine system within the Milltown Reservoir study area encompassed approximately 123 hectares that were composed of 18 hectares of scrub-shrub wetlands farmed for hay products, 70 hectares of relatively undisturbed scrub-shrub wetlands, 31 hectares of emergent wetlands, and 4 hectares of aquatic bed habitat (see USFWS 1991a).

Wildlife survey

Aquatic invertebrates, fish, birds, small mammals, and other vertebrates inhabiting MRW were surveyed in 1990 following Warren-Hicks et al. (1989) and other routine guidance for conducting wildlife surveys (Gysel and Lyon 1980; Davis 1982; Ohmart and Anderson 1986). These qualitative surveys were not sufficient to completely assess the presence or absence of species expected to occur in riverine, lake, or wetland habitats; however, 14 taxa of aquatic macroinvertebrates and 20 taxa of vertebrates other than birds were observed at the site. Species of small mammals and other terrestrial vertebrates were typical of riparian sites in western Montana.

A total of 89 bird species was observed in the area from April through October 1990. Most of the bird species observed at Milltown Reservoir were reported as either probable or confirmed breeders for this area. Canada geese (*Branta canadensis*) were the most abundant waterfowl breeding in the area, probably producing more young than all other waterfowl combined. Water bird and passerine bird species diversity was similar to avian communities that occupy similar habitats at nearby Lee Metcalf

National Wildlife Refuge, Stevensville, MT. Most of the bird species found at Milltown Reservoir could be characterized as either wetland or edge species (USFWS 1991b). Different wetland habitat types were highly interspersed at Milltown Reservoir, resulting in diverse vegetative structure.

Earthworm tests in laboratory and field

Earthworms expressed no acute toxicity in either laboratory or field tests during preliminary or definitive studies (see Linder et al. 1994). However, correlation analysis with both Spearman's rank and Kendall's rank correlation procedures indicated that subtle biological response data (e.g., behavioral, morphologic, and dermatopathologic effects) from field tests completed in 1991 were most significantly associated with soils that have elevated total and DTPA-extractable Cu (r_S, 0.37 [$P = 0.00658$] for total Cu; r_S, 0.36 [$P = 0.0756$] for DTPA-extractable Cu; r_S, 0.29 [$P = 0.0546$] for total Cu; r_S, 0.27 [$P = 0.0780$] for DTPA-extractable Cu).

Estimates of the bioaccumulation potential of metal in MRW soils were considered by analyzing earthworms for target analytes following their 14-d laboratory exposures. To make these data more relevant for evaluating wildlife risk (i.e., earthworms are consumed intact by predators in the field), earthworms were not purged prior to analysis. The extent to which metals are available for trophic-level transfer (either as metal incorporated into earthworm tissue through bioaccumulation or transferred through coincidental ingestion of gut contents) clearly will vary as a function of metal concentrations in soil (see Table 5-2).

Root elongation and groundwater phytotoxicity assessments

Phytotoxicity assessments available from root elongation tests with ground water indicated that samples collected with hand-driven well points were quite heterogeneous, as would be expected on the basis of other measurements (e.g., soil physical structure and metals content) taken across the site. Biological activity associated with ground water collected from sample units across MRW was relatively low; some biological effects were noted, but no samples consistently expressed acute toxicity (germination failure in the root elongation test). From the work with root elongation testing, phytotoxicity, although subtle in expression, may be linked to elevated metal concentrations in ground water collected from stations in Sample Units 7 and 8.

Root elongation tests on soil eluates

Five seeds (cucumber, lettuce, radish, red clover, and wheat) were tested with soil eluates, and no statistically significant reductions in root length were recorded. Some data presented biologically significant responses, however, and suggested that soil samples collected at certain MRW sampling locations (e.g., Sample Units 7 and 8) inhibited root elongation when seeds were exposed to soil-derived eluates. While these biological effects were not statistically significant, these trends were consistent with other tests (e.g., root elongation tests with ground water) used for the biological assessment at MRW.

Table 5-2 Range in total and DPTA-extractable metals in soil samples collected at MRW[1]

Sample Unit	Metal[2]									
	As		Cd		Cu		Pb		Zn	
	Total	Extractable	Total	Extractable	Total	Extractable	Total	Extractable	Total	Extractable
2	15–82	< dl–0.068	9–11	< dl–0.017	560–825	188–200	22–75	0.048–1.1	≥ 2700	304–416
3	39–81	0.058–0.07 0	5.0–9.0	3.2–3.8	350–712	144–264	53.0–92.0	4.2–17.4	840–1400	176–256
4	11.0–90.0	< dl–0.050	2.0–11.0	< dl	50–1066	< dl	23.0–110	4.5–4.7	150–2135	59.0–128
6	62–130	0.088	10.0–14.0	6.3	600–950	192	70.0–100	0.061	≥ 2200	400
7	110–125	< dl	13.0–14.0	4.3–9.6	875–1050	200–208	76.0–97.0	0.012–0.158	3400–4300	368–480
8	91–105	< dl–0.086	3.0–6.0	2.9–4.6	530–900	224–320	70–100	0.055–16.6	930–1440	216–224
9	79–107	< dl–0.047	6.0–7.0	3.5–4.3	505–650	184–240	50–66	0.014–0.052	1900–2000	296–360
10	70–95	< dl–0.210	7.0–12.0	4.6–5.6	530–720	176–232	65–75	0.027–0.119	1800–2800	296–384
11	62.0–84.0	< dl–0.066	4.0–6.0	2.9–4.5	480–700	168–280	58–79	0.023–0.091	1200–1550	240–392
12	47–64	< dl–0.049	3.0–8.0	3.4–4.6	340–620	144–152	49–65	0.016–9.8	1400–2400	256–408

[1] Sample Units 1 and 5 were not tested.
[2] Concentrations as μg analyte/gm dry weight soil (ppm); extractable metals derived from DPTA (0.025M) extractions on splits of MRW soil samples
< dl = less than detection limits: As, 20 ppb; Cd, 1 ppb; Cu, 36 ppb; Pb, 3 ppb; Zn, 4 ppb.

Metals accumulation in upland and terrestrial plants

As summarized in Table 5-3, vegetation samples collected coincident with soil and groundwater samples indicated that target metals did accumulate in vegetation growing at MRW. The extent of accumulation varied spatially, as well as among species and anatomically within plants. Emergent vegetation, e.g., cattail and sedge, appeared to accumulate the most metals, while upland vegetation appeared to accumulate metals, especially those having little nutrient value, to relatively low concentrations. Metals with known nutritional value to plants, e.g., Zn, were bioaccumulated many-fold relative to the concentration of metal in soil.

Table 5-3 Total metals in plant materials collected at MRW

	Metal (total)[1]									
	As		Cd		Cu		Pb		Zn	
Vegetation type[2]	Above ground	Below ground	Above ground	Below ground	Above ground	Below ground	Above ground	Below ground	Above ground	Below ground
Aquatic[3]	0.8–35.2	4.2–238.7	0.58–17.8 (908)[4]	5.38–370.5	9.4–17.8	21.9–370.5	3.2–14.8	22.9–46.6	41.7–203.4	73.8–>1800
Forbs	0.3–1.9	2.0–21.3	0.16–6.2	0.62–8.4	5.4–14.4	9.1–145.2	1.2–4.4	5.8–20.2	11.1–405.4	23.1–757.1
Grasses	0.5–17.2	6.4–324.7	0.42–2.22	1.53–23.3	4.9–46.5	14.4–737.7	3.2–11.1	12.8–77.5	36.2–247.4	71.8–>1800

[1] Range of metal residues as µg analyte/gm (dry weight; ppm); analytical detection limits; As, 20 ppb; Cd, 1 ppb; Cu, 36 ppb; Pb 3 ppb; Zn, 4 ppb
[2] Above ground = stem or foliar portions; below ground = rhizomes, roots, and tubers
[3] Rooted aquatic, floating vascular, and emergent vegetation
[4] Single sample of floating aquatic vegetation (*Lemna* sp.)

Soil physicochemical characterizations and metals analysis

As indicated by characterizations completed in the definitive studies, the soils at MRW are heterogeneous across the site (e.g., soil texture, soil pH, organic material [OM] and CEC) (Figure 5-6, Table 5-4). As suggested by Figure 5-6, variability within sample units was relatively limited compared to variability among sample units, which supported the initial stratification argument from a sampling design and analysis perspective. Similarly, the distribution of selected target metals—both total and DTPA-extractable—in soil varied spatially, but the variation within the sample unit appeared less than the variation among sample units in MRW (Figure 5-7). Statistically, a nonparametric analysis of variance (ANOVA), multiple comparison test (Friedman's, P = 0.05; see Linder et al. 1994) indicated that sample units ranked high-to-low for selected target analytes (Cd, Cu, and Zn) as follows: Sample Unit 6 > Sample Units 7, 10 > Sample Unit 2 > Sample Units 8, 9, 12 > Sample Units 3, 4, 11. When these target analytes rankings were evaluated relative to the biological tests (e.g., earthworm and plant tests) completed on co-located soil samples, an integrated assessment of risk to biological and, by inference, ecological targets was developed (see Table 5-5, as well as Pascoe, Blanchet, Linder, Palawski et al. 1994).

a)

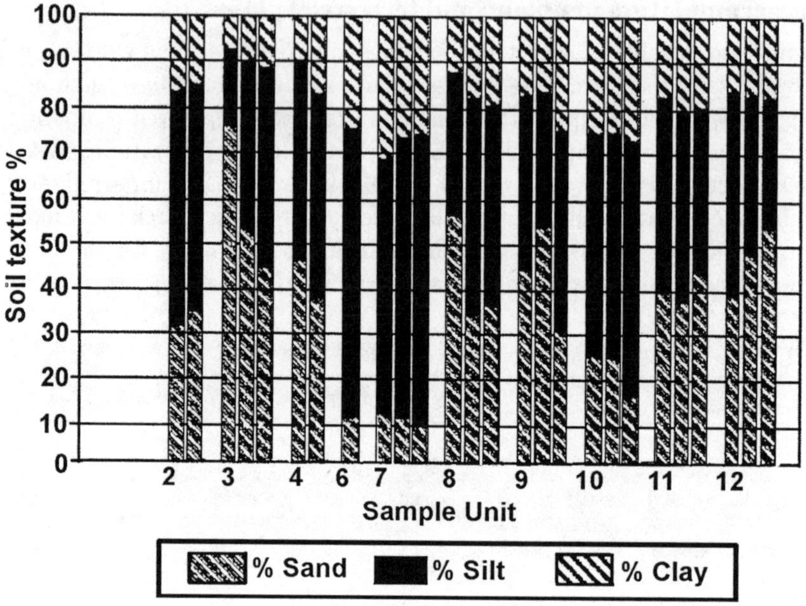

b)

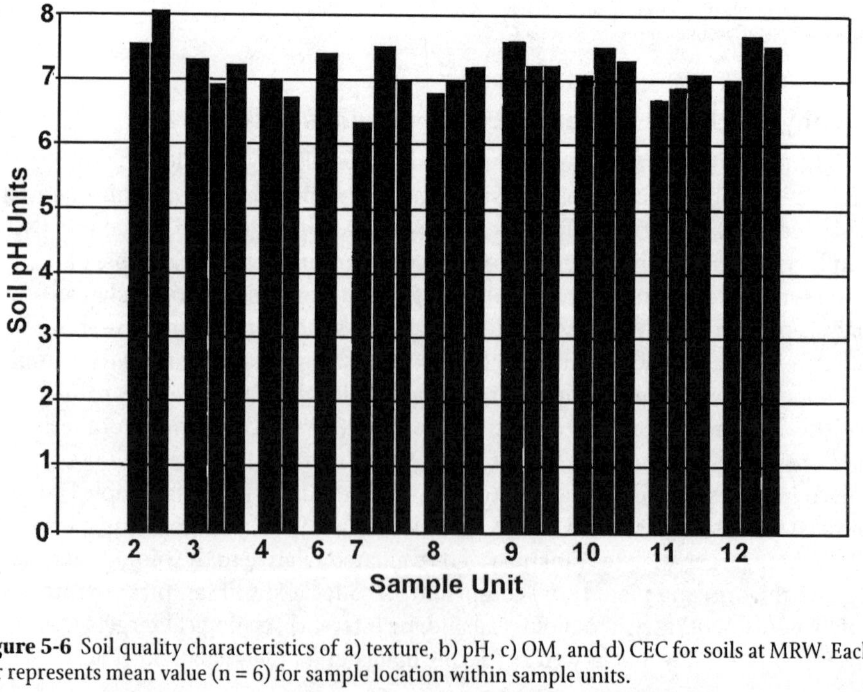

Figure 5-6 Soil quality characteristics of a) texture, b) pH, c) OM, and d) CEC for soils at MRW. Each bar represents mean value (n = 6) for sample location within sample units.

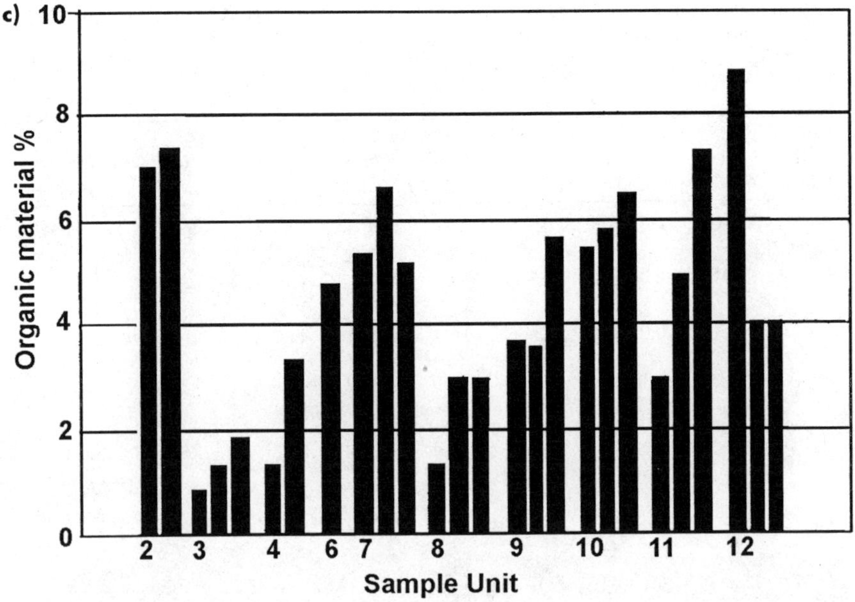

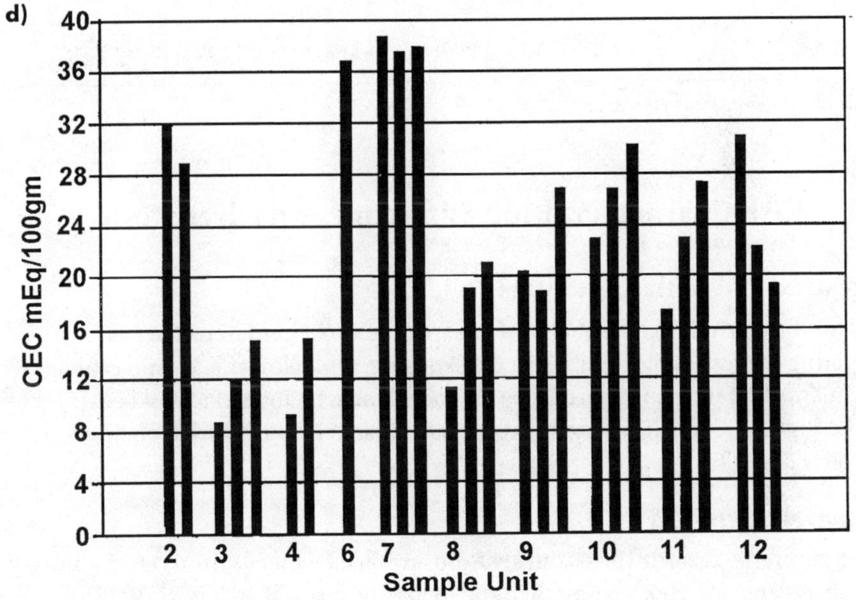

Figure 5-6 *continued*

Table 5-4 Soil analysis for MRW samples: pH, cation exchange capacity (CEC), total nitrogen (TN), organic matter (OM), and textural analysis[1]

	Soil analysis characteristic								
Sample Unit	pH (units)	CEC mEq/100g	TN (%)	OM (%)	Coarse (> 2mm)	Sand (2mm–50μm)	Silt (50–20μm)	Clay (< 2μm)	USDA textural classification
2	7.6–8.1	29.0–31.9	0.25–0.28	7.04–7.40	0.0	32.1–35.3	50.8–52.3	13.9–15.6	Silt loams
3	6.9–7.3	8.8–15.1	0.04–0.58	0.87–1.89	0.0	44.7–76.2	17.5–44.4	6.2–10.9	Sandy loams to loams
4	6.7–7.0	9.2–15.3	0.05–0.12	1.38–3.37	0.0–0.5	37.5–46.1	44.8–46.0	9.1–16.0	Loams
6	7.4	36.9	0.240	4.79	0.0	11.2	64.6	24.3	Silt loams
7	6.3–7.5	37.5–38.7	0.25–0.30	5.20–6.63	0.0	8.9–11.9	57.1–65.3	25.9–30.9	Silty clay loams to silt loams
8	6.8–7.2	11.5–21.1	0.07–0.14	1.38–3.01	0.0	33.7–55.9	31.9–48.1	12.2–19.9	Sandy loams to loams
9	7.2–7.6	18.8–26.9	0.16–0.23	3.57–5.66	0.0	29.5–52.8	30.3–44.9	16.9–25.6	Loams to sandy loams
10	7.1–7.5	22.9–30.2	0.25–0.27	5.46–6.48	0.0	14.7–24.0	499–57.2	26.0–28.1	Loams to silt loams to silty clay loams
11	6.7–7.1	17.3–27.2	0.11–0.25	2.96–7.29	0.0	35.7–42.4	36.6–42.4	18.4–21.8	Loams
12	7.0–7.7	19.3–30.9	0.16–0.27	4.03–8.83	0.0	45.9–51.8	29.2–36.7	17.4–19.0	Loams to sandy loams

[1] Sample Units 1 and 5 were not tested.

Risk Characterization Summary and Discussion

Terrestrial and wetland habitats

Risks for lower trophic components of the wetland ecosystem were assessed by integrating the results of the site-specific exposure, biological effects, and ecological assessments that were summarized by Pascoe, Blanchet, Linder, Palawski et al. (1994). Higher trophic-level organisms were evaluated through a food-chain model (Pascoe et al. 1996).

Soil macroinvertebrates

Sublethal effects to earthworms during exposures to soil metals from certain units were observable with both laboratory and field exposures (Linder et al. 1994). Sublethal effects were limited to a variety of malformations, including segmented swelling, segmental constriction, coiling, rigidity, flaccidity, cutaneous lesions, and behavioral patterns.

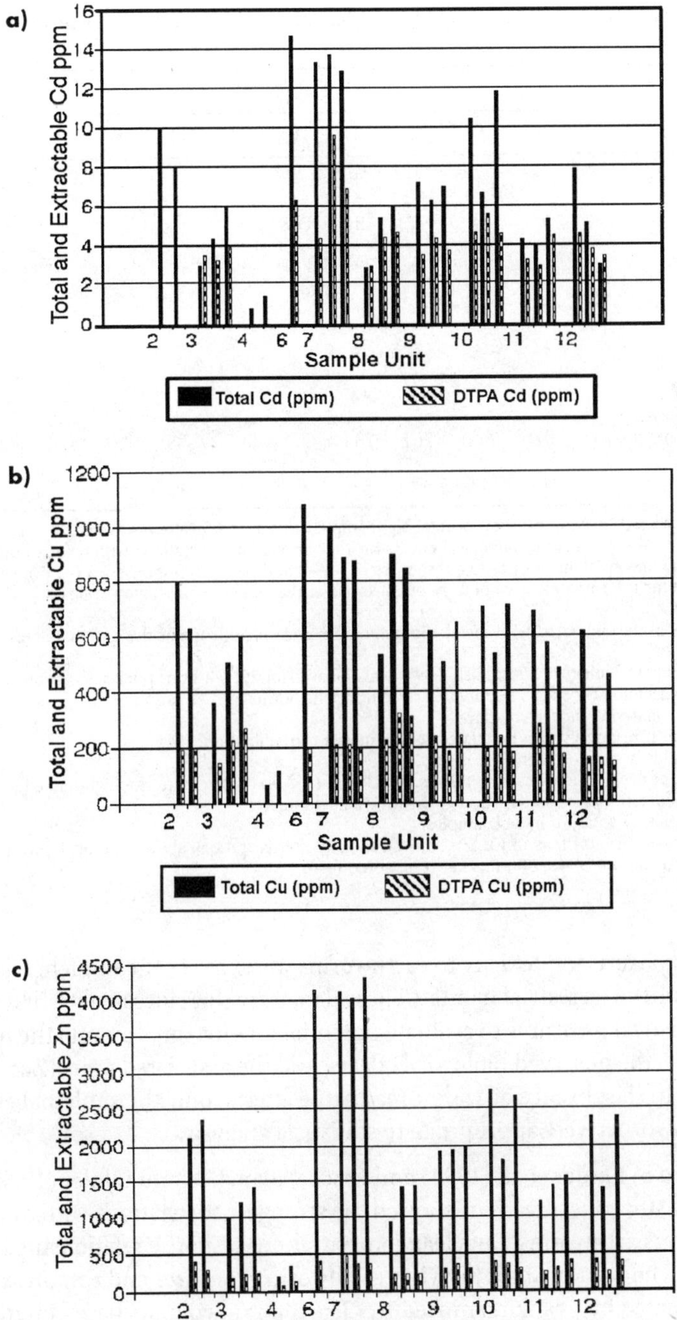

Figure 5-7 Selected metals in soils at MRW: a) total and DTPA-extractable Cd, b) Cu, and c) Zn. Each bar represents mean value (n = 6) for sample location within sample units.

Table 5-5 Summary of wetland studies at MRW: integration of biological and chemical aspects of the ecological triad

	Sample Units[a]									
Biological test[b]	7[c]	6[d]	8[c]	2[c]	10[e]	9[e]	11	3[e]	12	4[f]
Earthworm (field)	+	–	+	+	–	–	–	+/–	–	+/–
Earthworm (lab)	+/–	+	+	+	+/–	–	–	+	–	++
Root elongation	+		+	+	+/–	–	–	+	–	–
Seed germination				+						–
Biomass	+			+						
Sum biological[g]	++	+	++	++	+	+	–	+	–	++
Cu concentration (µg/g)[h]	975	870	761	734	654	595	585	529	470	244
Sum chemistry[i]	++	++	++	++	+	+	+	+	–	–

[a] Units are rank-ordered by concentration of total Cu; Sample Units 1 and 5 were not tested.
[b] Consistent statistical differences in biological effects for the various sample stations within each unit are graded as (+), inconsistent but positive responses as (+/–), and negative responses as (–). Unit 4 was scored (++) for the earthworm laboratory test because of the exceptionally high responses relative to other samples.
[c] Biological effects likely associated with metal contamination; units include major depositional areas of wetland.
[d] Inconsistent results in biological tests; likely low metals bioavailability; however, poor association was observed between biological effects and metals concentrations normalized to cation exchange capacity, organic material, or percent clay.
[e] Moderate biological responses may be related to low metals contamination.
[f] Biological effects likely due to other than metals.
[g] Relative ranking of overall biological test results. A value of (++) was assigned to the high-ranked units, (+) the moderate-ranked units, and (–) the low-ranked units.
[h] Mean concentration of total Cu in soil samples.
[i] Relative ranking of concentrations of Cu, Zn, and Cd in soils; concentrations above 500 mg/kg were scored (+), concentrations above 700 mg/kg were scored (++).

The data on exposure and toxicity to earthworms were the most complete relative to other studies of the terrestrial habitat. These data were therefore analyzed by a variety of statistical measures to evaluate potential relationships among the metal concentrations, the observed biological effects, and the associated units (Zar 1986; Sprent 1989). In the absence of widespread acute effects, only the sublethal effects noted in earthworms were appropriate to statistical analysis.

As summarized in Linder et al. (1994) and Pascoe, Blanchet, and Linder (1994), total and extractable Cu concentrations showed the strongest correlations with morphological effects in earthworms, but clear concentration–response relationships were not observed. The relationships between earthworm exposures and responses were therefore evaluated by a ranking procedure. The top-ranked units based on morphological endpoint measurements were Units 2, 8, 7, and 4. The top units ranked by total Cu concentration were Units 7, 6, 8, and 2. Qualitative comparison of the ranking results suggested a fairly good correlation by unit of sublethal effects and total metals or total Cu concentrations, with the exceptions of Units 4 and 6. Control responses with on-site reference soils ranged from 0 to 6.67%, and results of the ranking suggest an association of elevated earthworm responses with soil Cu concentrations exceeding 800 mg/g in Units 2, 7, and 8.

In an attempt to understand the factors that govern bioavailability of metals in MRW soils, further statistical analyses compared concentration–response relationships with physical and chemical characteristics of the soils. Regression analyses and nonparametric ANOVA tests consistently demonstrated a lack of correlation between sublethal effects in earthworms and CEC, percent OM, and percent clay of soils (Pascoe, Blanchet, Linder, Palawski et al. 1994). Normalization of metal concentrations to these variables failed to show correlations to sublethal effects that were any stronger than those with total Cu alone. Despite these poor correlations, the marked differences in soil characteristics between Units 4 and 6, for which biological responses differed greatly (Linder et al. 1994), suggest that unexamined properties of the soils of these units likely govern metals bioavailability and, hence, biological responses in wetland soils.

Terrestrial vegetation

The root zone study at the wetland operable unit demonstrated subtle biological effects from exposure to rhizosphere water and soil eluates in certain sampling units (Linder et al. 1994). Acute effects were not observed, but significant inhibition of root growth was observed in multiple species with root zone water from Units 7 and 8 when compared to control samples and samples from Units 9, 10, 11, and 12. Because of the preliminary nature of these studies, data on soil characteristics from these stations were unavailable to evaluate potential factors governing bioavailability of metals in the rooting zone.

In Pascoe, Blanchet, Linder, Palawski et al. (1994), possible threshold ranges for inhibitory effects on root growth were identified at Cd concentrations at 3 to 4 mg/L and of Zn at 1500 to 9000 mg/L in rooting zone water. Exceedance of these ranges was associated with root growth inhibition in samples from Units 7 and 8. In preliminary studies, root elongation also was inhibited in plants exposed to eluates of soil from Units 2 and 3. In general, the results suggested that the higher concentrations of metals in soils and rooting zone water from Units 2, 3, 7, and 8 were related to root growth inhibition under laboratory exposures.

Risks to primary consumers and higher-trophic-level organisms

Evaluation of risks to primary consumers and higher trophic-level organisms in the wetland habitat was performed by a food-chain evaluation. Exposures, expressed as daily intake, were compared to dose–response information (i.e., no-observed-adverse-effects levels [NOAELs] in mg/kg-d) from the scientific literature (Pascoe et al. 1996). The lack of toxicity information on most metals for many of the exposed species necessitated the use of dose-response data from rodents as surrogate toxicity criteria. Exposures were modeled from the results of field measurements in vegetation and other lower trophic biota as well as sediments, soils, and water (Pascoe et al. 1996).

Since the limited dataset for metals concentrations in vegetation and invertebrates at the site did not show correlations among concentrations and geographic locations on a unit basis (Linder et al. 1994; Pascoe, Blanchet, Linder, Palawski et al. 1994), site-wide average concentrations of metals in biota were used to model their trophic transfer. Receptors were assumed to be exposed to site-wide contaminants on a random basis. Given the limited habitat in upland areas of the site and the presence of the dam at the downstream end, it was assumed that all exposures, except for migrating species, occurred at the site for the receptors of concern (see Pascoe and DalSoglio 1994).

Complete results of the food-chain analysis are reported in Pascoe, Blanchet, and Linder (1994) and Pascoe et al. (1996), but the site-specific data on body burden measurements of As, Cd, Cu, Pb, and Zn in the meadow vole *(Microtus pennsylvanicus*) and deer mouse (*Peromyscus maniculatus*) suggested that soil metals bioavailability was limited to < 0.1% at the MRW (Pascoe, Blanchet, and Linder 1994). A conservative estimate of 10% was assumed for soil and sediment metals absorption by deer, waterfowl, and predatory birds. For all small mammals, regardless of modeled territory size, the highest estimated daily doses for As, Cd, Cu, and Zn were below the surrogate toxicity criteria (Pascoe et al. 1996). However, for muskrat (*Ondatra zibethicus*), consumption of aquatic vegetation from the depositional areas of the wetland (i.e., Units 2 and 7 in Figure 5-4) where metals concentrations were 2- to 10-fold greater than site-wide concentrations, the calculated Pb intake rate (0.23 mg/kg-d) exceeded the toxicity criterion. This was largely influenced by the preference of muskrat for cattails as the primary food source, which had elevated tissue concentrations of Pb in these areas.

Intake rates of metals calculated for waterfowl were below surrogate toxicity criteria (Pascoe et al. 1996). Similarly, intake rates of metals calculated for deer (*Odocoileus hemionus*), assuming partial forage time at the wetland, did not exceed surrogate toxicity criteria (Pascoe et al. 1996).

Summary of terrestrial risk characterization

A relative ranking scheme (Pascoe, Blanchet, Linder, Palawski et al. 1994) was used to summarize and integrate exposures and biological effects for the terrestrial habitat (Table 5-5). In this procedure, where consistent statistical differences in biological effects for the sample stations within each of the 10 sample units are observed, the unit is graded as a plus (+), inconsistent but positive responses as a plus/minus (+/–), and negative responses as a minus (–). (Unit 4 was scored as ++ for the earthworm laboratory test because of the exceptionally high responses relative to other samples.) Units were then ranked by the sum of ranks for the biological responses and by the concentrations of total Cu. For this ranking, a rating of "++" depicts the high-ranked units, "+" the moderate-ranked units, and "–" the low-ranked units. This comparison demonstrates the apparent association between total Cu concentrations and a variety of biological effects across the site, with Units 2, 7, and 8 standing out as having highest rankings for both chemistry and biological responses. For Units 4 and 6, normalizing for soil physical and chemical characteristics could not readily explain the observed inconsistencies between chemistry and biological response rankings.

The results of this comparison are depicted on a map of the wetland sampling units in Figure 5-8. Concentrations of total Cu and the sum of biological responses are shaded for moderate (+) and high (++) values (i.e., "+" is shaded with single lines and "++" with double lines, with the chemistry ranking depicted by vertical lines and the biological ranking by horizontal lines; the triangular representations are described below for sediment ranking).

The graphical depiction in Figure 5-8 illustrates the spatial correlation of biological responses with metals concentrations in the reservoir wetland soils. This type of presentation also demonstrates the higher concentrations of Cu and greater biological effects in sediments that have accumulated directly behind the dam in the old river channel (i.e., Unit 2) and behind the old railway berm (i.e., Units 7 and 8).

The sediment evaluations were critical to the evaluation of habitats at risk in the wetland. The weight of evidence from the sediment quality triad of chemistry, ecology, and toxicity studies suggests that benthic invertebrate communities in the reservoir are at risk in sediments where metal concentrations are elevated and acid-volatile sulfide (AVS) concentrations are low. Elevated metals in oxidizing environments are found in sediments of the old river channel (Unit 2) and upstream of the railroad berm (Unit 7) in the MRW (Ingersoll et al. 1994; Figure 5-8). Oxidizing environments at risk in the reservoir and upper CFR have been observed in shallow or fast-moving waters in depositional areas where metals concentrations are elevated. Sediment toxicity was generally observed where molar simultaneously extracted metal (SEM) Cu/AVS ratios exceeded unity, consistent with observations of others (refer to Ingersoll et al. 1994 for additional details).

The scaled ranking for the chemistry, toxicity, and benthos variables are plotted on maps of the reservoir operable unit as tri-axial graphs in Figure 5-8, as per Chapman et al. (1991). The tri-axial graphs depict geographic trends and the magnitude of the differences among station responses. A symmetrical triangle indicates similar chemistry, toxicity, and benthos responses; a larger triangle indicates a more severely degraded station. As an example of the utility of this type of presentation, the sediment sampling station MR-11 has large and relatively symmetrical triangles, representative of the elevated chemistry, toxicity, and impacted benthos which suggest metal-induced degradation of the sediment habitats in this area.

The food-chain study indicated that minimal risks to the health of primary consumers and higher trophic organisms are expected from the metals present in the wetland soils, vegetation, and lower trophic biota at the site. Any potential risks

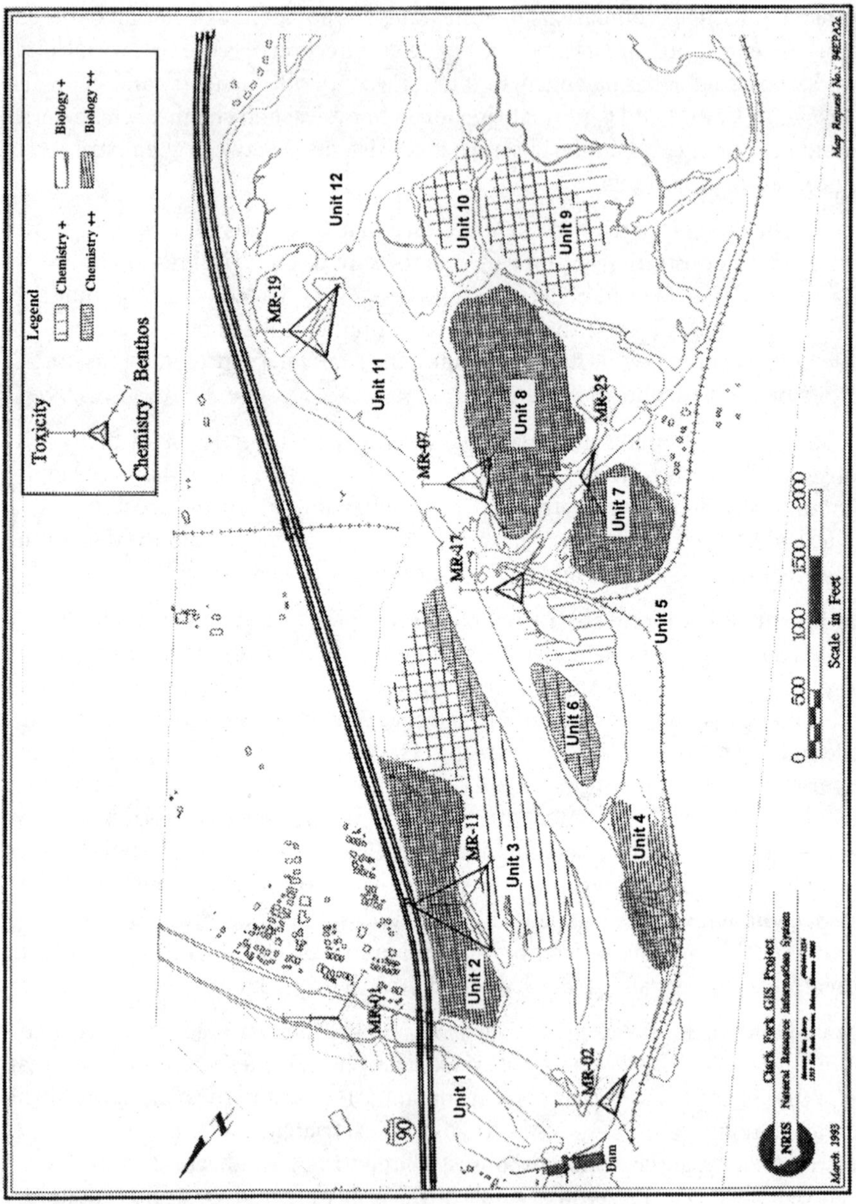

Figure 5-8 Geographic distribution of relative ecological risks at MRW

predicted from the site-specific toxicity tests do not appear to be expressed in ecological impacts, as suggested by the results of the wildlife survey and vegetation studies during the wetland delineation. Thus, although toxicity studies may suggest that elevated metals concentrations pose potential risks to the health of individual ecological receptors in the wetland habitats, risks to wetland populations and communities are likely minimal. The likelihood of limited metals bioavailability at the site, as suggested by results of small mammal studies (Pascoe, Blanchet, and Linder 1994) and soil chemistry studies described previously, further supports lower ecological effects than predicted by soil-contaminant data alone.

In summary, integrating information from the exposure, biological effects, and ecological assessments suggests that the soils of the old river channel near the interstate highway and the depositional area just upstream of the abandoned railroad berm pose the greatest risk for biological effects to terrestrial receptors.

Aquatic vegetation

Available evidence suggests that aquatic plants are not at risk for community or ecosystem impacts at moderately elevated metals concentrations, but because of the limited number of stations, observed biochemical effects suggestive of potential chronic effects may be due to the presence of elevated ammonia, metals, or other chemicals in the sediments at MRW (Linder et al. 1994). The correlation of aquatic plant effects and amphipod toxicity in the same sediments also suggests that emergent plants are good indicators of chemical contamination in the wetland at Milltown Reservoir (Pascoe, Blanchet, Linder, Palawski et al. 1994). For example, responses of emergent macrophytes to whole sediment exposures were significant for test locations that were also characterized by the highest concentrations of simultaneously extracted Cu and exceeded the toxicity criterion in the benthic analyses (Ingersoll et al. 1994).

The ecological component of the aquatic plant evaluations was based on qualitative observations during the wildlife survey and other field activities (USFWS 1991b; Linder et al. 1994). Although community structure analyses were not performed, field observations suggested that aquatic plant communities were healthy and widespread throughout the reservoir. Impacts to emergent plant communities were not observed, suggesting that subtle indications of stress to aquatic plants may not be associated with readily apparent risks to the aquatic ecosystem at Milltown Reservoir (Linder et al. 1994; Pascoe, Blanchet, Linder, Palawski et al. 1994)

Amphibians

The sublethal responses observed in amphibians during preliminary studies at Milltown Reservoir were insufficient for statistical analysis (Linder, Wyant et al. 1991). However, a possible association was noted between an increasing incidence of malformations from laboratory exposures to reservoir surface waters with increasing metals concentrations (Pascoe, Blanchet, Linder, Palawski et al. 1994). For example, no-effect concentrations (NECs) of metals in surface water at < 6% effects were associated with concentrations of Cd and Zn at 1 mg/L and 6 mg/L, respectively, and NECs in whole sediments associated with these water samples ranged from 300 to 450 mg/g for Cu and 650 to 1060 mg/g for Zn. Above these ranges, amphibian malformations in laboratory studies were > 20%. The NECs for amphibian responses are similar to the NEC values for simultaneously extracted Cu at 325 mg/g and Zn at 1064 mg/g based on amphipod responses (Pascoe, Blanchet, Linder, Palawski et al. 1994).

Results of preliminary studies on amphibian responses to surfacewater exposures were consistent with those of the sediment benthic analyses. Concentrations of metals in sediments at stations that were toxic to amphibians were in the range of concentrations where benthic invertebrate toxicity was observed (i.e., 300 to 450 mg/g for total Cu and 650 to 1060 mg/g for Zn). Although normalization of extractable metals concentrations to AVS was not completed in the preliminary year's work, the results of the amphibian studies support the estimated thresholds for risks to sediment biota.

Ecological Significance of Risk Assessment Findings

Understanding the ecological significance of the risk assessment results is essential to evaluating the overall risks to the wetland ecosystem. Risk managers rely on an adequate description of the significance of the risk findings when they make decisions about managing a contaminated ecosystem or watershed. Answering the question of ecological significance of the findings, however, depends on defining the relationships among different types of "significance." In general, the better the quality and the higher the quantity of data, the easier the determination of statistical significance. However, as pointed out by Barnthouse et al. (1989), very precise data can result in statistical significance even with biologically inconsequential results or low biological importance. Conversely, biologically significant trends and field observations should not be dismissed because they lack significance in a classical statistical analysis. Thus, biologically important impacts are defined as those that, as evaluated in toxicity bioassays, affect populations, communities, and ecosystems, rather than individuals. This definition is based on the understanding that measurement of impacts to individuals does not necessarily indicate impacts to the ecosystem. Biologically significant results, (e.g., impaired reproduction or teratogenicity) are the focus in setting long-term management goals for the site.

The definition of ecological significance can be further addressed by a relative ranking of impacts, as outlined by Duinker and Beanlands (1986):

- Major impact: Affects an entire population or species in sufficient magnitude to cause a decline in abundance and/or change in distribution beyond which natural recruitment (reproduction, immigration from unaffected areas) would not return that population or species, or any population or species dependent upon it, to its natural level.

- Moderate impact: Affects a portion of a population and may bring about a change in abundance and/or distribution over one or more generations but does not threaten the integrity of that population or any population dependent upon it.
- Minor impact: Affects a specific group of localized individuals within a population over a short period of time but does not affect other trophic levels or the population itself.
- Negligible impact: Any impacts below the minor category are considered negligible.

For the MRW/CFR risk assessment, the inclusion of quantitative studies on chemical exposures, biological effects assessment, and ecological studies was designed to help determine the ecological significance of the results by providing a link among these 3 legs of the risk assessment triad (Pascoe, Blanchet, Linder, Palawski et al. 1994).

Wetland and upland habitat findings

For the lower-trophic-level organisms, the sublethal effects observed in the toxicity studies could suggest subtle ecological impacts. The study of rooting zone impacts can illustrate the potential significance of sublethal effects measured in biological test systems. The rooting zone study demonstrated the inhibition of root growth in plants exposed to rhizosphere water from areas of high metals concentrations (i.e., Units 2, 7, and 8). An inhibition in root elongation in this bioassay suggests that lateral root growth may be inhibited in certain plant types in those units. Such inhibition could result in decreased absorption of nutrients, including Fe, and an imbalance in such nutrients as Cu and Zn. These alterations in turn could affect biomass above ground, as was demonstrated during the greenhouse study with soils from Units 2 and 7, and result in iron-deficiency chlorosis. Thus, the risks to wetland vegetation in depositional areas of the reservoir operable unit can be considered minor to moderate.

For the terrestrial habitats (i.e., the wetland and adjoining uplands viewed within a larger landscape setting), the findings of the exposure and biological effects assessments need to be placed in context with those of the ecological assessment to identify the significance of ecological risk. For example, results of the wildlife survey and wetland delineation study suggested a healthy wetland ecosystem on a site-wide basis. Thus, integration of the results of the ecological studies with the subtle effects observed in the bioassays suggests that the wetland ecosystem on a site-wide basis does not show substantial adverse ecological effects despite possible local impacts. Because community structure analyses of soil invertebrates were not performed, the link connecting the toxicity studies to the apparently healthy wildlife on a site-wide basis is missing. Also, the lack of community studies on smaller discrete areas of the wetland, such as those units identified as exhibiting biological effects, precludes their identification as ecologically impacted. In other words, whether the subtle effects observed in the earthworm and vegetation studies may be observable at the ecosystem level in smaller subunits of Units 2, 7, and 8 has not been studied.

The scientific literature provides little to form a basis for translating the subtle toxicity test results, such as earthworm morphological changes, to impacts on site ecology. Terrestrial community structure analyses would provide more definitive answers to the ecological significance of the subtle effects observed in the toxicity bioassays.

The foodweb analysis demonstrated that primary consumers and higher-trophic-level organisms like predatory birds, waterfowl, and deer are not at high risk from exposures to site-related contaminants. This conclusion was supported by the finding of low bioavailability of soils metal. The only potential concern was the effect of the modeled intake of metals on muskrat. Given the uncertainties in the modeled intake and the lack of toxicity data on muskrat, it is unlikely that the exposures would be expressed in population or ecosystem impacts. In addition, the waterfowl survey at the wetland suggested that the populations of Canada geese and various duck species are healthy and reproducing. No evidence was observed of contaminated sediment-dwelling invertebrates affecting the health of waterfowl in the wetland. Similarly, the food-chain transfer study did not suggest that metals in invertebrates or aquatic plants would impact muskrats, beaver, or mink in the wetland.

In summary, the biological assessment studies and food-chain analysis suggested that overt acute toxic effects were lacking from the terrestrial or wetland soils exposures and that the sublethal effects observed would not likely increase ecosystem risks. From this, risks to the terrestrial habitat can best be characterized as minor (Pascoe, Blanchet, Linder, Palawski et al. 1994; Pascoe et al. 1996).

Aquatic habitat findings

For the aquatic habitats, including those emergent zones of the wetland, elevated exposures to sediment metals correlated with toxicity to benthic invertebrates and impacted benthic community structure. The finding of increased number of genera of Chironomidae in sediments exhibiting toxicity to benthic invertebrates suggests an imbalance in the benthic community that is due to the metals contamination. Overt effects, such as the decreased abundance or loss of taxa observed in major groups of biota in contaminated Great Lakes sediments, are not apparent in Milltown Reservoir or CFR sediments. However, as described in Canfield et al. (1994), the type of imbalance seen in benthic community structure at the site has been observed in other studies of sediments with high metals concentrations and can be explained by a disturbance in population competition dynamics.

The significance of the risk assessment findings for the sediment benthic habitat can be described as moderate for the benthic communities in oxidizing environments. Although sediment ecology is imbalanced at contaminated stations under oxidizing conditions, it is unknown whether other ecological parameters, such as predator–

prey relationships, are subsequently affected by this imbalance. The impacted benthic invertebrates in both the upper CFR and the reservoir operable units are likely of greater significance to trout populations through the transfer of metals during feeding.

While the wetlands at Milltown Reservoir presented few high-risk characteristics, the baseline risk assessment for the MRW-CFR clearly suggested that the upper river and wetlands were interconnected and could not be viewed as disjointed features in the landscape. A number of lines of evidence indicated that severe impacts of contaminant metals on the fishery of the upper CFR were likely. For example, concentrations of various metals in surface water of the upper CFR have exceeded water quality criteria, and metals concentrations are elevated in invertebrates from riffle and depositional areas. Toxicity tests have demonstrated that fish health is adversely affected following exposure to water and sediment at metals concentrations typical of the upper CFR, and trout behavior in toxicity tests suggests avoidance of elevated metals concentrations is likely to occur. Fish with reduced growth rate and health could be eliminated from natural populations where metals stresses are present, and their potential avoidance of CFR water may prevent adequate access to suitable habitat and food sources. The weight of evidence from fishery studies indicates that the health of trout populations and the fishery ecology of the upper CFR are at major risk from the metals contamination. Furthermore, one of the concerns for evaluating MRW was the potential for chronic impacts from metals releases during such episodic events as spring snowmelt and summer thunderstorms (Pascoe and DalSoglio 1994). Because the ecological and in situ biological assessments were performed during summer and fall, the results of the studies could be representative of conditions after the spring snowmelt. Because spring flows of the upper CFR prior to the risk assessment sampling program were high enough to increase metals concentrations in surface waters, the study results may be reflective of conditions during recovery from acute impacts (Pascoe, Blanchet, Linder, Palawski et al. 1994).

Conclusions

The ecological risk assessment at MRW suggests that no acute toxicity or adverse biological effects are occurring at present. Consistently, and regardless of the field or laboratory test methods used, biological assessments at MRW were unable to demonstrate acute toxicity; however, evidence of subtle biological effects was noted in samples collected from depositional areas. Future remediation plans should weigh the potential biological and ecological impacts associated with remediation efforts against the current impacts associated with elevated metals in soils and sediments. While the current subtle effects and potential effects should not be understated in the ecological risk assessment for MRW, currently any widespread physical alteration of wetland habitats may be neither beneficial nor technically justified. Future site monitoring should address problems that may occur with remediation at MRW and at upstream operable units and, in particular, should consider the long-term effects of metal exposures on vegetation in the depositional areas. Also, indirect effects resulting from site management (e.g., habitat alteration associated with reduced vegetative growth that may result from "walk-away" [no remedial action] or sediment-dredging decisions) should be considered as a potential consequence of the metals that presently occur in the soils and sediments at MRW.

References

[ASTM] American Society for Testing and Materials. 1997. Annual book of ASTM standards. Volume 11.05, Biological effects and environmental fate; biotechnology, pesticides. West Conshohocken PA: ASTM.

Barnthouse LW, Suter GW, Rosen AE. 1989. Inferring population level significance from individual-level effects: an extrapolation from fisheries science to ecotoxicology. In: Suter GW, Lewis MA, editors. Aquatic toxicology and environmental fate. Volume 11. Philadelphia PA: American Society for Testing and Materials. ASTM STP 1007.

Brumbaugh WG, Ingersoll CG, Kemble NE, May TW, Zajicek JL. 1994. Chemical characterization of sediments and pore water from the upper Clark Fork River and Milltown Reservoir, Montana. *Environ Toxicol Chem* 13:1971–1983.

Canfield TJ, Kemble NE, Brumbaugh WG, Dwyer FJ, Ingersoll CG, Fairchild JF. 1994. Use of benthic invertebrate community structure and the Sediment Quality Triad to evaluate metal-contaminated sediment in the upper Clark Fork River, Montana. *Environ Toxicol Chem* 13:1999–2012.

Chapman PM, Power EA, Dexter RN, Andersen HB. 1991. Evaluation of effects associated with an oil platform, using the sediment quality triad. *Environ Toxicol Chem* 10:407–424.

Cowardin LM, Carter V, Golet FC, Blake E. 1979. Classification of wetlands and deepwater habitats of the United States. Washington DC: Biological Services Program. Fish and Wildlife Service, U.S. Department of the Interior. FWS/OBS-79/31.

Davis DE. 1982. Handbook of census methods for terrestrial vertebrates. Boca Raton FL: CRC Press. 397 p.

Duinker PN, Beanlands GE. 1986. The significance of environmental impacts: an exploration of the concept. *Environ Manage* 10(1):1–10.

Farag AM, Boese CJ, Woodward DF, Bergman HL. 1994. Physiological changes and tissue metal accumulation in rainbow trout exposed to foodborne and waterborne metals. *Environ Toxicol Chem* 13:2021–2029.

[FICWD] Federal Interagency Committee for Wetland Delineation. 1989. Federal manual for identifying and delineating jurisdictional wetlands. Washington DC: U.S. Army Corps of Engineers, U.S. Environmental Protection Agency, U.S. Fish and Wildlife Service, and USDA Soil Conservation Service. Cooperative technical publication.

Greene JC, Bartels C, Warren-Hicks W, Parkhurst B, Linder G, Peterson S, Miller W. 1989. Protocols for short term toxicity screening of hazardous waste sites. Corvallis OR: USEPA Environmental Research Laboratory. EPA/600/3-88/029.

Gysel LW, Lyon LJ. 1980. Habitat analysis and evaluation. In: Schemnitz S, editor. Wildlife management techniques manual. 4th ed. Washington DC: The Wildlife Society. p 305–327.

Ingersoll CG, Brumbaugh WG, Dwyer FJ, Kemble NE. 1994. Bioaccumulation of metals by *Hyallela azteca* exposed to contaminated sediments from the upper Clark Fork River, Montana. *Environ Toxicol Chem* 13:2013–2020.

Kaputska L. 1989. Vegetation assessment. In: Warren-Hicks W, Parkhurst B, Baker Jr S, editors. Ecological assessment of hazardous waste sites. Corvallis OR: U.S. Environmental Protection Agency. EPA/600/3-89/013.

Kemble NE, Brumbaugh WG, Brunson EL, Dwyer FJ, Ingersoll CG, Monda DP, Woodward DF. 1994. Toxicity of metal-contaminated sediments from the upper Clark Fork River, Montana, to aquatic invertebrates and fish in laboratory exposures. *Environ Toxicol Chem* 13:1985–1997.

Klute A. 1986. Methods of soil analysis, Part 1. Physical and mineralogical methods. 2nd ed. Madison WI: American Society of Agronomy and Soil Science Society of America. 1188 p.

Linder G, Bollman M, Wilborn D, Nwosu J, Baune W, Smith S, Ott S, Callahan C. 1991. Final technical report for the preliminary field survey and on-site, in situ and laboratory evaluations completed at Milltown Reservoir. Prepared for U.S. Environmental Protection Agency, Region 8, Helena, Montana. Corvallis OR: ManTech Environmental Technology, Inc.

Linder G, Hazelwood R, Palawski D, Bollman M, Wilborn D, Malloy J, DuBois K, Ott S, Pascoe G, DalSoglio J. 1994. Ecological assessment for the wetlands at Milltown Reservoir, Missoula, Montana: characterization of emergent and upland habitats. *Environ Toxicol Chem* 13:1957–1970.

Linder G, Ingham E, Henderson G, Brandt CJ. 1992. Evaluation of terrestrial indicators for use in ecological assessments at hazardous waste sites. EPA 600/R-92-183. Corvallis OR: U.S. Environmental Protection Agency, Environmental Research Laboratory.

Linder G, Wyant J, Meganck R, Williams B. 1991. Evaluating amphibian responses in wetlands impacted by mining activities in the western United States. In: Fifth Biennial Symposium on Issues and Technology in the Management of Impacted Wildlife. Boulder CO: Thorne Ecological Institute. p 17–25.

Lipton J. 1993. Aquatic resources injury assessment, Upper Clark Fork River Basin. Prepared for the State of Montana, Helena, MT. Boulder CO: RCG/Hagler, Bailly, Inc.

McBee K. 1989. Field surveys: terrestrial vertebrates. In: Warren-Hicks W, Parkhurst B, Baker Jr S, editors. Ecological assessment of hazardous waste sites. Corvallis OR: U.S. Environmental Protection Agency. EPA/600/3-89/013.

Montana Power Company. 1992. Milltown fisheries protection, mitigation, and enhancement plan. Butte MT: Montana Power Company.

Moore JN, Luoma SN. 1990. Hazardous waste from large-scale metal extraction: the Clark Fork waste complex, MT. In: Watson V, editor. Proceedings of the Clark Fork River symposium. Missoula MT: University of Montana.

Ohmart RD, Anderson BW. 1986. Riparian habitats. In: Inventory and monitoring of wildlife habitat. Cooperrider AY, Boyd RJ, Stuart HR, editors. Denver CO: U.S. Dept. Inter., Bur. Land Manage. Service Center.

Page AL, Miller RH, Keeney DR. 1982. Methods of soil analysis, Part 2. Chemical and microbiological properties. Madison WI: American Society of Agronomy and Soil Science Society of America.

Pascoe GA. 1993. Wetland risk assessment. *Environ Toxicol Chem* 12:2293–2307.

Pascoe GA, Blanchet RJ, Linder G. 1994. Bioavailability of metals to small mammals at a metals-contaminated wetland. *Arch Environ Contam Toxicol* 27:44–50.

Pascoe GA, Blanchet RJ, Linder G. 1996. Food-chain analysis of exposures and risks to wildlife at a metals-contaminated wetland. *Arch Environ Contam Toxicol* 30:306–318.

Pascoe GA, Blanchet RJ, Linder G, Palawski D, Brumbaugh WG, Canfield TJ, Kemble NE, Ingersoll CG, Farag A, DalSoglio JA. 1994. Characterization of ecological risks at the Milltown Reservoir/Clark Fork River Sediments Superfund Site, Montana. *Environ Toxicol Chem* 13:2043–2058.

Pascoe GA, DalSoglio JA. 1994. Planning and implementation of a comprehensive ecological risk assessment at the Milltown Reservoir/Clark Fork River Superfund Site, Montana. *Environ Toxicol Chem* 13:1943–1956.

[SCS] Soil Conservation Service. 1951. Soil survey manual. Washington DC: U.S. Department of Agriculture. Handbook No. 18. 503 p.

Sprent P. 1989. Applied nonparametric statistics. New York: Chapman and Hall. 259 p.

Stollar RL. 1990. Groundwater monitoring. In: Devinny JS, Everett LG, Lu JCS, Stollar RL, editors. Subsurface migration of hazardous wastes. New York: Van Rostrand Reinhold. p 169–266.

Suter GW. 1993. Ecological risk assessment. Chelsea MI: Lewis. 538 p.

Suter GW, Loar JM. 1992. Weighing the ecological risk of hazardous waste sites: the Oak Ridge case. *Environ Sci Technol* 26:432–438.

[USEPA] U.S. Environmental Protection Agency. 1986. Testing methods for evaluating solid waste. Washington DC: USEPA Office of Solid Waste and Emergency Response. SW-846.

[USEPA] U.S. Environmental Protection Agency. 1992. Framework for ecological risk assessment. Washington DC: Risk Assessment Forum. EPA/630/R-92-001.

[USEPA] U.S. Environmental Protection Agency. 1997. Ecological risk assessment guidance for Superfund. Process for designing and conducting ecological risk assessments. Interim final report. Washington DC: USEPA. EPA/540/R-97/006.

[USFWS] U.S. Fish and Wildlife Service. 1991a. Milltown Reservoir sediments site endangerment assessment wetland delineation and classification. U.S. Fish and Wildlife Service, Fish and Wildlife Enhancement, Montana State Office, Helena, MT. Prepared for U.S. Environmental Protection Agency, Region 8, Montana Office, Helena MT (Interagency Agreement No. DW 14953503-01-0).

[USFWS] U.S. Fish and Wildlife Service. 1991b. Milltown Reservoir sediments site endangerment assessment wildlife survey. U.S. Fish and Wildlife Service, Fish and Wildlife Enhancement, Montana State Office, Helena, MT. Prepared for U.S. Environmental Protection Agency, Region 8, Montana Office, Helena, MT (Interagency Agreement No. DW 14953503-01-0).

Warren-Hicks W, Parkhurst B, Baker Jr S. 1989. Ecological assessment of hazardous waste sites. Corvallis OR: USEPA, Environmental Research Laboratory. EPA/600/3-89/013.

Wilborn DC, Bollman MA, Gillett CS, Ott SL, Linder GL, Callahan CA. 1997. A field screening method using the earthworm (*Eisenia foetida andrei*) to evaluate contaminated soils. In: Dwyer FJ, Doane TR, Hinman ML, editors. Environmental toxicology and risk assessment: modeling and risk assessment. 6th ed. Philadelphia PA: American Society for Testing and Materials. STP 1317. p 490–517.

Woessner WW, Moore JM, Johns C, Popoff M, Sartor L, Sullivan M. 1984. Arsenic source and water supply remedial action study, Milltown, Montana. Missoula MT: Univ Montana.

Woodward DF, Brumbaugh WG, DeLonay AJ, Little EE, Smith CC. 1994. Effects on rainbow trout fry of a metals-contaminated diet of benthic invertebrates from the Clark Fork River, Montana. *Trans Am Fish Soc* 123:51–62.

Woodward DF, Farag AM, Bergman HL, DeLonay AJ, Little EE. 1994. Metals contaminated benthic invertebrates in the Clark Fork River, Montana: Determining effects of early life stage rainbow trout and brown trout. *Can J Fish Aquat Sci* 52(9):1994–2004.

Zar JH. 1986. Biostatistical analysis. Englewood Cliffs NJ: Prentice-Hall. 620 p.

CHAPTER 6

Case Study: Contaminant Impacts on Freshwater Wetlands: Kesterson National Wildlife Refuge, California

A. Dennis Lemly

Limited availability of water was one of the major obstacles to early settlement of many arid regions in the western U.S. (Reisner 1986). The shortage of water and perceived need to homestead on desert lands led to the establishment of the U.S. Bureau of Reclamation (then named the Reclamation Service) in 1902. The primary mission of this agency was to "reclaim" unproductive lands by bringing water to arid regions and turning desert into farmland. This reclamation began in earnest with the completion of the Newlands Water Project in Nevada in 1915 and reached a peak with the building of such massive projects as Hoover Dam on the Colorado River, the California Aqueduct across the Mojave Desert, and the Central Valley Irrigation Project in California (Reisner 1986). However, the price for this reclamation and associated increase in agricultural production was a sharp reduction in the amount of water available to native wetlands. Battles for water rights between settlers, farmers, urban developers, and water authorities in the west have raged for well over 100 years (Reisner 1986), but only in the last few decades have the water needs of remnant native wetlands gained significant attention. Private conservation groups and the U.S. Fish and Wildlife Service (USFWS) now consider the issue of water quantity and quality for wetlands to be a priority concern throughout the western states (Rude 1989; USDOI 1991).

CHAPTER PREVIEW

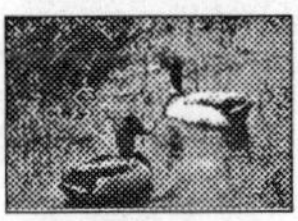

Ecotoxicology and Risk Assessment for Wetlands. Michael A. Lewis et al., editors.
 ISBN 1-880611-16-3

Water quantity is an issue because massive amounts of water have been diverted for human use. For example, most of the historic flows of the upper and middle reaches of the San Joaquin River, CA, are impounded and diverted for agricultural irrigation (Clifton and Gilliom 1989; State of California 1990). Native fishes and aquatic communities have disappeared and the once important runs of Chinook salmon (*Oncorhynchus tshawytscha*) no longer take place (Moyle 1976; Moore et al. 1990). About 90% of the historic wetlands in California's Central Valley is gone, and more than 60% of the entire waterfowl population in the Pacific flyway is now channeled into the remaining wetlands during migration (Flayer et al. 1989). The potential for contaminant impacts under these circumstances is maximized because large numbers of birds are crowded into small areas, where they may be more susceptible to disease outbreaks brought on by contaminant-related stress (Gilmer et al. 1982). A similar situation exists in Nevada, where native wetlands along the Carson River have declined in response to a 90% reduction in freshwater inflows (Rowe and Hoffman 1987; Thompson and Merritt 1988; Hoffman, Hallock et al. 1990; Hallock et al. 1992).

Water quality was recognized as a priority issue in the early 1980s when contamination was discovered at Kesterson National Wildlife Refuge in California. Agricultural irrigation water applied to nearby farmlands leached naturally occurring trace elements from the soil and carried these contaminants to the refuge in return flows (subsurface drainwater) used as part of the water supply for wetland management within the Kesterson Reservoir portion of the refuge. The contaminants, particularly Se, accumulated in aquatic food chains and resulted in massive poisoning of fish and wildlife (Tanji et al. 1986; Presser and Ohlendorf 1987; Ohlendorf et al. 1989). Although not as well known or publicized as Kesterson Reservoir, similar episodes of contamination from irrigation drainage have occurred at other locations (Stephens et al. 1988; Sylvester et al. 1988; Hoffman, Hallock et al. 1990; Hallock et al. 1992: Seiler and Skorupa 1995).

Trace elements, pesticides, and salts associated with agricultural irrigation drainwater pose a serious contaminant threat to wetlands in arid regions of the western United States (USDOI 1986; Sylvester et al. 1988; Moore et al. 1990; Seiler and Skorupa 1995). In the mid-1980s, the U.S. Department of the Interior (USDOI) began extensive field and laboratory studies to identify and evaluate the toxicological significance of contaminants in irrigation drainage (USDOI 1990a, 1990b). The initial research focused on aquatic habitats and wildlife resources in California (Moore et al. 1990) but later included many other wetlands throughout the western states (USDOI 1986; Sylvester et al. 1988; Seiler and Skorupa 1995). This paper examines the history and implications of the irrigation drainage problem by presenting a case history of Kesterson Reservoir on the Kesterson National Wildlife Refuge.

The Kesterson Story

Water development and irrigation drainage

In response to concerns about reliability of water supplies, a major federal water delivery and irrigation project was proposed for California's Central Valley in the mid-1930s (Moore et al. 1990). The Central Valley Project (CVP) was proposed for a variety of purposes including navigation, flood control, land reclamation, water storage and delivery, and public recreation, but today about 85% of the total consumptive use of water from the CVP is for irrigation of agricultural crops (State of California 1990). Although remarkable in its ability to stimulate agricultural production, intensive irrigation of this arid valley has detrimentally affected the land for many years. By 1940, substantial San Joaquin Valley farm acreage was abandoned because of salt buildup and poor drainage (California Department of Water Resources 1974).

In 1949, the U.S. Bureau of Reclamation (USBR) submitted a status report to the U.S. Congress, recommending additional water development in the San Joaquin Valley. The USBR also noted that because subsurface soils on the west side of the valley consisted of impervious clay that prevented deep infiltration of water, continued intensive irrigation would eventually demand that drainage systems be installed to collect and convey return flows to the Sacramento–San Joaquin River Delta, San Francisco Bay, and the Pacific Ocean (Moore et al. 1990). The first subsurface drainage systems were installed in the 1960s, concurrent with the construction of the San Luis Unit of the CVP (Beck 1984). Irrigation drainwater was dealt with on a piecemeal basis until the late 1970s, when the San Joaquin Valley Interagency Drainage Program was formed to review drainage needs for the valley. That program recommended construction of a valley-wide master drain with a series of flow-regulating reservoirs to be operated as wetlands for wildlife (IDP 1979).

The master San Luis Drain was originally designed to be operated in conjunction with adjacent regulating reservoirs to seasonally discharge subsurface irrigation wastewater into the San Joaquin–Sacramento River Delta during periods of high outflow, thereby ensuring drainage water dilution. Kesterson Reservoir (a series of 12 shallow ponds) was the first regulating reservoir to be built (Moore et al. 1990). In 1970, the USFWS and the USBR signed a cooperative agreement for management of Kesterson Reservoir and associated wetlands. That agreement formally established 2390-ha Kesterson National Wildlife Refuge (NWR) and specified that the USFWS manage the area for wildlife and associated recreational values, but retained the right for USBR to use the reservoir for management of irrigation drainwater (Zahm 1986). By 1972, only 132 km of the intended 302 km of the master drain were finished, and project funds were depleted. The 520-ha Kesterson Reservoir became the terminus of the drain, and its 12 shallow ponds functioned as an evaporation and seepage basin (Zahm 1986; Moore et al. 1990).

Through the mid-1970s, the master drain conveyed a mixture of operational spillage from valley water projects, agricultural surface runoff, and subsurface drainage. In 1978 the proportion of subsurface drainwater increased, and by 1981 almost all of the flows discharged into Kesterson Reservoir were composed of subsurface drainage generated by 3240 ha of irrigated agricultural lands in the Wetlands Water District of the San Luis Unit (Zahm 1986). In 1980–1981, samples of water from the drain and Kesterson Reservoir were found to be highly saline and contained elevated concentrations of Se, other trace elements, and metals (Saiki 1986a). In 1982–1983, greatly elevated concentrations of selenium were detected in aquatic invertebrates, fish, and wildlife at Kesterson Reservoir (Saiki 1986b; Ohlendorf 1986; Ohlendorf, Hoffman et al. 1986). By 1985, death and deformities had affected thousands of aquatic birds, and the "poisoned" refuge became highly publicized (Marshall 1985; Popkin 1986). Although irrigation drainwater was strongly implicated as the cause of the problem, data available at the time were not sufficient to positively link contaminants in the drainwater to observed toxic effects. In 1986, the USFWS and the USBR entered into an agreement to fund studies on the effects of agricultural irrigation drainwater on fish and wildlife populations. That agreement initiated a multi-year research effort conducted by USFWS research centers.

Field studies of contaminant bioaccumulation and toxicity

Beginning in 1982, 4 years before the formal USFWS–USBR research agreement was signed, biological surveys were conducted by the USFWS to determine the extent and severity of contamination in aquatic food chains at Kesterson Reservoir and to identify the primary contaminants of concern for further study (Saiki 1986a, 1986b; Ohlendorf, Hoffman et al. 1986). Extensive chemical analyses of 12 trace elements, 23 pesticides, nutrients, and ionic composition revealed that Se concentrations were greatly elevated in the water, detritus, and organisms present in the reservoir. It was apparent that Se was the most important constituent for detailed toxicological study. Some of the highest concentrations of Se ever reported for fish tissues (370 μg/g dry weight) were found in these early studies. Aquatic invertebrates and forage fish contained from 1000 to 5000× the concentrations of Se present in the water, which clearly illustrated bioaccumulation. Aquatic birds (e.g., grebes, coots, waterfowl, and shorebirds) that fed on these aquatic organisms similarly showed significant bioaccumulation of Se.

Later surveys confirmed high selenium concentrations and identified boron as another constituent of concern, particularly in regard to avian reproduction (Saiki and Lowe 1987; Hothem and Ohlendorf 1989; Schuler et al. 1990; Ohlendorf et al. 1990). Elevated Se concentrations were found in all animal types living in Kesterson Reservoir, including fish, birds, insects, frogs, snakes, and small mammals (Saiki 1986a; Clark 1987; Ohlendorf, Hothem, and Aldrich 1988; Ohlendorf et al. 1989). The finding of high Se concentrations in food organisms of predatory birds and endangered species such as the San Joaquin kit fox (*Vulpes macrotis mutica*) resulted in additional emphasis being placed on rapid, thorough assessment of the toxic threat of irrigation drainage.

Although farmers in the valley used many kinds of agricultural chemicals, these potentially toxic compounds were absent in drainwater and biological samples. Irrigation surface runoff can contain high concentrations of pesticides and herbicides (Presser and Barnes 1985; Moore et al. 1990), but the natural biological and chemical filter provided by the soil effectively degrades and removes these materials as irrigation water percolates downward to form subsurface drainage (Neil 1987; Fujii 1988; Nishimura and Baughman 1988). At the same time, naturally occurring trace elements in the soil, such as Se and B, are leached out under the alkaline, oxidizing conditions prevalent in the valley and are carried in solution in the drainwater (Presser and Ohlendorf 1987; Deverel and Millard 1988).

The concentrations of Se identified in the biological samples were of great concern because field studies indicated a high frequency of mortality and developmental deformities, a known symptom of Se poisoning, in the embryos and hatchlings of waterfowl and other aquatic birds nesting at Kesterson Reservoir (Ohlendorf, Hothem et al. 1986; Ohlendorf et al. 1989; Williams et al. 1989). Congenital malformations were often multiple and consisted of missing eyes and feet, protruding brains, and grossly deformed beaks, legs, and wings (Ohlendorf, Hoffman et al. 1986; Ohlendorf, Kilness et al. 1988; Hoffman et al. 1988). Four species of ducks (mallard, *Anas platyrhynchos*; pintail, *A. acuta*; cinnamon teal, *A. cyanoptera*; and gadwall, *A. strepera*), coot (*Fulica americana*), avocet (*Recurvirostra americana*), grebe (*Podiceps nigricollis*), and stilt (*Himantopus mexicanus*) were affected. The deformities observed in these wild birds closely matched those seen in experimental studies of Se toxicity in domestic chickens, and the amount of selenium in food organisms eaten by aquatic birds at Kesterson equaled or exceeded concentrations known to cause mortality and deformities in chicken embryos (Hoffman et al. 1988; Hothem and Ohlendorf 1989). Several pathological and biochemical indicators of Se toxicosis were also found in the adult wild birds (Ohlendorf, Kilness et al. 1988). Other field studies documented a massive fish kill in the San Luis Drain near at Kesterson Reservoir in 1983 (Saiki 1986a), followed by a high frequency (30%) of stillbirths in mosquitofish (*Gambusia affinis*), the only fish species remaining in the reservoir (Saiki et al. 1991). Tissue concentrations of Se in these mosquitofish were greater than those associated with reproductive failure in fish populations of reservoirs impacted by Se from coal-fired power plants in the eastern U.S. (Lemly 1985). Collectively, the field evidence strongly implicated Se as the cause of mortality and reproductive failure in fish and wildlife populations at Kesterson Reservoir. However, detailed laboratory studies were also conducted to identify specific cause–effect relationships and establish toxicity thresholds for Se and other trace elements of concern.

Laboratory evaluation of contaminant fate and effects

Laboratory studies with aquatic organisms were conducted using 1.0-L closed-system aquatic microcosms to determine how different environmental conditions affected the chemical speciation of selenium in water and sediments and bioaccumulation in food chains (Besser et al. 1989, 1993). Dissolved Se was removed from the water column in 3 ways: uptake by biota, sorption onto sediments, and transformation into volatile Se compounds with subsequent diffusion into the atmosphere. Fine, organic-rich sediments caused a more rapid flux of Se into the substrate than did coarse sand. The net movement and bioaccumulation of Se was unaffected by the concentration of dissolved S (80 to 180 mg/L), which has been found to affect Se uptake in studies that did not use closed-system microcosms. Inorganic forms of (selenate, selenite) were more persistent in the water column than organic (selenomethionine), but the organic form was bioaccumulated to a much greater degree than the inorganic forms (Besser et al. 1989). Dissolved organic Se concentrations as low as 0.04 µg/L were bioaccumulated up to 382,000 times, resulting in food-chain Se residues sufficient to poison predatory species of fish and wildlife (5 to 15 µg/g dry weight) (Besser et al. 1993; Lemly 1993). Comparable food-chain residues were not attained with inorganic Se until waterborne concentrations reached 10 µg/L (selenite) to 100 µg/L (selenate), indicating that organoSe compounds may contribute disproportionately to Se bioaccumulation and toxicity in aquatic ecosystems (Besser et al. 1993).

Another series of studies was conducted to determine toxic effects of dietary and waterborne Se on growth, survival, behavior, and reproduction of invertebrates, fish, and waterfowl. Some of the representative data are summarized in Table 6-1. The major conclusions of these investigations were as follows:

1) Organic Se is generally much more toxic than inorganic Se to fish and wildlife, both in waterborne and dietary exposures (relative toxicity: selenomethionine = 100 to 1000, selenite = 10, selenate = 1).
2) Reproductive effects were induced to a greater extent by organic Se (selenomethionine) than inorganic forms (selenate, selenite), and teratogenic effects like those observed in the field at Kesterson Reservoir were induced only by organic Se.
3) Significant sublethal physiological, biochemical, and behavioral effects were found that add to the overall toxic threat of Se.
4) Selenomethionine is a good experimental model for the forms of organic Se occurring naturally in food-chain organisms in the field.
5) The most sensitive indicator of Se toxicity in fish and waterfowl is reproductive failure.
6) Reproductive effects often occur with no mortality or visible toxic symptoms in the adults.

Table 6-1 Toxicity of Se to fish, wildlife, and invertebrates in studies conducted as part of the USDOI's Kesterson Reservoir irrigation drainwater investigations

Species and life stage	Exposure and duration	Toxic effect	Reference
Cladoceran (*Daphnia magna*) neonates[1]	Waterborne, 48-h acute		Ingersoll et al. 1990
	Selenate	LC50 = 2.56 mg/L	
	Selenite	LC50 = 0.70 mg/L[2]	
	6:1 Selenate/selenite mixture	LC50 = 1.79 mg/L	
	Seleno[L]-methionine	50 to 70% mortality at 4 to 8 µg/L	
	Waterborne, 21-d life cycle	Reproduction impaired at 348 µg/L[2]	
	6:1 Selenate/selenite mixture		
Midge (*Chironomus riparius*) neonates[1]	Waterborne, 48-h acute		Ingersoll et al. 1990
	Selenate	LC50 = 10.5 mg/L	
	Selenite	LC50 = 14.6 mg/L	
	6:1 Selenate/selenite mixture	LC50 = 14.3 mg/L	
	Seleno[L]-methionine	LC50 = 6.88 mg/L	
	Waterborne, 30-d life cycle		
	6:1 Selenate/selenite mixture	Reproduction impaired at 6.05 mg/L	
Rainbow trout (*Oncorhynchus mykiss*) sac fry	Waterborne, 90-d chronic		Hunn et al. 1987
	Selenite	35 to 70% mortality at 47 to 100 µg/L[2]	
Chinook salmon (*Oncorhynchus tshawytscha*) fry	Waterborne, 96-h acute		Hamilton and Buhl 1990
	Selenate	LC50 = 115 mg/L	
	Selenite	LC50 = 13.8 mg/L	
	6:1 Selenate/selenite mixture	LC50 = 50.9 mg/L	
	Seleno[DL]-methionine	No effect to 21.6 mg/L[3]	
Chinook salmon (*Oncorhynchus tshawytscha*) fry	Waterborne, 120-d chronic		USDOI 1990a
	Selenate	No effect to 139 µg/L	
	Selenite	No effect to 139 µg/L	
	6:1 Selenate/selenite mixture	No effect to 130 µg/L	

Table 6-1 *continued*

Species and life stage	Exposure and duration	Toxic effect	Reference
Chinook salmon (*Oncorhynchus tshawytscha*) fingerlings	Dietary, 60 to 100-d chronic		
	Natural Se[4]	30 to 50% mortality at 26 mg/kg[5]; reduced growth[2], impaired behavior, and reduced smolting at 6.5 mg/kg	Hamilton et al. 1986
		35 to 50% mortality at 9 to 35 mg/kg[2]; reduced growth at 5.3 mg/kg	Hamilton et al. 1990
	Seleno[DL]-methionine	5 to 50% mortality at 9.5 to 35 mg/kg2; impaired behavior at 18.2 mg/kg; seawater mortality at 35.4 mg/kg	Hamilton et al. 1990
Coho salmon (*Oncorhynchus kisutch*) fry	Waterborne, 96-h acute		Hamilton et al. 1990
	Selenate	LC50 = 32.5 mg/L	
	Selenite	LC50 = 7.80 mg/L	
	6:1 Selenate/selenite mixture	LC50 = 24.5 mg/L	
Striped bass (*Morone saxatilis*) fingerlings	Waterborne, 96-h acute		USDOI 1990a
	Selenate	LC50 = 39.0 mg/L	
	Selenite	LC50 = 1.0 mg/L[2]	
	6:1 Selenate/selenite mixture	LC50 = 15.0 mg/L	
	Seleno[L]-methionine	LC50 = 4 µg/L	
	Waterborne, 90-d chronic		
	Selenate	No effect to 3.0 mg/L	
	Selenite	No effect to 3.0 mg/L	
	6:1 Selenate/selenite mixture	No effect to 3.0 mg/L	
Bluegill (*Lepomis macrochirus*) juveniles[6]	Waterbone, 96-h acute		USDOI 1990a
	Selenate	LC50 = 98.0 mg/L	
	Selenite	LC50 = 7.8 to 13 mg/L	
	6:1 Selenate/selenite mixture	Mortality at > 13.0 mg/L	
	Seleno[L]-methionine	LC50 = 13 µg/L	
	Seleno[DL]-methionine	LC50 = 13 mg/L	
	Waterborne, 30 to 60-d chronic		
	6:1 Selenate/selenite mixture	50 to 97% mortality at 1.4 to 5.3 mg/L; abnormal behavior at 1.4 mg/L	
Bluegill (*Lepomis macrochirus*) juveniles	Dietary, 90-d chronic		USDOI 1990a
	Seleno[L]-methionine	Reduced growth at 16.7 mg/kg[5]; no mortality to 33.3 mg/kg	

Table 6-1 *continued*

Species and life stage	Exposure and duration	Toxic effect	Reference
Bluegill (*Lepomis macrochirus*) adults	Waterborne, 140-d chronic		Coyle et al. 1993
	6:1 Selenate/selenite mixture	No effect to 8 µg/L	
	Dietary, 140-d chronic Seleno[L]-methionine	No direct effect[7] to 33.3 mg/kg[5]; impaired reproduction at 33.3 mg/kg[2]; toxic threshold for reproductive effects = 16 to 33 mg/kg[2]	
Mallard (*Anas platyrhynchos*) ducklings	Dietary, 42-d chronic		Heinz et al. 1988
	Selenite	25 to 97% mortality at 40 to 80 mg/kg[5]; reduced growth at 20 mg/kg	
	Selenomethionine	12.5 to 100% mortality at 40 to 80 mg/kg[2]; reduced growth at 20 mg/kg	
	Dietary, 28-d chronic Seleno[DL]-methionine	100% mortality at 60 mg/kg[2]; reduced growth at 15 mg/kg; physiological effects at 15 mg/kg	Hoffman et al. 1991
Mallard adults	Dietary, 120-d chronic		
	Selenite	No direct effect[7] to 10 mg/kg; 95% mortality at 100 mg/kg; impaired reproduction at 25 mg/kg[2]	Heinz et al. 1987
	Seleno[DL]-methionine	No direct effect[7] at 10 mg/kg[5]; impaired reproduction at 10 mg/kg[2]; teratogenesis in young at 10 mg/kg[2]	Hoffman and Heinz 1988
Mallard adults	Dietary, 120-d chronic		
	Selenite	No direct effect[7] to 25 mg/kg[5]; impaired reproduction at 25 mg/kg	Hoffman and Heinz 1988
	Seleno[DL]-methionine	No direct effect[7] to 16 mg/kg; impaired reproduction at 8 mg/kg[2]; teratogenesis in young at 8 mg/kg[2]	Heinz et al. 1987
Mallard adults	Dietary, 120-d chronic		
	Seleno[DL]-cystine	No direct effect[7] at 16 mg/kg[5]; no reproductive effect at 16 mg/kg	Heinz et al. 1989
	Seleno[DL]-methionine	No direct effect[7] to 16 mg/kg; impaired reproduction at 8 mg/kg[2]; teratogenesis in young at 8 mg/kg[2]; toxic threshold for reproductive effects = 4 to 8 mg/kg[2]	
		Hepatotoxicity at 8 mg/kg[2]	Hoffman et al. 1992

1 All individuals were less than 24-h old at the initiation of tests.
2 For comparision, subsurface irrigation drainage contains as much as 1400 µg/L (1.4 mg/L) selenium and can result in fish and wildlife dietary intake of > 200 mg/kg Se.
3 The notation "no effect to" indicates no effect through the concentration indicated, which was a maximum of a range of concentrations tested in the study.
4 The source of selenium was selenium-contaminated fish collected from the field.
5 Dietary selenium concentration on a dry weight basis.
6 Individuals were 5 months old at the initiation of tests.
7 Effects on growth, condition factor, gonado-somatic index, survival, physiology, and apparent health of adults.

7) Selenium is biochemically transferred from parents to the offspring in eggs, where it causes teratogenesis and mortality as the yolk and albumin are absorbed during early development and hatching.
8) Selenium has the ability to bioaccumulate in aquatic food chains and, thereby, contaminate the diet and induce reproductive effects in fish and waterfowl even though total waterborne concentrations are far below levels of concern for direct toxicity.
9) Concentrations of Se in subsurface irrigation drainage typically range from 75 to 1400 μg/L (Presser and Ohlendorf 1987; Fujii 1988; Barnum and Gilmer 1988), yet concentrations of only 1 to 3 μg/L may be sufficient to load aquatic food chains with residues that reduce the reproductive success of fish and wildlife.
10) Once in an aquatic system, Se is biologically accumulated, transformed, and cycled such that the ultimate toxic threat to fish and wildlife is similar regardless of whether the chemical form coming into the system is predominantly selenate or selenite.
11) The concentrations of Se present at Kesterson Reservoir were 10 to 500× greater than the toxic effect thresholds for fish and wildlife.

Other laboratory studies examined the toxicity of B (Smith and Anders 1989; Hamilton and Buhl 1990; Hoffman, Camardese et al. 1990; Hoffman et al. 1991), which is also commonly found at greatly elevated concentrations in drainwater environments. The findings indicated that B could be toxic to fish and wildlife at concentrations similar to those occurring at Kesterson Reservoir, from the standpoint of both direct toxicity and reproductive effects (effects due to teratogenesis were unique to Se). Moreover, the results showed that the combined toxicity of B–Se mixtures to ducklings was approximately additive, particularly when the nutritional status of birds was compromised because of reduced protein in the diet (Hoffman et al. 1991). Arsenic was also determined to be a drainwater contaminant with the potential to poison wildlife by interacting with Se and B (Camardese et al. 1990; Whitworth et al. 1991; Hoffman et al. 1992). Studies of whole and diluted irrigation drainwater indicated that direct waterborne toxicity to fish was caused by atypical ratios of major ions (Ca, chloride, Mg, Na) and sulfate, in addition to trace elements such as Se and B (Saiki et al. 1992). Collectively, these findings indicated that the overall toxicity observed at Kesterson Reservoir was not caused exclusively by Se; several other factors contributed to the problem by degrading water quality and affecting the nutritional status and health of fish and wildlife.

Cleanup costs and implications for managing wetlands

Soon after the toxic threat of contaminants in irrigation drainage was verified (1984–1985), the Secretary of the Interior, citing concerns over possible violation of the Federal Migratory Bird Treaty Act, officially closed Kesterson NWR to the public, began a hazing program to scare waterfowl and other wildlife away from the reservoir, and issued an order for the San Luis Drain to be plugged (USGAO 1987). By June 1986, all irrigation drainage flows into Kesterson ponds had stopped. In 1987, USBR implemented a cleanup plan that called for drainage of the contaminated wetlands, excavation and on-site disposal of contaminated soil and plant material in a lined and capped containment area, and long-term site monitoring to detect possible seepage of contaminated water (USGAO 1987). The cost of the cleanup was about $50 million (USGAO 1987; San Joaquin Valley Drainage Program 1988). The lands comprising Kesterson Reservoir were removed from the national refuge system and placed under the jurisdiction of USBR for management as a contaminated landfill. To offset this loss of wetlands, some 9500 ha of private lands adjoining the refuge were purchased and developed into waterfowl and upland wildlife habitat (USGAO 1987; San Joaquin Valley Drainage Program 1990). The total cost of mitigating Se contamination at Kesterson was about $60 million (1987 dollars), not including the ongoing cost of long-term site monitoring.

Agricultural irrigation drainwater clearly has the potential to severely impact fish and wildlife populations. Moreover, once the aquatic environment is contaminated, cleanup is extremely expensive. Kesterson NWR is a classic example of what can happen if irrigation drainwater is used to support wetlands in an arid environment without careful evaluation of the drainwater constituents and other important factors. The conditions at Kesterson—geological sources of Se, mobilization and transport mechanisms, concentrating mechanisms, sites for bioaccumulation—and the resulting biogeochemical pathway for Se have been termed the "Kesterson effect." The Kesterson effect is present at some locations throughout the western states (Presser and Ohlendorf 1987; Presser 1994), which points to the need for wetland managers throughout the West to identify and evaluate water sources and biota that could be contaminated with irrigation drainage. This is particularly important for public lands because 200 wildlife refuges and management areas in the western U.S. receive water from more than 400 USDOI water projects, most of which consist of agricultural irrigation-drainage facilities constructed by the USBR (1981). Concerns voiced by the news media, environmentalists, politicians, and scientists about the health and well-being of other wildlife refuges and arid wetlands became persistent following the Kesterson episode (Harris 1991). In 1986 the USDOI established a federal multi-agency program headed by the U.S. Geological Survey to investigate irrigation-related drainwater problems throughout the western U.S. To date, this program has identified numerous sites where irrigation drainwater contaminants threaten wetland biota (Lemly et al. 1993; Presser et al. 1994; Seiler and Skorupa 1995).

Conclusions

Since the mid-1800s, development of agriculture-based economies in the western United States has taken a tremendous toll on wetlands. The quantity and quality of these historic natural areas have been severely reduced, and many of the remnant wetlands that remain are being contaminated by agricultural drainwater. The Kesterson episode marked the turning point in understanding the extent and severity of this threat to fish and aquatic birds throughout the western U.S. Subsurface irrigation drainage is the most widespread and biologically significant source of contaminants to wetlands in arid regions and threatens waterfowl populations in both the Pacific and Central flyways. The public is also at risk, and human health warnings have been issued in drainwater-affected areas.

The quantity of water reaching most of the remaining wetlands has been severely reduced because historic freshwater inflows have been diverted for agricultural and municipal use. In some cases, the loss of inflows has been partially replaced by irrigation return flows, but drainwater is highly saline and contaminated. Freshwater inflows will determine the ultimate fate of wetlands in the arid western U.S. It is not realistic to expect agriculture to cease for the benefit of wetlands, but a better balance must be achieved in the way water is allocated between agriculture and wildlife. Otherwise, many wetlands will be degraded as salts and contaminants build up, a process that is already well underway at several important national wildlife refuges. Federally subsidized irrigation has supported agriculture at the expense of wetlands for nearly 100 years in the western U.S. This trend must be reversed if the wetlands and their associated fish and wildlife populations are to survive.

References

Barnum DA, Gilmer DS. 1988. Se levels in biota from irrigation drainwater impoundments in the San Joaquin Valley, California. *Lake Reservoir Manage* 4:181–186.

Beck LA. 1984. Case history: San Joaquin Valley. *California Agriculture* 38:16–17.

Besser JM, Canfield TJ, LaPoint TW. 1993. Bioaccumulation of organic and inorganic Se in a laboratory food chain. *Environ Toxicol Chem* 12:57–72.

Besser JM, Huckins JN, Little EE, LaPoint TW. 1989. Distribution and bioaccumulation of Se in aquatic microcosms. *Environ Pollut* 62:1–12.

California Department of Water Resources. 1974. Status of San Joaquin Valley drainage problems. Bulletin No. 127-74. Sacramento CA: California Department of Water Resources. 66 p.

Camardese MB, Hoffman DJ, LeCaptain LJ, Pendleton GW. 1990. Effects of arsenate on growth and physiology in mallard ducklings. *Environ Toxicol Chem* 9:785–795.

Clark Jr DR. 1987. Se accumulation in mammals exposed to contaminated California irrigation drainwater. *Sci Total Environ* 66:147–168.

Clifton DG, Gilliom RJ. 1989. Sources and concentrations of dissolved salts and Se in the San Joaquin River and its tributaries, California, October 1985 to March 1987. Water-Resources Investigations Report 88-4217. Sacramento CA: U.S. Geological Survey. 33 p.

Coyle JJ, Buckler DR, Ingersoll CG, Fairchild JF, May TW. 1993. Effect of dietary Se on the reproductive success of bluegills (*Lepomis macrochirus*). *Environ Toxicol Chem* 12:551–565.

Deverel SJ, Millard SP. 1988. Distribution and mobility of Se and other trace elements in shallow groundwater of the western San Joaquin Valley, California. *Environ Sci Technol* 22:697–702.

Flayer WE, Peters DD, Pywell HR. 1989. Wetlands of the California Central Valley: status and trends—1939 to mid-1980s. Portland OR: U.S. Fish and Wildlife Service. 29 p.

Fujii R. 1988. Water-quality and sediment-chemistry data of drainwater and evaporation ponds from Tulare Lake Drainage District, Kings County, California, March 1985 to March 1986. Open-File Report 87-700. Sacramento CA: U.S. Geological Survey. 19 p.

Gilmer DS, Miller MR, Bauer RD, LeDonne JR. 1982. California's Central Valley wintering waterfowl: concerns and challenges. *Trans North Am Wildlife Nat Resources Conf* 47:441–452.

Hallock RJ, Hoffman RJ, Thompson SP, Burge HL. 1992. Irrigation drainage in and near Stillwater, Humboldt, and Fernley wildlife management areas and Carson Lake, West-Central Nevada, 1988–1990. Part II. Effects on wildlife. Carson City NV: U.S. Geological Survey. Water-Resources Investigation Report 92-401.

Hamilton SJ, Buhl KJ. 1990. Acute toxicity of boron, molybdenum, and Se to fry of Chinook salmon and coho salmon. *Arch Environ Contam Toxicol* 19:366–373.

Hamilton SJ, Palmisano AN, Wedemeyer GA, Yasutake WT. 1986. Impacts of Se on early life stages and smoltification of fall Chinook salmon. *Trans North Am Wildlife Nat Resources Conf* 51:343–356.

Hamilton SJ, Buhl KJ, Faerber NL, Wiedmeyer RH, Bullard FA. 1990. Toxicity of organic Se in the diet to Chinook salmon. *Environ Toxicol Chem* 9:347–358.

Harris T. 1991. Death in the marsh. Covelo CA: Island Press. 245 p.

Heinz GH, Hoffman DJ, Gold LG. 1988. Toxicity of organic and inorganic Se to mallard ducklings. *Arch Environ Contam Toxicol* 17:561–568.

Heinz GH, Hoffman DJ, Gold LG. 1989. Impaired reproduction of mallards fed an organic form of Se. *J Wildlife Manage* 53:418–428.

Heinz GH, Hoffman DJ, Krynitsky AJ, Weller DMG. 1987. Reproduction in mallards fed Se. *Environ Toxicol Chem* 6:423–433.

Hoffman DJ, Camardese MB, LeCaptain LJ, Pendleton GW. 1990. Effects of boron on growth and physiology in mallard ducklings. *Environ Toxicol Chem* 9:335–346.

Hoffman RJ, Hallock RJ, Rowe TG, Lico MS, Burge HL, Thompson SP. 1990. Reconnaissance investigation of water quality, bottom sediment, and biota associated with irrigation drainage in and near Stillwater Wildlife Management Area, Churchill County, Nevada, 1986–1987. Water-Resources Investigations Report 89-4105. Carson City NV: U.S. Geological Survey. 150 p.

Hoffman DJ, Heinz GH. 1988. Embryotoxic and teratogenic effects of Se in the diet of mallards. *J Toxicol Environ Health* 24:477–490.

Hoffman DJ, Ohlendorf HM, Aldrich TW. 1988. Se teratogenesis in natural populations of aquatic birds in central California. *Arch Environ Contam Toxicol* 17:519–525.

Hoffman DJ, Sanderson CJ, LeCaptain LJ, Cromartie E, Pendleton GW. 1991. Interactive effects of boron, Se, and dietary protein on survival, growth, and physiology in mallard ducklings. *Arch Environ Contam Toxicol* 20:288–294.

Hoffman DJ, Sanderson CJ, LeCaptain LJ, Cromartie E, Pendleton GW. 1992. Interactive effects of arsenate, Se, and dietary protein on survival, growth, and physiology in mallard ducklings. *Arch Environ Contam Toxicol* 22:55–62.

Hothem RL, Ohlendorf HM. 1989. Contaminants in foods of aquatic birds at Kesterson Reservoir, California, 1985. *Arch Environ Contam Toxicol* 18:773–786.

Hunn JB, Hamilton SJ, Buckler DR. 1987. Toxicity of sodium selenite to rainbow trout fry. *Water Res* 21:233–238.

[IDP] San Joaquin Valley Interagency Drainage Program. 1979. Agricultural drainage and salt management in the San Joaquin Valley: final report including recommended plan and first-stage environmental impact report. Fresno CA: IDP.

Ingersoll CG, Dwyer FJ, May TW. 1990. Toxicity of inorganic and organic Se to *Daphnia magna* (Cladocera) and *Chironomus riparius* (Diptera). *Environ Toxicol Chem* 9:1171–1181.

Lemly AD. 1985. Toxicology of Se in a freshwater reservoir: Implications for environmental hazard evaluation and safety. *Ecotoxicol Environ Safety* 10:314–338.

Lemly AD. 1993. Guidelines for evaluating Se data from aquatic monitoring and assessment studies. *Environ Monitor Assess* 28:83–100.

Lemly AD, Finger SE, Nelson MK. 1993. Sources and impacts of irrigation drainwater contaminants in arid wetlands. *Environ Toxicol Chem* 12:2265–2279.

Marshall E. 1985. Se poisons refuge, California politics. *Science* 229:144–146.

Moore SB, Winckel J, Detwiler SJ, Klasing SA, Gaul PA, Kanim AR, Kesser BE, DeBevec AB, Beardsley A, Puckett LK. 1990. Fish and wildlife resources and agricultural drainage in the San Joaquin Valley, California. Sacramento CA: San Joaquin Valley Drainage Program. 867 p.

Moyle PB. 1976. Inland Fishes of California. Berkeley CA: Univ California Pr. 405 p.

Neil JM. 1987. Data for selected pesticides and volatile organic compounds for wells in the western San Joaquin Valley, California, February to July 1985. Sacramento CA: U.S. Geological Survey. 10 p. Open-File Report 87-48.

Nishimura GH, Baughman S. 1988. Agricultural drainage conditions in the San Joaquin Valley. Technical Report. Sacramento CA: San Joaquin Valley Drainage Program. 40 p.

Ohlendorf HM. 1986. Aquatic birds and Se in the San Joaquin Valley. In: Howard AQ, editor. Se and agricultural drainage: implications for San Francisco Bay and the California environment (Se II). Tiburon CA: The Bay Institute of California. p. 14–24.

Ohlendorf HM, Hoffman DJ, Saiki MK, Aldrich TW. 1986. Embryonic mortality and abnormalities of aquatic birds: apparent impacts of Se from irrigation drainwater. *Sci Total Environ* 52:49–63.

Ohlendorf HM, Hothem RL, Aldrich TW. 1988. Bioaccumulation of Se by snakes and frogs in the San Joaquin Valley, California. *Copeia* 1988:704–710.

Ohlendorf HM, Hothem RL, Bunck CM, Aldrich TW, Moore JF. 1986. Relationships between Se concentrations and avian reproduction. *Trans North Am Wildlife Nat Resources Conf* 51:330–342.

Ohlendorf HM, Hothem RL, Bunck CM, Marois KC. 1990. Bioaccumulation of Se in birds at Kesterson Reservoir, California. *Arch Environ Contam Toxicol* 19:495–507.

Ohlendorf HM, Hothem RL, Welsh D. 1989. Nest success, cause-specific nest failure, and hatchability of aquatic birds at Se-contaminated Kesterson Reservoir and a reference site. *Condor* 91:787–796.

Ohlendorf HM, Kilness AW, Simmons JL, Stroud RK, Hoffman DJ, Moore JF. 1988. Se toxicosis in wild aquatic birds. *J Toxicol Environ Health* 24:67–92.

Popkin R. 1986. Kesterson: nonpoint nightmare. *EPA Journal* 12:13–14.

Presser TS. 1994. The Kesterson effect. *Environ Manage* 18:437–454.

Presser TS, Barnes I. 1985. Dissolved constituents including Se in waters in the vicinity of Kesterson National Wildlife Refuge and the west Grassland, Fresno and Merced counties, California. Water-Resources Investigations Report 85-4220. Menlo Park CA: U.S. Geological Survey. 73 p.

Presser TS, Ohlendorf HM. 1987. Biogeochemical cycling of Se in the San Joaquin Valley, California, USA. *Environ Manage* 11:805–821.

Presser, TS, Sylvester MA, Low WH. 1994. Bioaccumulation of Se from natural geologic sources in the western states and its potential consequences. *Environ Manage* 18:423–436.

Reisner M. 1986. Cadillac desert: the American West and its disappearing water. New York: Viking Penguin. 582 p.

Rowe TG, Hoffman RJ. 1987. Wildlife kills in the Carson Sink, western Nevada, winter 1986–1987. *U.S. Geological Survey Water-Supply Paper* 2350:37–40.

Rude, K. 1989. Squeezing out water for wildlife. *Ducks Unlimited Magazine*. March/April 1989: 30–32.

Saiki MK. 1986a. A field example of Se contamination in an aquatic food chain. Fresno CA: California Agricultural Technology Institute. Publication No. CAT1/860201. p 67–76.

Saiki MK. 1986b. Concentrations of Se in aquatic food-chain organisms and fish exposed to agricultural tile drainage water. In Howard AQ, editor. Selenium and agricultural drainage: implications for San Francisco Bay and the California environment (Se II). Tiburon CA: The Bay Institute of California. p. 25–33.

Saiki MK, Jennings MR, Hamilton SJ. 1991. Preliminary assessment of the effects of Se in agricultural drainage on fish in the San Joaquin Valley. In: Dinar A, Zilberman D, editors. The economics and management of water and drainage in agriculture. Boston MA: Kluwer Academic. p 369–385.

Saiki MK, Jennings MR, Wiedmeyer RH. 1992. Toxicity of agricultural subsurface drainwater from the San Joaquin Valley, California, to juvenile Chinook salmon and striped bass. *Trans Am Fish Soc* 121:78–93.

Saiki MK, Lowe TP. 1987. Se in aquatic organisms from subsurface agricultural drainage water, San Joaquin Valley, California. *Arch Environ Contam Toxicol* 16:657–670.

San Joaquin Valley Drainage Program. 1988. Status Report 10. Sacramento CA: San Joaquin Valley Drainage Program. p 1–3.

San Joaquin Valley Drainage Program. 1990. Status Report 17. Sacramento CA: San Joaquin Valley Drainage Program. p 1.

Schuler CA, Anthony RG, Ohlendorf HM. 1990. Se in wetlands and waterfowl foods at Kesterson Reservoir, California, 1984. *Arch Environ Contam Toxicol* 19:845–853.

Seiler RL, Skorupa JP. 1995. Identification of areas at risk for Se contamination in the western United States. In: Water resources at risk. Denver CO: American Institute of Hydrology. p LL-85–LL-94.

Smith GJ, Anders VP. 1989. Toxic effects of boron on mallard reproduction. *Environ Toxicol Chem* 8:943–950.

State of California. 1990. Irrigation water use in the Central Valley of California. Sacramento CA: California Department of Water Resources. 58 p.

Stephens DW, Waddell B, Miller JB. 1988. Reconnaissance investigation of water quality, bottom sediment, and biota associated with irrigation drainage in the Middle Green River Basin, Utah, 1986–1987. Water-Resources Investigations Report 88-4011. Salt Lake City UT: U.S. Geological Survey. 70 pp.

Sylvester MA, Deason JP, Feltz HR, Engberg RA. 1988. Preliminary results of the Department of the Interior's irrigation drainage studies. In: Symposium proceedings: planning now for irrigation and drainage. Reston VA: Irrigation Division, American Society of Civil Engineers. p 665–677.

Tanji K, Lauchli A, Meyer J. 1986. Selenium in the San Joaquin Valley. *Environment* 28:6–39.

Thompson SP, Merritt KL. 1988. Western Nevada wetlands—history and current status. *Nevada Public Affairs Review* 1:40–45.

[USBR] U.S. Bureau of Reclamation. 1981. Water and power resource services project data. Washington DC: U.S. Bureau of Reclamation. 1496 p.

[USDOI] U.S. Department of the Interior. 1986. Contaminant issues of concern on national wildlife refuges. Washington DC: U.S. Fish and Wildlife Service, Division of Refuge Management. 162 p.

[USDOI] U.S. Department of the Interior. 1990a. Agricultural irrigation drainwater studies in support of the San Joaquin Valley Drainage Program—final report. Columbia MO: U.S. Fish and Wildlife Service, National Fisheries Contaminant Research Center. 309 p.

[USDOI] U.S. Department of the Interior. 1990b. Effects of irrigation drainwater contaminants on wildlife—summary report. Laurel MD: U.S. Fish and Wildlife Service, Patuxent Wildlife Research Center. 38 p.

[USDOI] U.S. Department of the Interior. 1991. Vision for the future. Washington DC: U.S. Fish and Wildlife Service. 12 p.

[USGAO] U.S. General Accounting Office. 1987. National refuge contamination is difficult to confirm and clean up. Publication GAO/RCED-87-128. Washington DC: USGAO. 84 p.

Whitworth MR, Pendleton GW, Hoffman DJ, Camardese MB. 1991. Effects of dietary boron and arsenic on the behavior of mallard ducklings. *Environ Toxicol Chem* 10:911–916.

Williams M, Hothem RL, Ohlendorf HM. 1989. Recruitment failure in American avocets and black-necked stilts nesting at Kesterson Reservoir, California, 1984–1985. *Condor* 91:797–802.

Zahm GR. 1986. Kesterson Reservoir and Kesterson National Wildlife Refuge: history, current problems, and management alternatives. *Trans North Am Wildlife Nat Resources Conf* 51:324–329.

Chapter 7

Workgroup III Synopsis: Contaminant Fate and Effects in Coastal and Estuarine Wetlands

Donald F. Boesch, chair
Michael A. Lewis, William H. Mckee, Douglas Morrison, Pasquale F. Roscigno, Geoffrey I. Scott, J. Kevin Summers

Wetlands of the ocean coasts and estuaries are characterized by the influence of frequent water-level fluctuations as effected by astronomic tides as well as by meteorologically forced changes in the level of coastal waters. Some coastal wetlands experience extremely wide water-level fluctuations (several meters) predictably twice a day, while others experience only micro tides, and wind events may be the dominant control of water level. Coastal and estuarine wetlands also contain variable concentrations of dissolved salts from the ocean. Tidal flooding and salinity result in profound differences in the structure and function of coastal and estuarine wetlands in comparison to inland, freshwater wetlands. In addition to tidal wetlands, this chapter addresses those wetlands in the upper reaches of estuaries that are influenced by the tides but do not experience measurable salinity (i.e., tidal freshwater wetlands). Here we consider coastal and estuarine wetlands inhabited by emergent, vascular plants, including salt and brackish marshes and mangrove swamps.

Chapter Preview

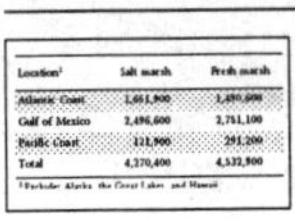

Ecotoxicology and Risk Assessment for Wetlands. Michael A. Lewis et al., editors.
 ISBN 1-880611-16-3

Coastal wetlands are of exceptional importance to human society and have been the focus of active protection, management, and restoration efforts. In the U.S., rates of wetland losses due directly to human activities, such as dredging and filling, have been reduced significantly as a result of more effective regulatory control. However, coastal wetlands are still under great pressure as a result of the rapid population growth in coastal regions in the U.S. and around the world and because of the rising demand for access to the coast for recreation (Dahl 1990; Dahl and Johnson 1991). Estuarine areas are densely populated: an estimated 45% of the U.S. population lives in these areas (Culliton et al. 1990). The population has increased by almost 30 million over the last 3 decades. It is predicted that the U.S. coastal population will increase to 127 million persons by 2010.

In addition to the direct human impacts associated with coastal development (e.g., dredging, filling, and bulkheading), coastal wetlands are confronted by changing environmental conditions, which result in their loss or degradation. These conditions include erosion, subsidence, sea-level rise, changing salinity conditions, and sedimentation or lack thereof. Some of these conditions are changing as a result of the natural evolution of coastal and estuarine ecosystems, but many result from human activities. For example, soil erosion, damming, water consumption and diversion, and stream channelization within a catchment can affect the sediment supply and freshwater input to the receiving estuary, with potentially significant consequences to the coastal wetlands. The U.S. Army Corps of Engineers received over 27,000 proposals to alter coastal wetlands in 14 coastal states between 1981 and 1985 (Mager and Thayer 1986). On an even larger scale, the accelerated rise in global sea level, predicted to result from global climate warming caused by the buildup of greenhouse gases in the atmosphere, portends significant changes in coastal wetlands.

In addition to these physical impacts, coastal ecosystems, and wetlands in particular, experience heavy loadings of potentially toxic contaminants and nutrients as a result of direct waste discharges and diffuse human activities on land. For example, significant amounts of pesticides enter the coastal zone as a result of river runoff. Approximately 29.4 million pounds of 35 pesticides were applied to the nation's estuarine drainage areas in 1987 (Pait et al. 1992).

Coastal wetlands represent 5% of the total wetland acreage in the United States. Coastal wetlands comprise about 16% of the nation's coastal area and over 4.4 million hectares (Feld et al. 1991). Coastal wetland acreage in the continental U.S. is shown in Table 7-1. The average annual loss of coastal wetlands between the mid-1950s and mid-1970s was about 7200 hectares (USEPA 1988a). Despite stricter regulatory control, it is estimated that there was a net loss of 28,700 hectares of estuarine intertidal emergent wetlands in the U.S. over the decade following the mid-1970s (Dahl and Johnson 1991), representing about 1.7% of the coastal wet-

Table 7-1 Coastal wetland acreage in the continental United States

Location[1]	Salt marsh	Fresh marsh	Forested wetlands[2]	Total wetlands
Atlantic Coast	1,651,900	1,490,600	8,410,900	11,553,400
Gulf of Mexico	2,496,600	2,751,100	8,211,800	13,459,500
Pacific Coast	121,900	291,200	757,100	1,170,200
Total	4,270,400	4,532,900	17,379,800	26,183,100

[1] Excludes Alaska, the Great Lakes, and Hawaii
[2] Includes mangroves
Source: Watzin and Gosselink 1992

lands that existed at the beginning of that period. These losses were the result of natural processes and human activities such as

- drainage,
- dredging and stream channelization,
- deposition of fill material,
- diking and damming,
- tilling for crop production,
- grazing by domesticated animals,
- discharge of pollutants,
- mining, and
- alteration of hydrology.

Wetlands were frequently seen as a nuisance in the early development of coastal regions, preventing direct access to the waterfront and harboring mosquitoes and mosquito-borne diseases. These wetlands are now appreciated for their significant values to society, including vital nurseries for fish and shellfish; habitat for waterfowl and other wildlife; protection against floods and destructive storm surges; trapping of sediments, contaminants, and human pathogens that might otherwise degrade water quality; and aesthetic serenity. Attempts to quantitatively estimate these values, using rather conservative accounting assumptions, indicate that coastal wetlands have a value to society of between $6,000 and $22,000 per hectare (Costanza et al. 1989).

Although there has been less focus on using coastal and estuarine wetlands for treatment of point- and nonpoint-source contamination than on nontidal wetlands, contaminant fate and effects are nonetheless important issues in coastal environmental protection and natural resource management. The ebb and flow of the tides, coupled with the tendency for materials to be captured in the backwaters of wetlands, result in many contaminants, ranging from floating oil to toxic contaminants associated with fine sediments, being concentrated in wetlands. Furthermore, efforts to rebuild or rehabilitate wetlands introduce questions about the fate of contaminants associated with sediments or inflows used for these purposes. For example, the creation or enhancement of coastal wetlands as a constructive use of dredged materials introduces questions about the fate and effects of chemical contaminants that may be contained in these materials. Finally, because of bidirectional tidal flows, coastal wetlands are generally very interactive with nearby open-water systems that may be subject to inputs of potentially toxic chemicals or nutrients. Understanding the fate and effects of these exchanges is critical to assessing risks to the greater coastal ecosystem.

This chapter is neither a treatise on the geochemistry and ecology of coastal wetlands nor an in-depth review of ecotoxicological methods or what is known about the fate and effects of contaminants in these ecosystems. Rather, it attempts to point out the salient features of coastal and estuarine wetland systems, particularly those that differ from freshwater wetlands, which should be taken into account in risk assessments based on the fate and effects of chemical contaminants (potentially toxic organic and inorganic chemicals and phytostimulants) related to those environments. Toward that end, this chapter has the primary focus on reviewing the characteristics and processes that are unique or of unusual importance in coastal and estuarine wetlands, and the implications to contaminant fate and effect are highlighted. Following that overview, approaches to risk assessment and its management implications for coastal wetlands are considered. Finally, this chapter concludes with a series of recommendations for further research and scientific assessment.

Distinguishing Characteristics of Coastal Wetlands

Salinity and biogeochemistry

Salinity effects on wetland organisms

Vascular plants evolved in terrestrial and freshwater environments, and relatively few forms have developed physiological mechanisms that allow them to tolerate the high salinity conditions of marine, or even estuarine, conditions. Consequently, coastal wetlands characteristically have much lower diversity of vascular plant species than freshwater wetlands. Some of these halophyte plants are able to exclude salts at the roots (e.g., the red mangrove *Rhizophora*), while others (e.g., *Spartina*) take up salts through the roots but have specialized salt glands embedded in the leaves (Mitsch and Gosselink 1993). Such halophytes are generally able to survive and grow in freshwater conditions but usually lose in competition with less salt-tolerant species. As a result of this interaction of physiological tolerance and competition, wetland plant communities change both vertically and along the estuarine salinity gradient. The most salt-tolerant species dominate under fully marine conditions and in high marsh, where evaporation can often raise soil salinity. As salinity approaches freshwater conditions along an estuarine gradient, more and more vascular plant species are able to maintain populations, and the relatively high salinity-tolerant species such as *Spartina alterniflora* are excluded.

Salinity also affects the distribution of other organisms inhabiting coastal wetlands. For invertebrates and fishes, the trend is typically the reverse of that of the vascular plants, with more species present under marine conditions and few species under very low salinity or highly variable salinity conditions.

Biogeochemical effects on wetland organisms

In addition to its major dissolved ions (e.g., Na^+ and Cl^-), seawater contains other ions at far higher concentrations than they are found in fresh water. Particularly important is sulfate, which serves as an electron acceptor for bacterial metabolism in the absence of oxygen in wetland sediments. Sulfate reduction dominates anaerobic respiration in most coastal wetland sediments and may even dominate over aerobic respiration. As much as 70% of the energy of net primary productivity may flow through reduced inorganic S compounds (Howarth et al. 1983). Sulfate is reduced to sulfide, which quickly reacts with reduced Fe to first form ferrous sulfide (FeS). Other sulfide products include pyrite (FeS_2), elemental sulfur, and organic sulfur compounds. Other metals in addition to Fe, including Cd, are precipitated as sulfides by this process and are unavailable to salt marsh species (Gambrell and Patrick 1988). Mercury is also precipitated by this process as a sulfide, but under low sulfate concentrations such as in oligohaline estuarine wetland sediments, it may be methylated by sulfate reducers, thereby greatly increasing its bioavailability. Sulfides also interact with organic matter (OM) to form gas products such as dimethyl sulfide (Vernberg 1993). The concentration of sulfides in wetland sediments is dependent on the availability of sulfate, organic substrate for the bacterial respiration, and the extent of tidal flushing. The highly reducing conditions, lack of oxygen, and high concentrations of sulfide in coastal wetland sediments have pervasive consequences for the fate, degradation, and bioavailability of contaminants and for the wetland organisms that are exposed to anoxic conditions and highly toxic sulfide (Mitsch and Gosselink 1993).

Soils of coastal wetlands have poorly developed profiles, represented by fluvaquents, sulfiquents, and histisols. Coastal wetlands with highly sulfitic soils are found worldwide but are more extensive in warmer regions. The formation of sulfitic soil horizons in marsh sediments appears related to major inputs of sediments. Ponds (1988) indicates that, on a world scale, many sulfitic deposits were formed 5 to 6 thousand years ago, representing young Holocene deposition with changes in sea level. Under flooded conditions, saline wetlands have a near-neutral pH and favor immobilization of metals, although some histic soils may be moderately to strongly acid (Gambrell 1994). However, oxidation of these pyrite-containing soils as a result of draining wetlands or placing dredged sediments subaerially produces large amounts of sulfuric acid, decreases pH, and solubilizes metals (McKee and McKevlin 1993). When dredged materials are placed in an upland position, appreciable quantities of Cd and Zn are released through oxidation of sulfides and breakdown of OM (Gambrell 1994). The sulfur dynamics can mobilize sediment P to diffuse from the sediment.

Many other geochemical differences exist between saline and freshwater wetland soils and among coastal wetland types. For example, it is worthwhile to note here that there are significant differences for carbonate sediments that form under tropical conditions (e.g., within some mangroves) because of the lower partial pressure of dissolved CO_2 in warm waters.

Limiting nutrients

Differences in the geochemistry in marine and brackish wetlands compared to freshwater wetlands affect the cycling and availability of major plant nutrients. Whereas P is typically the limiting nutrient in freshwater systems, it is generally not limiting in salt marshes because of the accumulation of P in marine clays and the rapid remineralization of phosphate (Whitney et al. 1981). Rather, N has been shown to limit salt marsh plant growth (Smart and Barko 1980). However, growth may be nitrogen limited only under well-drained conditions experienced in high marsh or in low marsh along tidal creeks. In poorly drained interior marshes, ammonium-N may actually build up as a result of the decomposition of OM and the prevalence of reducing conditions, but stresses related to low redox potential (lack of oxygen and high sulfide concentration) may decrease the assimilation of ammonium by the plants (Mendelssohn et al. 1982; Morris 1984).

Along the estuarine gradient, as the geochemical environment changes in response to total salinity and concentration of important ions such as sulfate, one can expect that P would become more limiting to plant growth. Tidal freshwater marshes, therefore, may be P limited, and low salinity (oligohaline) marshes may experience both N and P limitation, depending on specific environmental conditions. Mangroves rooted in carbonate sediments rather than mineral clays experience a completely different geochemical environment because P again may be limiting, even under high salinity conditions.

The flux of nutrients in coastal wetlands is not only of interest to the ecology of the wetland but also to the assessment of the interrelationship between the wetlands and the larger coastal ecosystem and to the evaluation of the degree to which the wetlands may serve to remove anthropogenic nutrient inputs. This phenomenon is complex because many factors are at work:

1) the geomorphology and tidal exchange of the wetland;
2) the inputs of nutrients from tidal flooding, ground water, and the atmosphere; and
3) the biotic uptake and transformations of nutrients (including shifts between particulate and dissolved and organic and inorganic phases and microbial nitrification and denitrification) in the wetland.

Studies of these fluxes in salt marshes have produced highly variable results because of this complexity and the differences among the marshes studied. In a review of studies conducted at that time, Nixon (1980) found that dissolved organic N and dissolved P are generally exported, and nitrite and nitrate tend to be imported.

The differences in plant nutrition among freshwater wetlands, salt marshes, and mangroves have considerable implications for the fate and effects of contaminants, particularly when the contaminants are excess nutrients. Will the nutrient input stimulate plant production? To what degree will the wetland trap nutrients, serving to remove them from the coastal system, where they may otherwise induce undesirable effects such as algal blooms and depletion of dissolved oxygen? How will the nutritional status of vascular plants and microbes affect the uptake, processing, and effects of trace metals and organic contaminants in wetlands? At what level of contamination will the assimilative capacity of the wetland be compromised?

Changing freshwater inflows

The quantity, quality, timing, and distribution of freshwater flow into coastal wetlands greatly influence physicochemical and biological processes in these ecosystems. Freshwater inflow, tidal processes, and geomorphology determine salinity gradients in coastal wetlands. Freshwater inflow to coastal wetlands influences the input and distribution of materials (e.g., nutrients and contaminants), sedimentation and erosion, the flux of materials between coastal wetlands and estuarine or marine open-water habitats, the distribution and movement of biota, biotic productivity, and biodiversity.

Differences in natural freshwater inflow patterns or hydrology (e.g., stream versus sheet flow) can influence the susceptibility of coastal wetlands to contaminant impacts. For example, assessments of the effects of oil spills on mangroves in Florida and Puerto Rico found that riverine mangroves were protected from oil spilled in coastal waters by freshwater inflow (Getter et al. 1981).

Alterations of natural freshwater flow patterns into coastal wetlands caused by water management practices (e.g., flood control, water use), dredging and filling, and other human activities are widespread in the United States. These alterations usually affect biotic and physicochemical processes. Well-known examples include Florida Bay (McIvor et al. 1994), the Mississippi River delta (Costanza et al. 1990; Boesch et al. 1994), and San Francisco Bay (Nichols et al. 1986). Ecotoxicologists must consider these effects of variable freshwater inflow when assessing contaminant impacts on coastal wetlands.

Hydrology affects sediment biogeochemistry in coastal wetlands (reviewed by Vernberg [1993] and Gambrell [1994]). The effects of changing salinity on contaminant release from sediments and bioavailability to flora and fauna vary among contaminants (Gambrell et al. 1977). As discussed above, S reduction is an important geochemical process affecting metal contaminant availability in coastal wetlands. Salinity changes from hydrological alteration do not greatly affect the mobility and availability of sulfide-bound metals (Gambrell 1994). However, increased freshwater inflow (e.g., channelization) can cause scouring and resuspension of sediments, resulting in the oxidation and the release of toxic metals. Drainage and water loss from incompressible sediments can lead to aeration, oxidizing sulfide metals and releasing the metals (Bradley and Morris 1990). Changes in freshwater inflow can cause changes in pH, which can affect the retention and release of contaminants (Gambrell 1994).

Clarke and McFarland (1991) reviewed metal bioaccumulation from sediments, addressing the influence of varying salinity on uptake. It was found that Se bioavailability increases with decreasing salinity; however, Zn uptake is unrelated to salinity. Cu uptake is particularly influenced by complexation with organics, and its uptake dependence on salinity is variable. Pb uptake may increase with increasing salinity, and Hg bioavailability may not be affected by salinity changes because of its tight binding with particulates. Overall, factors other than salinity are usually more important in affecting the biological uptake of metals.

Reducing freshwater inflow can diminish the capacity for estuaries to dilute, flush, and/or transform contaminant inputs. This is demonstrated in San Francisco Bay, where freshwater inflow has been reduced to less than 40% of historic levels (Nichols et al. 1986). Reduced freshwater inflow to the Nile River delta following construction of the Aswan High Dam, coupled with inputs of nutrient-laden urban wastewater and agricultural runoff, threatens the coastal wetlands in the delta (Stanley and White 1993).

Altering freshwater inflow patterns affects sediment deposition in coastal wetlands. Construction of levees and other human activities along the Mississippi and Atchafalaya rivers have practically eliminated riverine sediment inputs to many Louisiana coastal marshes, resulting in substantial wetland fragmentation and loss (Costanza et al. 1990; Boesch et al. 1994). Changing the natural freshwater input from sheet to channelized flow into wetlands in the Charlotte Harbor, FL estuary has caused increased deposition of dredged sediments (Morrison et al. 1990). In another example, the majority of the freshwater flow of the Santee River, SC was diverted to the Cooper River to enhance water flow through Charleston Harbor and promote its port facilities. As a result of this diversion, salt marshes and oyster reefs were established in the lower Santee River. However, due to the enhanced estuarine circulation caused by the greater flows down the Cooper River, sediments and their associated contaminants were deposited in Charleston Harbor, requiring extensive dredging. A decision was eventually made to divert much of the flow back down the Santee, thereby causing a shift in the estuarine salinity gradient down the lower Santee River, changing the distribution of wetland communities and eliminating oyster reefs.

Changing freshwater inflow can affect the timing and distribution of contaminant inputs. Channelization results in more localized and concentrated freshwater and sediment, and thus in more contaminant input (i.e., becoming more of a point-source input). Channelization can also cause contaminants in tidal waters to be transported further into coastal wetlands. Water-control structures (e.g., dams, locks) and their release schedules result in high-volume, pulsed discharges of variable timing to estuarine ecosystems. This can result in the sudden release of large quantities of poor quality water that previously had been held upstream of the water-control structure. Furthermore, the high flow rate with these releases can scour the bottom, resuspending sediments, and potentially releasing bound contaminants.

Altering freshwater inflow can cause changes in the species composition, distribution, and abundances of emergent and submerged plants. In the Charlotte Harbor, FL estuary, changing the natural freshwater input from sheet to channelized flow by constructing canals has resulted in cattails invading a mangrove wetland (Morrison et al. 1990). Mangrove distribution and productivity varies with differing salinity regimes (Odum et al. 1982). The natural freshwater flow patterns into Florida Bay wetlands have been altered by flood-control canal systems. Varying water management practices can greatly alter salinity in these wetlands, resulting in substantial and often rapid changes in plant composition and abundance (Montague and Ley 1993). Wetland plant species differ in their abilities to uptake toxic metals (Gambrell 1994). Short-term, seasonal, and longer-term variation in plant composition, distribution, and productivity due to varying freshwater inflow patterns may complicate ecotoxicological risk assessment.

Altering freshwater inflow can greatly affect secondary productivity and the abundance of these species. The decline in fisheries in San Francisco Bay is partially attributed to a > 50% reduction in historic freshwater inflow volumes (Nichols et al. 1986). Decreases in salmon populations in the Columbia River estuary are correlated to alteration of the timing of freshwater inflow (Simenstad et al. 1992). Substantial decreases in pink shrimp harvest in south Florida are correlated with reduced freshwater flow into Florida Bay and the Everglades coastal ecotone (McIvor et al. 1994).

Wading-bird nesting in south Florida was historically concentrated in the coastal wetlands (Ogden 1994). Many of these colonies collapsed after the natural freshwater flow into these wetlands was altered (Ogden 1994), likely because reduced freshwater inflow reduced the birds' food supply (Powell et al. 1989; Walters et al. 1992; Ogden 1994; Bjork and Powell 1994). The productivity, distribution, and species composition of bird-prey fishes is related to freshwater inflow patterns (Lorenz 1995). In Florida Bay wetlands, shifts in nesting location of the endangered American crocodile and lower juvenile survival relative to nearby areas are likely due to reduced freshwater inflow (Mazzotti and Brandt 1994).

Actions to restore more natural freshwater flow into coastal wetlands are proposed for several ecosystems around the United States. Evaluating potential contaminant problems must be part of these efforts. Reestablishing freshwater flow (hydropattern restoration) through the coastal Everglades to Florida Bay is an essential component of Florida Bay restoration (SFWMD 1995). Flooding former agricultural lands is a proposed strategy in this effort. These farmlands had the greatest application of the highly toxic pesticide endosulfan in the southeastern U.S. (Pait et al. 1992); the potential for endosulfan and nutrient inputs with freshwater flow restoration therefore needs to be evaluated and monitored. If these contaminants are found to impact the coastal wetlands, then constructed treatment wetlands, such as those used in the north Everglades for P removal, may be needed. Proposed restoration of the flow of sediment-laden Mississippi River water to Louisiana coastal marshes to abate wetland loss (Boesch et al. 1994) has potential contaminant impacts. These fresh waters and sediments may contain contaminants from upstream industrial and urban discharges.

Tidal influences

Consequences of tidal water exchange

Tides can result in the complete inundation and drainage of the coastal wetland soil surface twice a day where there are semidiurnal tides (or daily where the tides are diurnal). In reality, wetland flooding and drainage may be more complex than this, as coastal regions vary in tidal range, spring-neap tidal range differences, attenuation of tidal range up an estuary, and importance of wind forcing on sea level. However, in any case, variations in water level at a high frequency characterize coastal and estuarine wetlands. These variations have substantial consequences to wetland geochemistry and ecology, interactions between the wetland and the larger aquatic ecosystem, and the transport and effects of contaminants.

The cycle of flooding and drainage affects nutrient supply, the introduction of sediments needed for soil building, soil salinity, and the concentrations of important constituents such as oxygen and sulfate and sulfide. Tidal flooding and drainage essentially provide a subsidy that allows plants to survive in the face of the buildup of toxic soil conditions caused by high sulfide (caused by anaerobic microbial metabolism) and high salinity (caused by evapotranspiration). Rapid tidal drainage of tidal wetlands means that not all runoff is on the surface, and there may be significant subsurface runoff from wetland soils into tidal creeks. This complicates the traditional concepts of geochemical exchange based on soil profiles and vertical fluxes alone, with obvious effects on the fate of contaminants. In addition, this effect may result in short-term exposure to contaminant levels, which is difficult to quantify or replicate in effects studies.

Tides result in a bidirectional exchanges of chemicals, sediments, and organisms. In this way, coastal and estuarine wetlands are affected not only by land runoff and upstream drainage but also by downstream aquatic systems. Tides act to remove partially degraded organic material, distribute nutrients, and disperse plankton, nekton and dispersal-phase benthic organisms throughout the estuarine ecosystem. Tidal flooding brings in suspended sediments from the estuary or coastal waterbody, and the stilled conditions and baffling by plant stems and roots result in the trapping of sediments. At the same time, tidal action may also play a major role in scouring of salt marsh tidal creek banks and may lead to erosion and block slumping of marsh vegetation. In contrast to nontidal freshwater wetlands, material that leaves the wetland with outflows may return on subsequent flood tides.

Conditions of exposure

Tidal exchange affects the exposure conditions and assimilative capacity for contaminants. On a volume basis alone, contaminant discharges into coastal wetlands with a large tidal range would be expected to have reduced impacts compared to similar discharges into a microtidal (tidal range < 1m) wetland due to the greater dilution potential and shorter resident times within each tidal system. Current contaminant and nonpoint-source runoff models have not addressed this issue adequately. In a mesotidal (tidal range 1 to 3m) South Carolina salt marsh, Scott et al. (1992) found that agricultural pesticide runoff following periods of significant precipitation resulted in a pulsed exposure period of only 6 h because of the semidiurnal tidal mixing in that region. Additionally, they found that the higher-salinity, flood tide waters acted as a physical barrier to the dispersion of the pesticide-laden freshet until the tide receded. This resulted in periods of intense freshwater runoff at ebb tide with concomitant low salinity and heavy sedimentation rates.

Many species of fish and shellfish have life histories and reproductive behavior linked to tidal rhythms and wetland areas. In the Gulf of Mexico and southeastern Atlantic coast, estuarine-dependent species account for the overwhelming majority of the harvest of commercial and recreational fisheries. Spawning of the Atlantic silverside is clearly related to lunar periodicity of early morning, high spring tide, and egg hatchability may peak at nightly spring tides. In addition, the hatching of the eggs of the fiddler crab *Uca* is intimately tied to nocturnal spring tides. Dispersion of fish and invertebrate larvae is initially dependent on both tidal dispersion and the response of the larvae to light, temperature, salinity, and other factors (Vernberg and Vernberg 1974).

Longer-term changes in water level

The existence, extent, and zonation of coastal wetland vegetation are dependent on sea level and its tidal and meteorological variations. Mean sea level is not static, but may vary (at least in microtidal areas) as a function of year-to-year climatic variations, regional subsidence or uplift of the land surface, and longer-term global changes in climate. Coastal wetlands must adjust to these changes in order to maintain their extent and characteristics. Particularly important for some Gulf and Atlantic coast wetlands are the high rates of subsidence (as much as 1 cm/y or more) from downwarping of crustal material, compaction of thick Holocene sediments, or withdrawal of fluids (drinking water, oil, and formation waters) from the subsurface. Unless wetlands are able to raise the soil level through trapping mineral sediments, accreting organic debris, or adding root and rhizome volume, they succumb to increased tidal inundation, which exacerbates water logging, oxygen deficiency, and sulfide toxicity in wetland soils. In such rapidly subsiding wetlands with a deficiency in soil aggradation (e.g., Mississippi Delta wetlands and the Blackwater marshes of the Chesapeake Bay), wetland vascular plants may simply die.

Much concern has been directed to the effects on coastal wetlands of the accelerated rise in relative sea level due to global warming and expansion of ocean volume. In some cases, this may mean a retreat of coastal wetlands over fastlands, but where coupled with high rates of subsidence or "hardening" of shorelines by human activities (which prevents such wetland transgression) loss of coastal wetlands may be dramatic.

In addition to the obvious effects of changes in relative sea level on the ecology of coastal wetlands, changes in sea level may affect contaminant fates and effects in a number of ways, such as by flooding and exchange, sediment erosion, and mobilization of contaminants bound in wetland sediments, etc.

Production and habitat

Primary production

Coastal wetlands and mangrove swamps, with their attendant estuarine systems, are among the most productive in the world with respect to primary production (Keefe 1972; Turner 1976; Richardson 1979; Pomeroy et al. 1981; Maltby 1986) and secondary production (Chapman 1966; Burke and Mann 1974; Dame 1976; Wolff and de Wolf 1977; Dame et al. 1984; Lewis and Peters 1984; Day et al. 1988; Lana and Guiss 1992). An example of productivity in different types of mangrove wetlands appears in Table 7-2. Primary productivity of wetland flora includes significant portions of aboveground biomass (Dame and Kenny 1986), soil surface and epiphytic production (Vernberg 1993), and belowground biomass (da Cunha et al. 1991). As a result of this productivity, exposure of these plants to high inflows of contaminated waters (either tidal or freshwater inflow) or storage pools of contaminants or nutrients in marsh sediment can result in significant incorporation, dependent upon bioavailability, of these materials into plant biomass. The aboveground portions of this productivity serves multiple functions, including sediment trapping (Redfield 1972; Armentano and Woodwell 1975; Fleesa et al. 1977), production of a significant portion of the organic C base that fuels the detrital coastal marsh or estuarine ecosystem (Wiebe and Pomeroy 1972; Mitsch and Gosselink 1986; Pozo and Colino 1992), and habitat for wildlife (McIvor et al. 1994; Bjork and Powell 1994).

The architecture of monocultural or near-monocultural stands provides the perfect trap to sequester sediments that promote the building of marsh soils and to aid in filtering surface-flow-suspended solids before their export into coastal oceans. For coastal marshes to persist over time, sedimentation rates must be equal to or exceed sea-level rise. East Coast salt marshes and tropical mangrove swamps have been

Table 7-2 Comparison of productivity, respiration, and litter fall for several types of mangrove wetlands

	Mangrove wetland		
Activity	Riverine	Basin	Scrub
Gross primary productivity[a] kcal m^{-2} d^{-1}	108	81	13
Total respiration kcal $^{-2}$ d^{-1}	51	56	18
Net primary productivity[a] kcal $^{-2}$ d^{-1}	57	25	0
Litter production[b] kcal $^{-2}$ d^{-1}	14 ± 2	9.0 ± 0.4	1.5

[a] From several sites in Florida; based on CO_2 gas-exchange measurements; assumes 1 g OM = 4.5 kcal
[b] Average ± standard error from several sites in Florida and Puerto Rico; measured with litter traps; assumes 1 g OM = 4.5 kcal
Sources: Mitsch and Gosselink (1993) and data from Brown and Lugo (1982).

estimated to actively accrete material between 1.5 and 51.8 mm/y (Armentano and Woodwell 1975; Fleesa et al. 1977; Richard 1978; Sharma et al. 1987). In one study, Wolaver et al. (1988a, 1988b) determined that vegetated marshes and oyster reefs provided a sink for suspended sediments throughout the year but that the largest imports occurred during the summer months. Annual estimates of sedimentation showed approximately 65% of the inorganic and organic suspended solids that entered the marsh on a flood tide did not exit the marsh on the ebb tide (Wolaver et al. 1988a, 1998b). In conjunction with this sediment trapping, many of the contaminants bound to these particles will also be trapped in coastal wetlands. While this "filter" may work both ways in coastal tidal wetlands, the above sedimentation rate studies suggest the accretion of contaminants bound to inflowing sediments. In addition, nutrient-laden surface and subsurface flows can be stripped of nutrients that are subsequently incorporated in plant biomass. As a result, coastal wetland sediments can become storage pools for many contaminants. The contaminants in these storage pools generally may be unavailable to biota because of chemical bonding to sediment organics (unless the sediments are directly consumed).

Because of the high level of productivity of these grass-based (or mangrove-based) wetlands, significant amounts (thousands of g/y) of organic material become the base of the detrital pool in coastal wetlands. Through the processes of decomposition, this detritus is broken into smaller-sized particles through mechanical means and through colonization by bacteria, fungi, and protozoa. Egested materials from marsh macrofauna can provide rich media for microbial colonization. This production results in some export to estuarine waters and coastal oceans, but most of the production remains in the wetlands as part of the organic sediment matrix (Summers et al. 1980; Summers and McKellar 1981; Childers and McKellar 1987; Ausmus and McKellar 1990).

Organic matter and fate of contaminants

Understanding the flow of C between wetlands and estuaries is critical to understanding the movement of contaminants through the trophic structure of these systems. In particular, detrital matter plays a particularly prominent role, since 90% of the primary production of macroalgae, seagrasses, salt marshes, and mangroves is not grazed by herbivores (Mann 1982). This OM provides sites for the adsorption of metals and hydrocarbons and results in situations where these contaminants can be removed from one environment and transported to another for possible reintroduction in this new environment. While OM can be considered a contaminant in and of itself, in this chapter we consider the role of decomposition of OM as a function of wetlands.

Metals associated with OM are relatively bioavailable and are important contributors to interstitial water found in sediments. This pore water is the toxic fraction of the bulk sediment's contaminant concentration. Organic matter is an important component of sediments toxicity (which includes redox and sulfides) and is most often not reported with many datasets that attempt to report environmental contamination (Long and Morgan 1990), thus resulting in ambiguous toxicity results. Sediments contaminated with metals become sinks for the cycling of metals initially, but ultimately, they are sources for the subsequent redistribution of metals.

Polynuclear aromatic hydrocarbons (PAHs) are hydrophobic, with low aqueous solubility, which explains their rapid adsorption onto particulate organic matter (POM). While this results in sediment values that greatly exceed aqueous phase concentrations, equilibrium partitioning and biological activity (bioaccumulation, biotransformation, and biodegradation) can reintroduce PAHs into the aqueous phase. In anoxic bottom sediments, PAHs are stable and persistent. In more anoxic sediments, microbial degradation by bacteria and fungi does occur (Kennish 1992). The same saprophagic bacteria and fungi that naturally flourish on detritus regenerate minerals and convert POM into dissolved organic matter (DOM) (Valiela 1984) are critical to the degradation of PAHs and other hydrocarbons.

Polychlorinated biphenyls (PCBs) and other chlorinated hydrocarbons are another class of compounds whose affinity for sediment increases with increasing POM. However, these compounds are more difficult to degrade and consequently persist longer in the environment. In systems with high rates of sedimentation, rapid burial quickly removes them from the system (Bopp et al. 1981).

Dissolved organic matter provides binding sites for further uptake of metals and hydrocarbons. Equilibrium partitioning under steady-state conditions allows these contaminants to be bioavailable. Sources of POM are hypothesized to be associated with the "salinity-axis gradient" and the "marsh stream-order gradient" (Odum 1984). Terrestrial and riverine systems, along with phytoplankton, are associated with the salinity gradient. Marshes, mangroves, and wetlands produce the marsh stream-order gradient, which is our focus in this discussion. Consequently, it is difficult to identify the origins of the DOM in salt marshes (Wotton 1990).

Wind-induced resuspension may accelerate the release of DOM from the detritus (through leaching) and from sediment porewater entrainment. This is very common in Louisiana during winter, producing a winter maximum of DOC and net export to the Gulf of Mexico (Happ et al. 1977). For tidally driven systems, maxima of DOM are seen during flood tides, while minima are seen during slack high tide. Particulate organic matter has a greater range of variability. This seasonal and diel variability has toxicological implications, in that redistribution of DOM and POM, and the contaminants associated with them, result in exposure pathways for the biota that are variable and periodic. The anoxic conditions existing in sediments produce a microbially mediated anaerobic process by which methane, sulfide, and carbon dioxide are produced as the complex OM is reduced. Methanogenesis is the dominant pathway in freshwater systems, while sulfate reduction is characteristic of saline environments (Wotton 1990).

This marsh sediment organic matrix fuels the microbial decomposition pathways of the detritally based ecosystem. The bulk dissolved organic carbon pool in coastal wetland environments increases as marsh grass or mangrove lignocellulose degrades (Moran and Hodson 1990). Intensive microbial action on this decaying material results in the development of large pools of dissolved organic carbon with even larger and more diverse microbial populations. The populations of microbial organisms through their decompositional functions can mediate, modify, and enhance specific contaminant transformations. In addition, the dissolved organic carbon pools created through the decomposition process can provide a significant number of additional bonding sites for contaminants and contaminant transformations, thus altering the availability of these contaminants to biota. Obviously, not all of the contaminants are sequestered in sediments or made unavailable to biota. However, significant portions of incoming contaminants can be effectively removed. The remaining contaminant pools, if in appropriate chemical forms, are available and can be directly accumulated by marsh plants (primarily metals) and by surface algae. These plants can be grazed by herbivorous marsh biota (e.g., snails, insects) and incorporate contaminant loads that can be passed to higher trophic levels. Many secondary consumers such as invertebrates, birds, and fish feed on detritivores living on bottom sediments, resulting in complex trophic pathways and interactions that are essential for the recycling of this material. The body weight of copepods, for instance, may be composed of as much as 84% protein, fat, and carbohydrates (Wotton 1990).

Secondary production and habitat function

Estuaries and coastal wetlands provide unique habitats for a majority of coastal populations, including fish, shellfish, birds, and reptiles. A variety of fish and commercially important crustaceans need wetlands for their survival (Nelson et al.

1991, 1992). For example, about 90% of the Gulf Coast fishery depends on estuaries and wetlands during some point in their life cycles. These organisms may be more or less permanent inhabitants of the wetlands (e.g., forage fish, wading birds, ospreys, shellfish) or transient species living there for only part of their life cycle (e.g., migratory waterfowl and fish species). In many instances, coastal wetland and mangrove habitats represent a critical nursery and developmental ground during larval and juvenile life stages of many fish species (e.g., Atlantic croaker, weakfish, penaeid shrimp), critical spawning habitats for anadromous species (e.g., striped bass or white perch), or an overwintering habitat for some migratory species (e.g., waterfowl). However, coastal wetland and mangrove habitats also provide critical resident habitats for shellfish, reptiles, and many colonial bird species.

Estuaries and coastal wetlands provide the necessary environmental conditions to promote development of these species, and hence, year-class strengths for many fish species are often determined by the environmental conditions in these habitats. The incorporation of toxic contaminants in these habitats, as either surface films, sediment pools absorbed to suspended organic particles, or uptake by zooplankton provide a direct avenue of contact and/or ingestion by these early life stages. In some populations, elevated contaminant concentrations have contributed to the reduction of year-class strength.

Resident shellfish (e.g., oysters, clams, mussels) spend their entire life cycle exposed to whatever chemical environment characterizes their location. These populations are significant bioaccumulators of contaminants that are transported through or collected in coastal wetland environments. In addition, other shellfish populations spend significant portions of their life histories in coastal wetland and estuarine environments (e.g., blue crabs, penaeid shrimp). As a result, national coastal monitoring programs have used contaminant bioaccumulation by these shellfish as primary indicators of changes in exposure trends in estuarine environments (O'Connor and Beliaeff 1995).

Coastal wetlands provide nesting and foraging habitats for many wading birds, as well as ospreys and eagles (McIvor et al. 1994). Contaminant uptake of DDT through feeding pathways was a critical element in the severe population reductions experienced by brown pelicans in the 1960s and 1970s. Reductions in clutch size in many wading birds can be attributed to direct contaminant uptake, modifications in habitat size and quality (Powell and Powell 1986), and reduction in forage (Powell et al. 1989). Heavy metals have impaired reproduction in colonial wading birds in Texas (King and Cromartie 1986). Aquatic birds have also experienced embryonic mortality and abnormalities from exposure to metals from wetland sites (Ohlendorf and Fleming 1988). However, in many cases, the reduction in population size appears to be due to combinations of these factors. One example of this phenomenon is the hypothesis that increases in the uptake of endocrine-disrupting contaminants (e.g., Hg, endosulfan) through feeding mechanisms, combined with reduced habitat quality and quantity, have resulted in significantly reduced reproductive potential, and therefore significant reductions in populations of white ibis and great white heron in the Everglades. Similar hypotheses have been proposed concerning several fish populations. Another hypothesized cause of reproductive failure by wading birds is related indirectly to accumulations of OM. Increases in organic material stimulate the growth of oligochaete host species for *Eustrongylides* sp. These nematodes are ingested by forage fish (e.g., spot, mosquitofish), and the parasites grow within the gut of the fish. Subsequent ingestion of these fish by wading birds transfers the parasites to the gut of these birds, where they flourish. These parasites have been linked to significant mortality and reductions in reproductive success.

Because estuaries and coastal wetlands represent large congregations of early life stages of fish and shellfish, these habitats also represent primary feeding grounds for many adult and juvenile predators. While the majority of these predators are fish species, a number of these coastal predators include wading birds, piscivorous birds, and some small mammals. When elevated toxic contaminant concentrations exist in developmental estuarine and coastal wetland habitats, the uptake of these contaminants by larval and early juvenile life stages can easily be passed forward in the food chain and bioaccumulated by these predators.

Wetlands provide half the habitat for endangered species in the United States. These species are dependent entirely, or in part, on wetlands for food, reproduction, or protection (Sather and Smith 1984). For example, 57 threatened or endangered species inhabit the wetlands of south Florida. About one-half of the U.S. population of American crocodiles, a federally listed endangered species, nest in Florida Bay, a coastal mangrove swamp/sawgrass wetland (Mazzotti and Brandt 1994). Contaminants can impact endangered species by producing direct acute or chronic effects, by altering food chains, and by altering the habitat.

Assessing Risks

Hazard assessment for coastal wetlands

Water-quality criteria and biocriteria

Coastal wetlands have many unique physical, chemical, and biological conditions that can affect the loading rate, direction of cycling, and bioavailability of contaminants. For example, undisturbed wetlands have variable pH, lower dissolved oxygen, higher ammonia, high reducing conditions, greater photodegradation and biodegradation, and greater potential for chelation and organic complexation than do surface waters. Coastal wetlands often improve water quality of adjacent waters and those downstream by their assimilative capacity for removing and retaining sediments, nutrients, and toxicants from flood waters and surface runoff. However, the retained nutrients, toxicants, and possibly contaminated sediments may exceed toxic levels and adversely affect the structure and function of the wetland. The regulatory and scientific communities therefore are faced with a challenge to protect coastal wetlands from deterioration in sediment and water quality and also to allow the use of these wetlands for their natural bioremediative capabilities.

Designated uses for wetlands, such as the protection and propagation of fish, shellfish, and wildlife, must meet the goals of the Clean Water Act. Water quality standards and designated uses have been established by many states for rivers, lakes, and estuaries, and these may be applicable to wetlands. Although standards specifically designed for wetlands are uncommon, a national guidance document (USEPA 1990) and reviews of the current status of water-quality criteria and biocriteria development for wetland areas (Brown et al. 1989; Nelson 1990) are available.

Existing water-quality criteria are based primarily on aquatic animal species rather than on plants and wildlife, which comprise a greater component in wetlands. This is one of the major deficiencies in the development of water-quality criteria for coastal wetlands, since they are plant-dominated ecosystems. In addition, the animal species on which water-quality criteria are based may not be representative of those in coastal wetlands, and there is a need to determine whether the sensitivities of these species are relevant to those in coastal wetlands.

Biological criteria (biocriteria), unlike water-quality criteria, are based on site-specific water characteristics and biotic characteristics. Biocriteria are numeric values that describe the biological condition for a designated use. They are based on the comparison of the measurement of the biological community in unimpacted waters (reference condition) with that measured for a similar community at potentially affected test sites. Currently, only a few states, one of which is Florida (FDER 1988), have formulated biocriteria for coastal wetlands.

Risk assessment procedures for specific contaminants affecting coastal wetlands (estuarine and marine) currently follow those used for freshwater wetlands (USEPA 1992a, 1998). Exposure levels are compared with effect or toxic concentrations to determine the hazard. Risk assessment is then made, followed by risk management. The realism of this risk-assessment process depends upon the quality and quantity of the supporting technical data describing chemical toxicity and exposure, which are more often limited for coastal wetlands than for freshwater wetlands. The following discussion centers on the initial steps in the risk assessment process: problem identification and risk characterization for chemical toxicity in coastal wetlands.

A variety of factors affect the biotic diversity in coastal wetlands, including storm events, landscape modification, urbanization, water diversion, overexploitation of resources, and the presence of toxicants. Because of these factors, eutrophication, acidification, sedimentation, inundation, fragmentation of the habitat, and contaminant toxicity may occur. Chemical contaminants such as pesticides, oil, metals, and nutrients often enter wetlands from various point and nonpoint sources (Table 7-3). In some cases, their presence has adversely affected the biotic diversity (Mendelssohn et al. 1990; Kennish 1992). This is particularly true for pesticides and oil.

Table 7-3 Activities affecting wetlands in decreasing order

Point-source pollution	Nonpoint-source pollution
Industrial or municipal effluents	Land clearing or tillage
Mining	Channelization or dikes and levees
Energy development	Land drainage or irrigation
Hazardous waste sites	Urban runoff Municipal landfills Forest management

Source: Adamus 1989

The pH, temperature, vegetation density, and contaminant loading rate are several factors that impact the potential route and exposure duration as well as the environmental partitioning and speciation of the contaminant of concern. Some information on the exposure area and duration of impact of some contaminants has been reported (Table 7-4). The exposure duration of toxicants in wetlands can be constant because of leachates from treated structures (e.g., pilings), the discharge of effluents from municipal and industrial facilities, and continuous erosion from upland areas and the influx of contaminated groundwater. Intermittent exposures can occur as a result of seasonal applications of pesticides to upstream agricultural areas and from periodic spraying for nuisance insects.

Table 7-4 Scale of impact of pollutants in coastal wastewaters on receiving waters

Pollutant	Area of impact	Duration of impact
Ammonia toxicity	1 or 2 kilometers	Few hours
Other acute toxicity	Few kilometers	Less than 1 day
Coliforms	Up to 10 kilometers	Up to a week
Bacterial pathogens	Up to 10 kilometers	Up to a week
Viral pathogens	Up to 10 kilometers	Up to 4 months
Protozoan pathogens	Up to 10 kilometers	Up to 3 months
Deposition of organic matter	10 kilometers	Few days
Oil and grease	Few kilometers	Few days
BOD-caused DO decrease	Few kilometers	Few days
Nutrients (nitrogen)	Up to 100 kilometers	Months to a few years
Regional hypoxia	Up to 100 kilometers	Months to a few years
Heavy metals (sediments)	Few kilometers	Years to decades
Synthetic organics (sediments)	10s of kilometers	Decades

Source: NRC 1993

Exposure to toxicants is affected by salinity. Salinity stratification can have a significant effect on chemical toxicity to coastal wetland biota. Contaminants can be restricted to the less dense overlying water, reducing the bioavailability for toxicity to benthic life. However, if wind and water currents mix the less dense fresh water with the underlying, more dense saline water, the entire biota may be vulnerable. Therefore, the greater the tidal energy and wind exposure, the more likelihood of mixing and a toxicant impact (unless the mixing causes sufficient dilution to reduce toxicity). This factor is not a consideration in freshwater wetlands.

The bioavailability of chemicals in the sediments is more difficult to predict. Redox potential, organic carbon content and particle size are important factors controlling the amount of toxicity and bioaccumulation. As stated previously, salinity and the presence of sulfides may strongly influence the bioavailability of heavy metals.

Types of biota

The species at risk include many types of flora and fauna, several of which are of great economic value (e.g., shrimp, oysters). The diversity of biota and the relationship of their life cycles to the wetland are much more complex for coastal wetlands than for freshwater wetlands. The biotic composition is dynamic and largely influenced by seasonal environmental factors and life-history characteristics. In a broad sense, the types of biota include various invertebrates, fish, birds, and plants, including benthic (epibenthic and infaunal) and planktonic forms (phytoplankton and zooplankton). The species can be mobile and non-mobile, resident and migratory. Resident species may spend their entire life cycles in the wetland area or only part of their life cycles (e.g., to reproduce). Migratory species may enter a wetland area only briefly to feed. Based on these considerations, the life-history characteristics of wetland biota determine in part their potential for exposure to harmful pollutants.

Several representative species of animals and plants found in coastal wetlands have been used, although not commonly, in standard toxicity tests to determine the effects of specific chemical contaminants. In most cases, the test species are animal species that are more representative of estuaries. The techniques used in this process are briefly discussed next.

Water column toxicity tests

Specific assessment techniques for ecological risk assessments have been described on numerous occasions (USEPA 1986, 1988b, 1997; USACOE 1994). Acute and chronic toxicity tests have been conducted in the laboratory, using various species to determine the effects of toxicants on survival, growth, and reproduction. The laboratory tests are commonly conducted to meet regulatory compliance for the National Pollutant Discharge Elimination System permitting system; the Federal Insecticide, Fungicide and Rodenticide Act; and the Toxic Substances Control Act. The contaminants controlled by these regulations are often found in coastal wetlands as a result of several sources (Table 7-3). Common test species used in toxicity tests are mysids (*Mysidopsis bahia*), sheepshead minnows (*Cyprinodon variegatus*), and algae such as *Dunaliella tertiolecta* and *Skeletonema costatum*. These species were chosen in part for their sensitivity but more so because of their ease of culture and availability. The toxicity tests are conducted for 2 to 21 d under controlled environmental conditions of pH, temperature, salinity, and light. The endpoints are the LC50 value, the no-observed-effect concentration, and first-observed-effect concentration values. Methodologies for these tests are available from the USEPA (1992b) and several standard writing organizations such as ASTM (1993). To increase their relevance, the experimental conditions in some of the standardized laboratory tests have been altered to incorporate the simultaneous exposure of several species, the use of chemical mixtures, the variation of exposure duration, and the changing experimental conditions of pH and temperature.

Data summaries for specific chemicals and wetland flora and fauna do not exist because of the general lack of data, but several are available for estuarine biota (Mayer 1987). As stated earlier, current scientific understanding of toxicant effects on coastal and estuarine wetland biota has centered largely on determining the effects of pesticides (Kirby-Smith et al. 1992; Clark et al. 1993), and the database for these contaminants is larger than for any other.

In summary, single-species acute and chronic toxicity tests are seldom conducted with wetland species, particularly plants. Furthermore, there are only a few standardized phytotoxicity test methods and culture techniques, and there are few available estuarine test species indigenous to wetlands that have been identified as sensitive. There is uncertainty associated with extrapolating the sensitivities of commonly used estuarine test species to species that inhabit coastal wetlands. Therefore, the validity of using standard test species as surrogates for those in coastal wetlands is largely unknown and needs to be established.

Sediment toxicity tests

Animal species—Several types of sediment toxicity tests and test species have been used to determine the suitability of field-collected sediment to support benthic life (Traunspurger and Drews 1996). Tests have been developed largely in response to the disposal of dredged spoils, which can have a dramatic impact on sediment quality (Trent et al. 1976; Wakeman 1977; Saloman et al. 1982; Rice and White 1987), and for the derivation of sediment quality criteria and guidelines (Long et al. 1998). These tests are conducted with either whole sediment, elutriates, or interstitial water, usually for 10 to 30 d, depending upon the test species. The most frequently used estuarine test species in acute toxicity tests has been the amphipod, *Ampelisca abdita*. As with the water column toxicity tests, the use of wetland-specific benthic species is uncommon. Standard methods exist for whole sediment acute toxicity tests, which monitor survival over a 10-d exposure period (ASTM 1993; USEPA 1994). Chronic toxicity tests have not been standardized, although efforts are in progress for a 28-d test using the estuarine amphipod *Leptocheirus plumulosus* (USACOE 1996). Other test methods such as the sea urchin fertilization test have been used to assess the presence of contaminated sediment. The environmental relevance of the results of these and other sediment toxicity tests conducted with animal species has been questioned and remains an important issue. Current thinking is that these results should be used in combination with benthic community structure analysis and chemical quality determinations of the same sediment (the triad approach). Information concerning the toxicities of sediment-bound pesticides to wetland biota is available, such as that in Chandler (1990) and Chandler and Scott (1991).

Plant species—Wetlands are plant-dominated habitats. Several vascular plants (whole plant, seedlings, and seeds) have been used to assess the toxicity of coastal wetland sediments, but these are less frequently used than tests conducted with animal species. One of the more commonly used tests monitors the effects of contaminated sediment on early seedling growth of rooted macrophytic species (Wang 1992; Weber et al. 1995; Powell et al. 1996; ASTM 1997). These phytotoxicity tests have not been standardized for estuarine species and are in only the early stages of development. Walsh et al. (1990, 1991) describe one of the available test methodologies. The seeds of the plant (field-collected or obtained from a commercial source) are germinated, and the young seedlings are grown in the sediment of interest. A nutrient solution is added to the test species 2 to 3 times weekly. The test is conducted in an environmental growth chamber controlled for humidity, light, and temperature, usually for 20 to 30 d. Effects on root and shoot biomass are determined, as are the effects on whole plant biomass. The test species of choice have been *Spartina alterniflora* (smooth cordgrass), *Echinichloa crusgalli* (river grass), and *Sesbania macrocarpa* (water hemp), although various mangrove species can also be used. *S. alterniflora* is one of the more common test species and is found commonly in eastern U.S. coastal wetlands. If *S. macrocarpa* is used, effects of the sediment on nodule number and weight can also be determined.

A key limitation of the early seedling growth toxicity tests is the porewater salinity of the sediment. The salinity content of the wetland sediment limits the use of many potential test species, particularly if it exceeds 15%. Above this concentration, salinity may affect growth more than the effect of the chemical toxicants in the sediment. This limitation does not apply to those sediments collected from freshwater wetlands and is a major difference in conducting these types of tests. Other phytotoxicity tests have been used, such as those that determine effects on seed germination and root elongation and effects on plant physiology and metabolic activities. The determination of the relationship of peroxidase activity to chemical exposure is one example of attempts to develop stress bioindicators for plants, including several found in wetland areas (Byl and Klaine 1991). Chlorophyll deficiency in red mangroves may be an effective and relatively easy field bioassay for detecting mutagens such as PAHs in tropical coastal wetlands (Klekowski, Corredor, Morrell et al. 1994). Klekowski, Corredor, Lowenfield et al. (1994) have correlated chlorophyll-deficient mutations with in situ sediment PAH concentration.

In summary, sediment toxicity tests have been conducted with only a few organisms that represent those inhabiting coastal wetland areas. The tests have centered on determining acute effects on a few species of amphipods and chronic growth effects on a few vascular emergent plants. Additional information on the environmental relevance of the available data is needed; this can be obtained by conducting acute and chronic toxicity tests with additional species relevant to coastal wetlands.

Multispecies toxicity tests

The environmental significance of laboratory-derived toxicity results has been questioned on numerous occasions, and consequently, more relevant test designs have been utilized. For example, microcosms and mesocosms are ideal for developing experimental databases for model parameterization and hypothesis testing. Wetland microcosms and mesocosms are small samples of real-world coastal wetlands, designed to be representative of certain structural and functional attributes of wetland environments. The advantages of these experimental units are

1) they are reproducible (i.e., pseudoreplication) with measurable variability;
2) many of the important physical driving forces of coastal wetland systems can be controlled (e.g., salinity, nutrients, light, contaminant exposure);
3) experiments can be conducted at relatively low cost, at least compared to broader field studies; and
4) experiments that cannot be conducted in the field can be assessed using microcosms and mesocosms (e.g., high-level contaminant exposures).

Mesocosms are assumed to contain the relevant structural and functional aspects of the ecosystem of interest. Mesocosms have been used to simulate communities representative of streams, ponds, littoral zones of lakes, and estuaries. Mesocosms have been conducted outdoors and indoors for several days and up to several years. The test species have been field collected and also obtained from laboratory cultures. Intermittent and continuous dosing have been used.

The use of the mesocosm approach has been more common for freshwater wetland components. Their use to determine chemical effects on coastal wetlands is rare but a recognized need. The data from the more realistic mesocosm experiments have been compared to those from single-species tests for several chemicals. In most cases, the data trends are chemical specific, and no generalizations can be made. It should also be noted that there are difficulties associated with the use of mesocosms. The difficulty in maintaining the exposure concentration and the reduced level of replication are 2 of these negative factors. In addition to the use of mesocosms, other field-oriented techniques such as in-situ exposure or testing have occurred, examples of which can be found in Clark (1989).

Biomonitoring

The most realistic method of determining the impact of chemicals on coastal wetlands is the use of field biomonitoring techniques. The ecological condition of the biotic communities that inhabit coastal wetlands can be determined by using various sampling devices and analyzing the density and diversity of the community of interest. Routine techniques exist for this (ASTM 1993). In addition, information on a functional parameter, such as photosynthetic activity, and the growth and pigment content can be developed for the plant community and compared to the same parameters for the plant community in a reference wetland using the same analysis techniques. Bioaccumulation is also an assessment tool. Plants and bivalves have been used more often than other biota to determine the bioavailability of toxicants, particularly heavy metals and organics. The degree of uptake has been found to be dependent upon the species and the chemical of concern. Much work has been conducted with *Spartina,* but there appears to be no consensus on the ability of this species to serve as an indicator species because uptake and accumulation rates, particularly for metals, have varied widely. Overall, one of the primary difficulties with using bioaccumulation as an impact indicator is the lack of information for many toxicants on what constitutes a deleterious residue concentration to the organism and its significance to the population. However, it is still useful for evaluating contaminant mobilization into wetland food webs.

Models

Predicting the way in which coastal wetlands and estuaries will respond to anthropogenic modifications is the primary goal of ecosystem ecology as it relates to these types of systems. Adequately predicting ecosystem impacts requires sophisticated simulation models that represent the best available understanding of the way coastal wetland and estuarine systems function. Development of this capability is required for ecosystem management of potential impacts. Several recent developments make the use of these approaches possible. These include

1) accessibility of large spatial and temporal databases (e.g., remote sensing, aerial photography, large monitoring databases) through public access systems (e.g., the Internet),
2) advances in geographical information systems (GIS) technologies, and
3) availability of the computing power necessary to accomplish these models through desktop computing systems.

Current knowledge of spatial and temporal distributions of wetland fauna relative to contaminant burdens and storage pools is inadequate for developing mitigation, management, and restoration activities. Ecosystem-level spatial analyses using GIS formats can produce data-layered maps of spatiotemporal information on populations, communities, and physicochemical and contaminant relationships (e.g., overlays of plant species composition, biomass, density, reproductive indicators, faunal assemblages, body burdens, storage pools of contaminants).

Population, community, and ecosystem coastal wetland simulation models are necessary to evaluate observed laboratory, microcosm, and mesocosm results at these higher levels of ecological organization (Sklar et al. 1985). Ecosystem models tend to be more complex and realistic, while population models tend more toward generality and simplicity. However, both simulation approaches can provide useful tools for extrapolating experimental findings. A further complication, but a further advancement in ecological realism, is the use of spatial series of process-based models constructed into a spatial array to represent the fluxes of contaminants and/or nutrients through transport mechanisms among models. However, these spatially arrayed models require the collection of large amounts of field data for model construction and validation. Many of these models focus on contaminant exposure or bioaccumulation. Additional ecological process model development is needed to examine the effects of these exposures on populations of organisms, particularly on reproductive potential and its long-term effects on population abundance. As with field and laboratory observations, research should be focused on the sources and magnitudes of spatial and temporal variation in these models and their effects on model predictions. Finally, modeling efforts should evaluate model prediction variability due to structural uncertainties. These types of models, once calibrated and validated, can be used for scenario analysis—climate scenarios (e.g., changes in atmospheric forcing), management scenarios (e.g., impacts of site-specific manipulations), historical scenarios (e.g., system behavior without realized management of exposure scenarios), and boundary scenarios (e.g., changes in boundary conditions like sea-level rise) (Costanza et al. 1990).

Summary

Coastal wetlands behave in a manner similar to other ecosystems when they are stressed with contaminants. There is a change in species diversity and biotic density resulting in alteration of the trophic structure and function. However, current scientific information on what constitutes "normal" structure and function in coastal wetlands is limited, as is information on the relevance of current diagnostic tools used to detect these changes. Table 7-5 shows an evaluation of the usefulness of several of the assessment techniques.

Table 7-5 Suitability of biological indicators to detect wetland impacts

	Biological indicators				
Criteria	Bioaccumulation	Macroinvertebrates	Microbes	Bioassays	Biomarkers
Sensitivity	Fair	Good	Good	Good	Good
Common	Good	Good	Good	N/A	N/A
Integrative	Good	Good	Fair	Good	Good
Standardized	Good	Good	Good	Good	Good
Reliable	Fair	Fair	Fair	Good	Good
Predictive	Fair	Good	Good	Good	Good
Rigorous	Good	Good	Fair	Fair	Fair

Source: Adapted from Brown et al. (1989)

The research needs for coastal wetland ecotoxicology are similar to those for ecotoxicology in general. The relevance of the available test methods, toxicity data, and test species are important unknowns. Studies to date have been conducted in relatively short time periods, have used only a few test species, and do not address the effects of seasonal environmental fluctuations in physical, chemical, and biological conditions characteristic of wetlands. The development of criteria for reference wetlands and the determination of the natural variation in wetland structure and function versus that caused by anthropogenic stressors need additional research. Finally, in contrast to freshwater wetlands, the complexity of biota and the influence of salinity and tidal magnitude in coastal wetlands complicate current scientific understanding of most toxicant and nutrient impacts. These factors also complicate the derivation of water-quality criteria and biocriteria.

Contaminants and other risks

Risk assessments of contaminant effects (both potentially toxic chemicals and biostimulatory nutrients) on coastal wetland ecosystems must be placed in the context of the other natural variations, long-term changes, and human-induced physical changes that these wetlands experience. Perhaps as a result of tidal flushing, there are fewer well-documented cases in which anthropogenic contaminants have resulted in the loss or significant alteration of the vascular plant communities of coastal wetlands than there are for nontidal wetlands. The destruction of salt marshes exposed to chronic oil pollution and changes in species composition of heavily nutrient-enriched tidal freshwater wetlands are examples of such effects; however, in general, chemical contamination does not seem to have resulted in major changes in wetland vegetation, or at least, the effects of such contamination are overwhelmed by the effects of human alterations that directly (burning, filling, draining, or impounding wetlands) or indirectly (diverting or adding freshwater or increasing or decreasing sediment supply to an estuary) affect these wetlands.

Of course, contaminants may affect vascular plants in coastal wetlands in ways other than elimination of vegetation or change in species composition. Plant growth may be inhibited or stimulated and reproduction may be affected, and this may affect vegetation cover and composition over a longer period of time. Furthermore, the many other biotic components of coastal wetlands, including microbes, algae, invertebrates, fish, and other vertebrates, may themselves be affected by contamination. In this way, the structure and function of a wetland may be changed without obvious change in the characteristic vegetation. For example, in the South Carolina case described in Chapter 8, high mortality of grass shrimp, *Palaemonetes pugio*, following brief but lethal pesticide exposure, could diminish the food resources of the affected wetland for juvenile fish foraging there or, alternately, allow greater survival of juvenile penaeid shrimp because of reduced competition.

Consequently, it is important not only to quantify the risk posed by contaminant exposure but also to place risk assessment for contaminants in a relative-risk framework. This is necessary to determine the apportionment of regulatory, management, and restoration efforts between contaminant control and remediation and other activities, such as preventing or mitigating hydrological modifications. It is also important to consider that the same wetlands facing risks from chemical contaminants may also be experiencing effects from hydrological modification or other physical impacts that must be accounted for in both risk assessment and risk management. Moreover, some management options may have implications for contaminant risks that must be considered. For example, diversions of fresh water to wetlands facing saltwater intrusion may result in the introduction of potentially toxic chemicals and nutrients.

Constructed, rehabilitated, and managed wetlands

A number of issues regarding contaminants in constructed, rehabilitated, and managed wetlands merit some consideration here from the perspective of coastal wetlands. In particular, these include

1) construction of new wetlands or rehabilitation of deteriorating wetlands with the use of dredged material;
2) wetland creation or enhancement through river diversions;
3) remediation of wetlands damaged by contaminant spills, particularly oil spills; and
4) water-level management in coastal wetlands.

Wetlands constructed or enhanced by dredged material

The natural processes of infilling of coastal estuaries and embayments, coupled with increased soil erosion from human activities on the land, require extensive dredging of coastal ports and waterways in order to maintain navigational access. Most dredged material has no appreciable chemical contamination, but some contains elevated levels of chemical contaminants because of waste discharges into densely populated or heavily industrialized harbor regions and because of the tendency of chemical contaminants to associate with the fine sediments that tend to settle out in dredged channels. Chemical and biological criteria have been established (USACOE/USEPA 1991) to characterize dredged sediments as either contaminated or uncontaminated, and contaminated material must be subject to upland or confined disposal. However, things are not as simple as these 2 categories would suggest because there are intermediate levels of contamination, and toxicity and bioaccumulation are not always easily measured.

Although there may be a variety of effects from channel deepening (Nichols 1979) or subaqueous disposal of dredged materials (Wilson 1988), the risks of contaminants in dredged material used to create or enhance coastal wetlands are the focus of the following discussion. The use of dredged material to construct coastal wetlands has become popular as a form of mitigation to offset losses to wetlands caused by navigational access or coastal development or simply as a beneficial use of what otherwise may be considered as waste product. In addition, dredged material may be used to build or restore barrier islands and other coastal landforms that protect wetlands from erosion. In some cases where wetland subsidence is causing the deterioration of coastal wetlands, dredged materials have been distributed or sprayed over the wetland in order to build up the soil level and, thus, extend the life of the wetland.

Wetlands created or enhanced through river diversion

In the Mississippi Delta Plain, coastal wetlands are being created by diverting and managing the flow from the Mississippi and Atchafalaya rivers; the purpose is to introduce sediments that create new coastal wetlands and provide soil subsidy to sinking wetlands. Even more substantial diversions are being actively planned in an effort to restore the natural processes of active progradation in this delta system. Similarly, it is argued that restoration of freshwater flows through the Everglades is required in order to counter the encroachment of saline, mangrove wetlands into salt-intolerant, grassy wetlands.

Coastal wetland water-level management

Extensive areas of coastal wetlands in San Francisco Bay, south Louisiana, the east coast of Florida, and South Carolina are intentionally impounded (totally or partially) to enhance the production of waterfowl, facilitate aquaculture, reduce tidal erosion, maintain lower salinities, harvest salt, control mosquitoes, or simply as an artifact of a previous use (e.g., agriculture). There are many controversies over "marsh management" that involves water-level controls, including whether they have beneficial or negative effects on the long-term survival of the wetlands and the competing natural resource values that are affected by such management (e.g., waterfowl versus estuarine fisheries), but there obviously also must be differences in the fate and effects of contaminants in impounded (managed) versus unimpounded coastal wetlands. Impoundment affects

1) tidal mixing and, therefore, dilution and dispersion of the contaminant;
2) important biogeochemical processes that occur in wetland soils, which tend to drain less completely under these conditions;
3) the influx and retention of sediments; and
4) which species are exposed and the length of their exposure.

Workgroup Recommendations for Research and Assessment

Fate and effects research

1) Determine the effects of contaminant exposures and bioaccumulation on important birds, aquatic vegetation, fish, reptiles, mammals, and other species that reside in coastal wetlands for either part or all of their life cycle.

Information is needed on the effects on reproduction, growth, and survival. These data should be derived and used in the formulation of water quality standards for coastal wetlands.

2) Study the effects of changing environmental conditions (e.g., freshwater inflow and eutrophication) on the storage, bioavailability, and release of contaminants (particularly chlorinated hydrocarbons and other persistent organics), including assimilative capacity and releases from sediment sequestration.
3) Investigate the effects of contaminants, including both nutrients and potentially toxic contaminants, on the physical, chemical, and biological processes of wetland soil formation and soil remineralization processes.
4) Identify sensitive wetland plant test species and salt-tolerant, rooted vascular plants suitable for use in sediment toxicity testing.
5) Study the fate and effects of contaminants in relatively poorly studied coastal wetland types, including mangrove swamps, tidal freshwater marshes, and subarctic salt marshes.

Methods for interpretation and assessment

1) Develop a framework for reference conditions in salt marshes, brackish marshes, and mangroves, based on comparative synthesis and identifying the natural variability of physicochemical conditions.
2) Develop models and other methods to evaluate the changes in coastal wetlands on various spatial scales (specific wetland, coastal or estuarine ecosystems, watershed, regional, national, and global) in order to determine the significance of locally observed changes and to allow extension of results.
3) Develop interpretative models to translate results of contaminant fate and toxicity experiments to population-, community-, and ecosystem-level effects and methods to validate these models in the field. These models should consider both effects that are directly attributable to the contaminant and cascading effects that result from biotic interactions.

References

Adamus PR. 1989. Wetlands and water quality: EPA's research and monitoring implementation plan for the years 1989–1994. Corvallis OR: U.S. Environmental Protection Agency Environmental Research Laboratory, Office of Research and Development.

Armentano TV, Woodwell GM. 1975. Sedimentation rates in a Long Island marsh determined by 210-Pb dating. *Limnol Oceanogr* 20:452–456.

[ASTM] American Society for Testing and Materials. 1993. ASTM standards on aquatic toxicology and hazard evaluation. Philadelphia PA: ASTM.

[ASTM] American Society for Testing and Materials. 1997. Standard guide for conducting static, axenic, 14-day phytotoxicity tests in test tubes with submersed aquatic macrophyte

Myriophyllum sibiricum Komarov. Annual Book of ASTM Standards. West Conshohocken PA: ASTM. Volume 11.05. E 1913-97.

Ausmus ML, McKellar Jr HN. 1990. Network analysis of the North Inlet salt marsh ecosystem. In: Wulff J, Field JG, Mann KH, editors. Network analysis in marine ecology. Methods and applications. Coastal and Estuarine Studies. New York: Springer-Verlag. p 206–219.

Bjork RD, Powell GVN. 1994. Relationships between hydrological conditions and quality and quantity of foraging habitat for roseate spoonbills and other wading birds in the C-111 basin. Final Report to the South Florida Research Center, Everglades National Park, Homestead, FL, February 1994.

Boesch DF, Josselyn MN, Mehta AJ, Morris JT, Nuttle WK, Simenstad CA, Swift DJP. 1994. Scientific assessment of coastal wetland loss, restoration and management in Louisiana. *Journal of Coastal Research*, Special Issue. No. 20.

Bopp RF, Simpson HJ, Olsen CR, Kostyk N. 1981. Polychlorinated biphenyls in sediments of the tidal Hudson River, New York. *Environ Sci Tech* 15:210–216.

Bradley PM, Morris JT. 1990. Physical characteristics of salt marsh sediments: ecological implications. *Mar Ecol Prog Ser* 61:245–252.

Brown M, Brandt K, Adamus P. 1989. Potential indicators of ecological conditions in inland wetlands (Draft). Prepared for Environmental Monitoring Assessment Program (EMAP), U.S. Environmental Protection Agency, Office of Research and Development, Washington, DC, by University of Florida Center for Wetlands and NSI Technology Services Corporation (October). 77 p.

Brown SL, Lugo AE. 1982. A comparison of structural and functional characteristics of saltwater and freshwater forested wetlands. In: Gopal B, Turner RE, Wetzel RG, Whigham DF, editors. Wetlands—ecology and management. Jaipur, India: National Institute of Ecology and International Scientific Publications. p 109–130.

Burke MV, Mann KH. 1974. Productivity and production: biomass ratios of bivalve and gastropod populations in an eastern Canadian estuary. *J Fish Res Bd Can* 31:167–177.

Byl TD, Klaine SJ. 1991. Peroxidase activity as an indicator of sublethal stress in the aquatic plant, *Hydrilla verticillata* (Royle). In: Gorsuch JW, Lower RW, Wang W, Lewis MA, editors. Plants for toxicity assessment. Volume 2. Philadelphia PA: ASTM. ASTM STP 1115.

Chandler GT. 1990. Effects of sediment-bound residues of the pyrethroid insecticide fenvalerate on survival and reproduction of meiobenthic copepods. *Marine Environ Res* 29:65–76.

Chandler GT, Scott GI. 1991. Effects of sediment-bound endosulfan on survival, reproduction and larval settlement of meiobenthic polychaetes and copepods. *Environ Toxicol Chem* 10:375–382.

Chapman C. 1966. The Texas basins project. In: Smith R, Swartz A, Massman W, editors. Symposium on estuarine fisheries. Am. Fish. Soc. Spec. Publ. 3. p 83–92.

Childers DL, McKellar Jr HN. 1987. A simulation of saltmarsh water column dynamics. *Ecol Modell* 36:211–238.

Clark JR. 1989. Field studies in estuarine ecosystems: a review of approaches for assessing contaminant effects. In: Cowgall UM, Williams LR, editors. Aquatic toxicology and hazard assessment. Volume 12. Philadelphia PA: ASTM. STP 1027.

Clark JR, Lewis MA, Pait AS. 1993. Pesticide inputs and risks in coastal wetlands. *Environ Toxicol Chem* 12:2225–2233.

Clarke J, McFarland VA. 1991. Assessing bioaccumulation in aquatic organisms exposed to contaminated sediments. Vicksburg MS: Corps of Engineers, Waterways Experiment Station. Miscellaneous paper D-91-2.

Costanza R, Farber SC, Maxwell J. 1989. Valuation and management of wetland ecosystems. *Ecological Economics* 1:335–361.

Costanza R, Sklar FH, White ML. 1990. Modeling coastal landscape dynamics. *Bioscience* 40:91–107.

Culliton TJ, Warren MA, Goodspeed TR, Remer DG, Blackwell CM, McDonough III JJ. 1990. 50 years of population change along the nation's coasts. Coastal trends series, Report No. 2. Rockville MD: National Oceanic and Atmospheric Administration, Strategic Assessment Branch. 41 p.

da Cunha LP, Guiss C, Disaro ST. 1991. Seasonal variation of biomass and production dynamics for above- and belowground components of a *Spartina alterniflora* marsh in the euhaline sector of Paranagua Bay (SE Brazil). *Est Coast Shelf Sci* 32:231–241.

Dahl TE. 1990. Wetland losses in the United States 1780s to 1980s. Washington DC: U.S. Dept. of Interior. 13 p.

Dahl TE, Johnson CE. 1991. Wetland status and trends in the conterminous United States mid-1970s to mid-1980s. Washington DC: U.S. Department of the Interior, Fish and Wildlife Service. 21 p.

Dame RF. 1976. Energy flow in an intertidal oyster population. *Est Coast Mar Sci* 4:243–253.

Dame RF, Kenney PD. 1986. Variability of *Spartina alterniflora* primary production in the euhaline North Inlet estuary. *Mar Ecol Prog Ser* 32:70–80.

Dame RF, Zingmark RG, Haskin E. 1984. Oyster reefs as processors of estuarine materials. *J Exp Mar Biol Ecol* 83:239–247.

Day Jr JW, Hall CAS, Kemp WM, Yanez-Arancibia A. 1988. Estuarine ecology. New York: Wiley-Interscience. 588 p.

[FDER] Florida Department of Environmental Regulation. 1988. Chapter 17-6, Regulations for Wastewater Facilities. Tallahassee FL: FDER.

Feld DW, Reyer AJ, Genovese PV, Shearer BD. 1991. Coastal wetlands of the United States: a Special NOAA 20th Anniversary Report. Rockville MD: National Oceanic and Atmospheric Administration Strategic Assessment Branch.

Fleesa KW, Constantine KJ, Kushman MK. 1977. Sedimentation rates in a coastal marsh determined from historical records. *Ches Sci* 18:172–176.

Gambrell RP. 1994. Trace and toxic metals in wetlands—a review. *J Environ Quality* 23:883–891.

Gambrell RP, Collard VR, Reddy CN, Patrick Jr WH. 1977. Trace and toxic metal uptake by marsh plants as affected by Bh, pH, and salinity. Vicksburg MS: Dredged Material Res. Program, U.S. Army Corps of Eng. Waterway Exp. Station. Tech. Rep. D-77-40.

Gambrell RP, Patrick Jr WH. 1988. The influence of redox potential on the environmental chemistry of contaminants in soil and sediments. In: Hook DD, Crawford RMM, editors. The ecology and management of wetlands. Volume 1. Portland OR: Timber Pr. p 319–333.

Getter CD, Scott GI, Michel J. 1981. The effects of oil spills on mangrove forests: a comparison of five oil spill sites in the Gulf of Mexico and the Caribbean Sea. Reprint from Proceedings of the 1981 Oil Spill Conference, API Publ. No. 4334. Washington DC: American Petroleum Inst.

Happ G, Gosselink JK, Day Jr JW. 1977. The seasonal distribution of organic carbon in a Louisiana estuary. *Estuar Coast Mar Sci* 5.

Howarth RW, Giblin A, Gale J, Peterson BH, Luther III GW. 1983. Reduced sulfur compounds in the pore waters of a New England salt marsh. *Environ Biogeochem Ecol Bull* (Stockholm) 35:135–152.

Keefe W. 1972. Marsh production: a summary of the literature. *Contrib Mar Sci* 16:163–181.

Kennish MJ. 1992. Ecology of estuarines: anthropogenic effects. Boca Raton FL: CRC Pr.

King KA, Cromartie E. 1986. Mercury, cadmium, lead, and selenium in 3 waterbird species nesting in Galveston Bay, Texas, USA. *Colonial Waterbirds* 9:90–94.

Kirby-Smith WW, Eisenrich SJ, Howe JT, Luettich Jr RA. 1992. The effects in estuaries of pesticide runoff from adjacent farm lands. CR813415. Final Project Report. Gulf Breeze FL: U.S. Environmental Protection Agency.

Klekowski EJ, Corredor JE, Lowenfield R, Klekowski EH, Morell JM. 1994. Using mangroves to screen mutagens in tropical marine environments. *Mar Pollut Bull* 28:346–350.

Klekowski EJ, Corredor JE, Morrell JM, del Castillo CA. 1994. Petroleum pollution and mutation in mangroves. *Mar Pollut Bull* 28:166–169.

Lana PC, Guiss C. 1992. Macrofauna-plant-biomass interactions in a euhaline salt marsh in Paranagua Bay (SE Brazil). *Mar Ecol Prog Ser* 80:57–64.

Lewis VP, Peters DS. 1984. Menhaden—a single step from vascular plant to fishery harvest. *J Exp Mar Biol Ecol* 84:95–100.

Long ER, Field LJ, MacDonald DD. 1998. Predicting toxicity in marine sediments with numerical sediment quality guidelines. *Environ Toxicol Chem* 17:714–727.

Long ER, Morgan L. 1990. The potential for biological effects of sediment-sorbed contaminants tested. In: The National Status and Trends Program. Seattle WA: National Oceanic and Atmospheric Administration. NOAA Technical Memorandum NOS OMA 52. 215 p.

Lorenz JJ. 1995. Influence of hydrology on fish populations in the mangrove dominated zones of the C-111 and Taylor Slough basins. Report to Everglades National Park. Tavernier FL: National Audubon Society.

Maltby E. 1986. Waterlogged wealth: why waste the world's best places? Washington DC: Earthscan. 200 p.

Mann KH. 1982. Ecology of coastal waters: a system approach. Berkley CA: University of California Press.

Mager Jr A, Thayer GW. 1986. National Marine Fisheries Service habitat conservation efforts in the southeast region of the United States from 1981 through 1985. *Marine Fisheries Review* 48(3):1–8.

Mayer FL. 1987. Acute toxicity handbook of chemical to estuarine organisms. Technical Report. Gulf Breeze FL: U.S. Environmental Protection Agency. EPA 600/8-87-017.

Mazzotti FJ, Brandt LA. 1994. Ecology of the American alligator in a seasonally fluctuating environment. In: Davis SM, Ogden JC, editors. Everglades: the ecosystem and its restoration. Delray Beach FL: St. Lucie Pr.

Mendelssohn, IA, Flynn KM, Wilsey BJ. 1990. The relationship between produced water discharges and plant biomass and species composition in three Louisiana marshes. *Oil Chemical Pollution* 7:317–335.

Mendelssohn IA, McKee KL, Postek ML. 1982. Sublethal stress controlling *Spartina alterniflora* productivity. In: Gopal B, Turner RE, Wetzel RG, Whigham DF, editors. Wetlands ecology and management. Jaipur, India: National Institute of Ecology and International Science Publications. p 223–242.

McIvor CC, Ley JA, Bjork RD. 1994. Changes in freshwater inflow from the Everglades to Florida Bay including effects on biota and biotic processes: a review. In: Davis SM, Ogden JC, editors. Everglades: the ecosystem and its restoration. Delray Beach FL: St. Lucie Pr. p 117–146.

McKee Jr WH, McKevlin MR. 1993. Geochemical processes and nutrient uptake by plants in hydric soils. *Environ Toxicol Chem* 12:2197–2207.

Mitsch WJ, Gosselink JG. 1993. Wetlands. New York: Van Nostrand Reinhold. 722 p.

Montague CL, Ley JA. 1993. A possible effect of salinity fluctuation on abundance of benthic vegetation and associated fauna in Northeastern Florida Bay. *Estuaries* 16:703–717.

Moran MA, Hodson RE. 1990. Contributions of degrading *Spartina alterniflora* lignocellulose to the dissolved organic carbon pool of salt marsh. *Mar Ecol Prog Ser* 62:161–168.

Morris JT. 1984. Effects of oxygen and salinity on ammonium uptake by *Spartina alterniflora* Loisel and *Spartina patens* (Aiton). *J Exp Mar Biol Ecol* 78:87–98.

Morrison D, Malsi J, Renault P, Light P, Marx C. 1990. Effects of freshwater discharge from finger canals on estuarine seagrass and mangrove ecosystems in southwest Florida. In: Webb FJ, editor. Proceedings of 17th Annual Conference on Wetlands Restoration and Creation. Tampa FL: Hillsborough Community College. p 115–126.

Nelson DW, Monaco ME, Irlandi EA, Settle LR, Coston-Clements L. 1991. Distribution and abundance of fishes and invertebrates on Southeast estuaries. Rockville MD: National Oceanic and Atmospheric Administration. ELMR Report No. 9.

Nelson DW, Monaco ME, Williams CD, Czapla TE, Pattillo ME, Coston-Clements L, Settle LR, Irlandi EA. 1992. Distribution and abundance of fishes and invertebrates on Gulf of Mexico estuaries. Volume 1, Data summaries. Rockville MD: National Oceanic and Atmospheric Administration. ELMR Report No. 10.

Nelson RW. 1990. National guidance water quality standards for wetlands. Washington DC: U.S. Environmental Protection Agency, Office of Wetlands Protection.

Nichols FH, Cloern JE, Lourma SN, Peerson DH. 1986. The modification of an estuary. *Science* 231:567–573.

Nichols MM. 1979. The problem of misplaced sediment. In: Palmer HD, Gross MG, editors. Ocean dumping and marine pollution. Stroudsberg PA: Dowden, Hutchinson & Ross.

Nixon SW. 1980. Between coastal marshes and coastal waters—a review of twenty years of speculation and research on the role of salt marshes in estuarine productivity and water chemistry. In: Hamilton P, MacDonald KB, editors. Estuarine and wetland processes with emphasis on modeling. New York: Plenum. p 437–525.

[NRC] National Research Council. 1993. Managing wastewater in coastal urban areas. Washington DC: National Academy Pr.

O'Connor TP, Beliaeff B. 1995. Recent trends in coastal environmental quality: results from the mussel watch project 1986 to 1993. Rockville MD: National Oceanic and Atmospheric Administration.

Odum W, McIvor CC, Smith III TJ. 1982. The ecology of the mangroves of south Florida: a community profile. FWS/OSB-81/24. Washington DC: U.S. Fish and Wildlife Service, Office of Biological Services. 144 p.

Odum WE. 1984. Dual-gradient concept of detritus transport and processing in estuaries. *Bull Mar Sci* 35.

Ogden JC. 1994. A comparison of wading bird nesting colony dynamics (1931–1943 and 1974–1989) as an indication of ecosystem conditions in the southern Everglades. In: Davis SM, Ogden JC, editors. Everglades: the ecosystem and its restoration. Delray Beach FL: St. Lucie Pr.

Ohlendorf HM, Fleming WJ. 1988. Birds and environmental contaminants in San Francisco and Chesapeake Bays. *Mar Pollut Bull* 9:487–495.

Pait AS, De Souza AE, Farrow DRG. 1992. Agricultural pesticide use in coastal areas: a national summary. Rockville MD: National Oceanic and Atmospheric Administration.

Pomeroy LR, Darley WM, Dunn EL, Gallagher JL, Haines EB, Whitney DM. 1981. Primary production. In: Pomeroy LR, Wiegert RG, editors. The ecology of a salt marsh. New York: Springer-Verlag. p 39–67.

Ponds LJ. 1988. Wetland soils with high sulfide content. In: Hook DD, Crawford RMM, editors. The ecology and management of wetlands. Volume 1. Portland OR: Timber Pr. p 319–333.

Powell GVN, Bjork RD, Ogden JC, Paul RT, Powell AH, Robertson WB. 1989. Population trends in some Florida Bay wading birds. *Wilson Bull* 01:436–457.

Powell GVN, Powell AH. 1986. Reproduction by great white herons, *Ardea herodias*, in Florida Bay as an indicator of habitat quality. *Biol Conserv* 36:101–113.

Powell RL, Kimerle RA, Moser EM. 1996. Development of a plant bioassay to assess toxicity of chemical stressors to emergent macrophytes. *Environ Toxicol Chem* 15:1570–1576.

Pozo J, Colino R. 1992. Decomposition processes of *Spartina maritima* in a salt marsh of the Basque country. *Hydrobiol* 231:165–175.

Redfield AC. 1972. Development of a New England salt marsh. *Ecol Monogr* 42:201–237.

Rice C, White D. 1987. PCB availability assessment of river dredging using caged clams and fish. *Environ Toxicol* 6:259–274.

Richard GA. 1978. Seasonal and environmental variations in sediment accretion in a Long Island salt marsh. Estuaries 1:29–35.

Richardson MG. 1979. Esso Bernicia incident, Shetland. *Mar Pollut Bull* 10:97.

Saloman CH, Naughton SP, Taylor JL. 1982. Benthic community response to dredging barrow pits, Panama City Beach, Florida. Vicksburg MS: U.S. Army Corps of Engineers. Misc. Rep. No. 82-3. 138 p.

Sather JH, Smith RD. 1984. An overview of major wetland functions. Washington DC: U.S. Fish and Wildlife Service. FWS/OBS-84/18.

Scott GI, Fulton MH, Crosby MC, Key PB, Daughomah J, Waldren JT, Strozier ED, Louden CJ, Chandler GT, Bidleman RF, Jackson KL, Hampton TW, Hoffman T, Schulz A, Bradford M. 1992. Agricultural insecticide runoff effects on estuarine organisms: correlating laboratory and field toxicity tests, ecophysiology bioassays, and ecotoxicological biomonitoring. Final Project Report. Gulf Breeze FL: U.S. Environmental Protection Agency. CR813138-2.

[SFWMD] South Florida Water Management District. 1995. South Florida ecosystem restoration. Master Plan. Draft. Brooksville FL: SFWMD.

Sharma P, Gardner LT, Moore WS, Bollinger MS. 1987. Sedimentation and bioturbation in a salt marsh as revealed by 210-Pb, 137-Cs, and 7-Bi studies. *Limnol Oceanogr* 32:313–326.

Simenstad CA, Jay DA, Sherwood CR. 1992. Impacts of watershed management on land-margin ecosystems: the Columbia River estuary. In: Naiman RJ, editor. Watershed management: balancing sustainability and environmental change. New York: Springer-Verlag. p 266–306.

Sklar FH, Costanza R, Day Jr JW. 1985. Dynamic simulation modeling of coastal wetland habitat succession. *Ecol Modell* 29:261–281.

Smart RM, Barko JW. 1980. Nitrogen nutrition and salinity tolerance of *Distichlis spicata* and *Spartina alterniflora*. *Ecology* 61:630–638.

Stanley DJ, White AG. 1993. Nile delta: recent geological evolution and human impacts. *Science* 260:628–634.

Summers JK, McKellar Jr HN. 1981. The role of physical forcing functions in an estuarine model of carbon exchange with the sea. *J Int Soc Ecol Modell* 3:71–101.

Summers JK, McKellar Jr HN, Dame RF, Kitchens WM. 1980. A simulation model of estuarine subsystem coupling and carbon exchange with the sea. 2. North Inlet model structure, output, and validation. *Ecol Modell* 11:101–140.

Traunspurger W, Drews C. 1996. Toxicity analysis of freshwater and marine sediments with meio- and macrobenthic organisms: a review. *Hydrobiologia* 328:215–261.

Trent L, Pullen EJ, Proctor R. 1976. Abundance of macrocrustaceans in a natural marsh altered by dredging, bulkheading, and filling. *Fishery Bull* 74:192–200.

Turner RE. 1976. Geographic variations in salt marsh macrophyte production: a review. *Contrib Mar Sci* 20:47–68.

[USACOE] U.S. Army Corps of Engineers. 1994. Environmental quality risk assessment handbook. Volume 2, Environmental evaluation. Washington DC: USACOE. Manual No. 200-1-4.

[USACOE] U.S. Army Corps of Engineers. 1996. Preliminary protocol for conducting 28-day chronic sublethal sediment bioassays using the estuarine amphipod *Leptocheirus plumulosus* (Shoemaker). Vicksburg MS: USACOE. EEDP-01-36.

[USACOE/USEPA] U.S. Army Corps of Engineers/U.S. Environmental Protection Agency. 1991. Evaluation of dredged material proposed for ocean disposal. Washington DC: Office of Water. EPA-503/8-91-001.

[USEPA] U.S. Environmental Protection Agency. 1986. Hazard evaluation division: standard evaluation procedure—ecological risk assessment. Washington DC: Office of Pesticide Programs.

[USEPA] U.S. Environmental Protection Agency. 1988a. America's wetlands. Our vital link between land and water. Washington DC: Office of Wetlands Protection. OPA-87-016.

[USEPA] U.S. Environmental Protection Agency. 1988b. Review of ecological risk assessment methods. Washington DC: Office of Policy Analysis, Planning, and Evaluation. EPA/230/10-88/041.

[USEPA] U.S. Environmental Protection Agency. 1990. Water quality standards for wetlands. Washington DC: Office of Water. EPA/440/5-90/011.

[USEPA] U.S. Environmental Protection Agency. 1992a. Framework for ecological risk assessment. Washington DC: USEPA. EPA/630/R-92/001.

[USEPA] U.S. Environmental Protection Agency. 1992b. Short-term methods for estimating the chronic toxicity of effluents and receiving waters to marine and estuarine organisms. Washington DC: USEPA. EPA/600/4-91/021.

[USEPA] U.S. Environmental Protection Agency. 1994. Methods for assessing the toxicity of sediment-associated contaminants with estuarine and marine amphipods. Washington DC: USEPA. EPA/600/R-94/025.

[USEPA] U.S. Environmental Protection Agency. 1997. Ecological risk assessment guidance for Superfund: process for designing and conducting ecological risk assessments. Washington DC: Office of Solid Waste and Emergency Response. EPA/540/R-97/006.

[USEPA] U.S. Environmental Protection Agency. 1998. Guidelines for ecological risk assessment. Washington DC: USEPA. EPA/630/R-95/002F.

Valiela I. 1984. Marine ecological processes. New York: Springer-Verlag. 640 p.

Vernberg FJ. 1993. Salt-marsh processes: a review. *Environ Toxicol Chem* 12:2167–2195.

Vernberg FJ, Vernberg WB. 1974. Pollution and physiology of marine organisms. New York: Academic Pr. 492 p.

Wakeman TH. 1977. Release of trace constituents from sediments resuspended during dredging operations. In: Yen TF, editor. Chemistry of marine sediments. Ann Arbor MI: Ann Arbor Science. p 173–180.

Walsh GE, Weber DE, Brashers LK, Simon TL. 1990. Artificial sediments for use in tests with wetland plants. *Environ Exper Botany* 30:391–396.

Walsh GE, Weber DE, Simon TL, Brashers LK, Moore JC. 1991. Use of marsh plants for toxicity testing of water and sediments. In: Gorsuch JW, Lower WR, Lewis MA, Wang W, editors. Plants for toxicity assessment. Philadelphia PA: ASTM. STP 1115. p 341–354.

Walters C, Gunderson L, Holling CS. 1992. Experimental policies for water management in the Everglades. *Ecol Appl* 2(2):189–202.

Wang W. 1992. Use of plants for the assessment of environmental contaminants. *Rev Environ Contam Toxicol* 126:87–127

Watzin MC, Gosselink JG. 1992. Coastal wetlands of the continental United States. Baton Rouge LA: Louisiana Sea Grant College Program, Louisiana State University.

Weber DE, Walsh GE, MacGregor MA. 1995. Use of vascular aquatic plants in phytotoxicity studies with sediments. In: Hughes JS, Biddinger GR, Mones E, editors. Environmental toxicology and risk assessment. Third volume. Philadelphia PA: American Society for Testing and Materials. STP 1218. p 187–200.

Whitney DM, Chalmers AG, Haines EG, Hanson RB, Pomeroy LR, Sherr B. 1981. The cycles of nitrogen and phosphorus. In: Pomeroy LR, Wiegert RG, editors. The ecology of a salt marsh. New York: Springer-Verlag. p 164–181.

Wiebe WJ, Pomeroy LR. 1972. Microorganisms and their association with aggregates and detritus in the sea: a microscopic study. *Mem Ist Ital Idrobiol Dott Marco Marchi* 29(suppl.):325–352.

Wilson JG. 1988. The biology of estuarine management. London UK: Croom Helm.

Wolaver TG, Dame RF, Spurrier JD, Miller AB. 1988a. Bly Creek ecosystem study—inorganic sediment transport within an euhline salt marsh basin, North Inlet, South Carolina. *J Coast Res* 4:607–615.

Wolaver TG, Dame RF, Spurrier JD, Miller AB. 1988b. Sediment exchange between a euhaline salt marsh in South Carolina and the adjacent tidal creek. *J Coast Res* 4:17–26.

Wolff WJ, de Wolf L. 1977. Biomass and production of zoobenthos in the Grevelingen estuary, The Netherlands. *Est Coast Mar Sci* 5:1–24.

Wotton RS, editor. 1990. The biology of particles in aquatic systems. Boca Raton FL: CRC Pr. 336 p.

Chapter 8

Case Study: Ecotoxicological Assessment of Urban and Agricultural Nonpoint Source Runoff Effects on the Grass Shrimp, *Palaemonetes pugio*

Dana B. Finley, Geoffrey I. Scott, James W. Daugomah, Shawn L. Layman, LouAnn Reed, Marion Sanders, Scott K. Sivertsen, Erich D. Strozier

Estuaries have long been considered buffers for the detrimental effects of human waste and pollution on the world's oceans. Unfortunately, coastal areas are the most populated areas in many countries. It is estimated that by the year 2000, 75% of the U.S. population will reside within 100 km of the coast (Vernberg et al. 1992). This will result in significant changes in landscape ecology that may adversely affect estuarine ecosystem health. Ecological effects from increasing contamination due to nonpoint source (NPS) runoff in urbanized estuarine areas have not been adequately studied, although several studies (Vernberg et al. 1992; Fulton et al. 1993) have documented inputs of different components into the environment. For management practices to be employed, an understanding of the risk to fisheries production and human health must be discerned. This is particularly true in the southeastern U.S. There are over 300 small estuaries and tributaries from North Carolina through the eastern coast of Florida with substantial fisheries production at risk from the increase in urbanization within this region (NOAA 1994, 1995). It has been estimated that estuaries support 99% of the total world fish population even though they make up only 10% of the world's total oceanic environment (CEQ 1983).

Chapter Preview

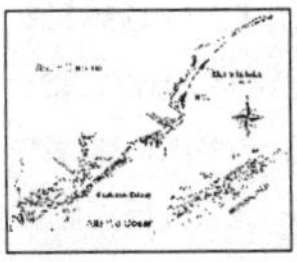

Ecotoxicology and Risk Assessment for Wetlands. Michael A. Lewis et al., editors.
 ISBN 1-880611-16-3

Nonpoint source release of polycyclic aromatic hydrocarbons (PAHs) into estuarine ecosystems may be due partly to anthropogenic sources such as atmospheric fallout, runoff from roadways, and boat emissions (USEPA 1979; Hoffman et al. 1983, 1985; Kucklick and Bidleman 1994; Pathirana et al. 1994). Natural processes such as volatilization, sedimentation, photochemical oxidation, and microbial degradation act to remove hydrocarbons from the water column (Zepp and Cline 1977; Lee et al. 1978; Gardner et al. 1979; USEPA 1979; Neely and Blau 1985) but in many environments, the removal processes are not fast enough to prevent significant exposure or accumulation by aquatic organisms (Gardner et al. 1979; Hoffman et al. 1983, 1985; Kucklick and Bidleman 1994; Pathirana et al. 1994). Many aromatic hydrocarbons settle to the bottom by adsorbing to fine-grain clays and organic matter (OM) (Lee et al. 1978). Such sedimentation allows intimate contact with estuarine epibenthic organisms such as the grass shrimp. Gardner et al. (1979) found marsh sediments conducive to only the slowest aromatic degradation because the oils become trapped and unavailable for microbial degradation. The acute and chronic effect of PAH interaction on faunal organisms and the extent to which bioaccumulation may occur is not completely understood. Bioaccumulation tends to occur with substances that have low vapor pressure, chemical stability, lipid stability, and a slow rate of biotransformation and degradation (Thomas and Colburn 1992).

Additional concern has been focused on agricultural NPS runoff effects on estuarine organisms within the southeastern U.S. (Scott et al. 1990, 1992), particularly since many agricultural areas will be transformed into urban landscape. Indeed, herbicide and fungicide usage may surpass agricultural insecticide usage in many southeastern coastal regions to meet demand for flawless golf courses and weed-free lawns and gardens (Colborn and Clement 1992). Earlier studies (Scott et al. 1990, 1992) of agricultural NPS runoff have established that discharges of insecticides occur with large pulsed exposures of freshwater as a result of rain events. This can create toxic conditions for grass shrimp (Baughman 1986), other crustaceans (Scott et al. 1990, 1992), fish (Fulton and Scott 1992), and other organisms (Chandler 1990). The primary insecticides applied to vegetables, the major agricultural crop in the coastal region of SC, are fenvalerate, azinphosmethyl, and endosulfan. Pyrethroids such as fenvalerate are detoxified quickly in mammals but have proved to be extremely toxic to aquatic organisms (96-h LC50 < 0.100 μg/L) (Chandler 1990). Azinphosmethyl, an organophosphate, is a slow, reversible acetylcholinesterase (AChE) inhibitor in mammals (Murphy 1986). *Palaemonetes pugio* exposure to the organochlorine endosulfan resulted in a 0.25 μg/L 96-h LC50 value (Scott et al. 1990). Initial effects of pulsed runoff events can be devastating, and chronic effects have been observed in benthic crustaceans as a result of sediment exposure to insecticides (Chandler and Scott 1991). Certainly, contaminant evaluation of NPS runoff is much more difficult than for point sources. For these reasons, it has become critical to understand the effects that high human-population densities may have on estuarine environments.

The grass shrimp, *Palaemonetes pugio,* is a common inhabitant of estuaries from Nova Scotia to the U.S. Gulf Coast (Williams and Wigley 1977). Although grass shrimp are of no direct commercial value, they are vital links in food chains by nutritionally supporting commercial and game fishes (Meehean 1936). One of the major roles of *P. pugio* is to accelerate the breakdown of the marsh grass and macroalgal detritus by releasing it as a heterogeneous mixture of fecal matter, grass shrimp biomass, and dissolved OM. These carbon sources are in turn channeled into the surrounding waters as a more readily available source of energy for the detrital food web (Welsh 1975; Buikema et al. 1980). The grass shrimp is uniquely adapted to the rigors of the dynamic environment of the estuary (Buikema et al. 1980). Of organisms found in small tidal creeks along the SC coast, the grass shrimp is the most abundant, with densities comprising > 50% of total stream annual abundance of pelagic macrofauna (> 15 mm) (Scott et al. 1992). In these areas, grass shrimp typically inhabit shallow marshes with emergent vegetation such as *Spartina alterniflora* (Buikema et al. 1980). Most of the energy in estuaries is contained in this vegetation, which is resistant to normal decomposition by microbes (Burkholder and Bornside 1956; Buikema et al. 1980).

Considerable variation in the life history of the grass shrimp has been reported to correlate with differences in environmental parameters (Anderson 1985). Alon and Stancyk (1982) have reported marked differences between 2 *P. pugio* populations and attributed the differences to salinity. These differences were not solely related to salinity but may also be due to the many variations between riverine and nonriverine estuaries where this study was conducted. This adaptability has allowed *P. pugio* to be recognized for its usefulness in acute laboratory toxicity tests for pesticides (van Dijk et al. 1977) and in situ toxicity tests (Scott et al. 1990, 1992), and it has also proved sensitive to many chemical contaminants (Sunda et al. 1978; Buikema et al. 1980; Fisher and Foss 1993). Because of *P. pugio's* abundance, sensitivity, and overall importance in southeastern estuaries of the U.S., it provides a useful ecotoxicological model to examine the effects of increasing NPS runoff pollution. To date, there have been many ecological studies on *P. pugio* to determine variation in life-history parameters (Wood 1967; Welsh 1975; Sikora 1977; Alon and Stancyk 1982), but none has attempted to use these differences to indicate the health of an estuary and its associated wetland areas and to correlate them with chemical contaminant inputs from urban and agricultural NPS runoff, as is our goal in this study.

Materials and Methods

Study sites

Ten sites along the SC coast were chosen that were affected by a wide range of urban and agricultural NPS runoff (Figure 8-1). The 2 agricultural watershed sites used were Kiawah (KWA) and treatment (TRT) sites. The KWA site is located on John's Island near Crab Haul Creek. This agricultural site does not use best management

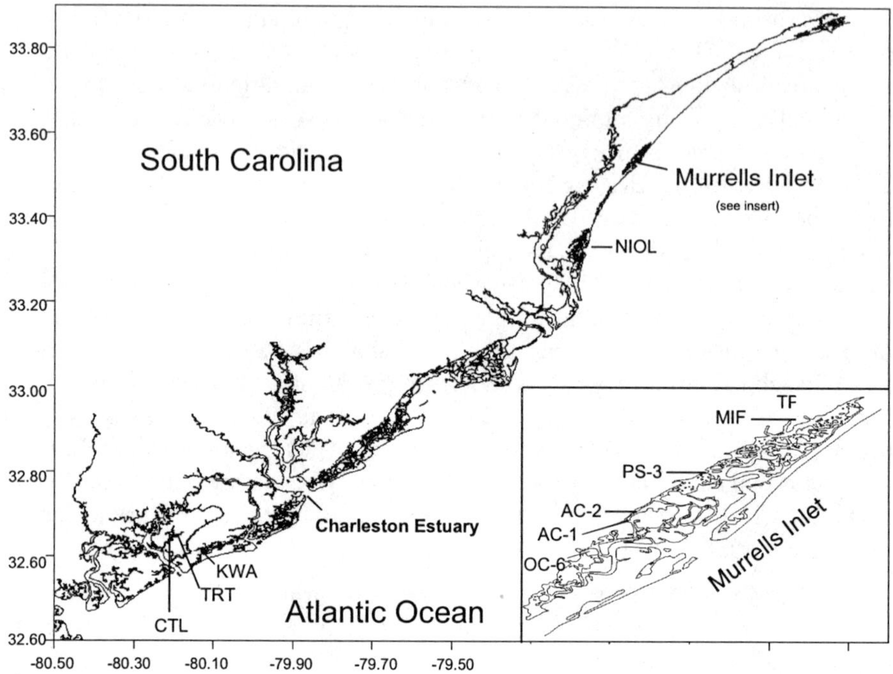

Figure 8-1 Map of SC indicating the locations of the 10 study sites. Main map: 1 cm = 3.4 km, Insert: 1 cm = 0.41 km

practices (BMPs), integrated pest management (IPM), or retention ponds (RPs) to control runoff. The TRT site, located on the eastern branch of Leadenwah Creek on Wadmalaw Island, is highly managed through the application of BMPs, IPM, and RPs to successfully reduce insecticide loading by > 89% (Scott et al. 1992). A reference site (CTL) was chosen near the agricultural watersheds. It is located on the western branch of Leadenwah Creek on Wadmalaw Island and is surrounded by deciduous forests and rural, single-family dwellings.

All of the urban watershed study sites are located in Murrells Inlet (MI), south of the Myrtle Beach "Grand Strand" in SC (Figure 8-1). Extensive urbanization from housing and service industries has resulted in the highest population density (> 600 residents/mi^2) in SC; however, there are no standard industrial codes for discharges into MI (Vernberg et al. 1992). The southernmost site selected in this area is OC-6 (Oak Creek), which is a small, private boat landing in an otherwise undeveloped area of MI. The next two sites, AC-1 (Alston Creek-1) and AC-2 (Alston Creek-2) are located in a small residential area (AC-1) and adjacent to a small seafood restaurant (AC-2). Parsonage Creek (PS-3) site is located in a large, public boat landing in a highly urbanized, impounded watershed in MI. The MIF site (Murrells Inlet Flo's Restaurant) is in an impounded watershed that has been dredged and significantly altered. Similarly, the TP-1 (Trailer Park-1) site is in a highly urbanized watershed, adjacent to the main causeway leading to Garden City beach, in a dredge canal draining a mobile home park. The reference site for the urbanized areas, North Inlet (NIOL), is located at Oyster Landing in North Inlet Estuary (NI) approximately 50 km south of MI. North Inlet Estuary is undeveloped and actively maintained as a National Estuarine Research Reserve and Sanctuary site by the National Oceanic and Atmospheric Administration (NOAA) and has been a long-term ecological research study site of the National Science Foundation.

Chemical analysis: agricultural insecticide runoff

To assess impacts of insecticide runoff at the CTL, TRT, and KWA sites, surfacewater (500 mL) samples were collected following periods of significant (> 1.27 cm/day) precipitation. The samples were extracted using C-18 solid phase extraction cartridges (Baxter #9006), eluted with ethyl acetate and analyzed by capillary column gas chromatography (CC-GC) (model HP-5890A) using electron capture and nitrogen phosphorous detectors (ECD and NPD, respectively) with methods described by Scott et al. (1990, 1992). The insecticides analyzed for were azinphos-methyl, endosulfan, and fenvalerate. Lower limits of detection for each insecticide ranged from 0.002 to 0.005 μg/L, and spiked recovery efficiencies were > 82%.

In addition, surface sediment samples were collected from each site and analyzed for insecticides using methods described by Scott et al. (1992) and USEPA (1980). The top 20 mm to 30 mm of surface sediments were collected and placed into a solvent-cleaned glass jar (0.5 L). All samples were then sealed and frozen (–30 °C) until analyzed. Samples were thawed and three 20-g aliquots of wet sediment were placed in aluminum weighing boats and dried at 60 °C for 24 h in a dry air incubator. After 24 h, samples were reweighed to determine % water content as described by USEPA (1980). Next, 7 g to 10 g of wet sediment from each sample was mixed with 100 g sodium sulfate. After they were dried, the samples were broken into a powder with a mortar and pestle and then placed in a solvent-cleaned glass thimble. Each sample was then Soxhlet-extracted for 14 h with dichloromethane (250 mL volume) at a rate of 1 cycle/h. Samples were then blown to 0.5 mL under a dry stream of nitrogen and added to 1 mL hexane (nanograde) before 0.5 mL of Hg (triple distilled) was added to each sample. Samples were vortexed for 30 s, allowed to settle, and vortexed again for another 30 s. The precipitate in each sample was allowed to settle, and the clean solvent (hexane) layer was decanted. Samples were transferred in a Florisil column and eluted into 3 separate fractions with 15 mL of 6%, 15%, and 50% ethyl ether in hexane, respectively. Each of the 3 fractions was evaporated under a dry stream of N to 1 mL and then diluted up to 5 mL with isooctane.

Sediment samples were analyzed by CC-GC (model HP-5890A) using USEPA (1980) methodologies and the same general procedure used in the analysis of water samples. The CC-GC used a DB-5 (5% phenyl, J & W Scientific) capillary column (25 m) and was equipped with either an ECD or an NPD. Samples were injected in the splitless mode with helium as the carrier gas at a flow rate of 1 mL/min. The injector temperature for the GC ECD was 220 °C, and the detector temperature for the ECD and NPD was 300 °C. A temperature program with a 20 °C/min ramp from 90 °C to 200 °C and then 10 °C/min ramp from 200 °C to 290 °C with a 15-min hold at 290 °C was used for the ECD and NPD. Analytes were quantified using single-point calibration and external standards. Results are reported in μg/kg dry weight for each insecticide detected. Lower limits of detection ranged from 0.1 μg/kg to 0.5 μg/kg dry weight, and spiked recovery efficiencies averaged 86.7%.

Chemical analysis: PAHs, chlorinated pesticides, and PCBs

Sediment samples were collected from each site in MI and NIOL. Sediment samples were analyzed for trace metals (Cr, Cu, Ni, Pb and Zn), PAHs [benzo(a)pyrene; benzo(g,h,i)perylene; benzo(k)fluoranthene; benzo(b)fluoranthene; chrysene; benzo(a)anthracene; pyrene; fluorene; anthracene; and phenanthrene], pesticides (4,4'-DDT, 4,4'- DDE, 4,4'- DDD, t-nonachlor, α-chlordane), and polychlorinated biphenyls (PCB congeners 52, 44, 66, 101, 118, 138, and 153) using methods described in the following section.

The analytical procedure for the quantification of PAHs, chlorinated pesticides, and PCBs in sediment was a modification of the methods of Krahn et al. (1988) and Schantz (1990). Briefly stated, the samples were removed from frozen storage and allowed to thaw at room temperature. For sediment, 8.5 g were placed into a glass mortar and mixed with 100 g of ashed (700 °C) anhydrous sodium sulfate. Any clumps that formed were broken with a glass pestle to form a dry powder. The sulfated samples were placed into glass Soxhlet thimbles, and 6 method internal standards (d-phenanthrene, d-fluoranthene, d-perylene, dibromooctafluorobiphenyl (DBOFBP), PCB congeners 103 and 198) were added to each sample and Soxhlet-extracted for 18 h with methylene chloride. Each extract was concentrated to 500 mL on an automatic concentrator (TurboVap). Initial cleanup began by injecting 400 mL of the extract into a semi-automated high performance-gel permeation chromatographic (HP-GPC) system equipped with an autosampler, fraction collector, UV detector, and 2 size-exclusion columns connected in series. High-molecular-weight compounds such as lipids were removed from the extract in the first 14-min fraction of the chromatogram. The fraction of interest was collected between 1 min before the retention time of DBOFBP and 2 min after perylene. The mobile phase was methylene chloride at 9.0 mL/min. The methylene chloride in the collected fraction was replaced with hexane and the volume reduced to 500 mL. Activated Cu was added to the hexane extract to remove S. The S-free extract was transferred onto a hexane-rinsed cyanopropyl solid-phase extraction (SPE) column and eluted with 12 mL of hexane. The hexane extract was reduced to 500 mL. An aliquot of 250 mL was taken for gel permeation chromatography (GPC) analysis. The hexane in the remaining 250 mL was replaced with acetonitrile for high performance liquid chromatography (HPLC) analysis.

PAHs

The 2 methods used to quantify PAHs (Table 8-1) were capillary gas chromatography–ion trap mass spectrometry (GC–ITMS), as described in Kucklick et al. (1997), and HPLC with fluorescence detection, utilizing a method reported by Sanders (1995), which was similar to Wise et al. (1988) and Schantz et al. (1990). Two fluorescence detectors (Perkin Elmer LC-240 and LS-4) connected in series at wavelengths specific to individual PAHs were used to monitor fluorescence. The separation between deuterated and nondeuterated PAHs was 0.44, 0.40, and 0.41 min for phenanthrene, fluoranthene, and perylene, respectively. Personal computer-based software (Perkin Elmer Omega II) was used for data collection. A National Institute of Standards and Technology (NIST) certified PAH standard solution and the deuterated PAH internal standards were used to calibrate the instrument. Retention times and fluorescence-specific wavelengths identified sample peaks.

Table 8-1 Recovery of PAHs from spiked matrices analyzed by HPLC with fluorescence detection[1]

Compound	Amount added (ng/g dry weight)	Amount recovered (ng/g dry weight)	Mean recovered (%)	Standard deviation (%)
Fluorene	12.8	7.8	61	14.8
Phenanthrene	12.9	13.1	102	7.0
Anthracene	9.8	7.6	78	29.6
Fluoranthene	12.9	13.2	102	15.2
Pyrene	12.9	14.0	109	18.6
Benzo(a)anthracene	11.1	12.5	113	14.4
Chrysene	12.9	14.3	111	18.6
Perylene	9.7	9.0	93	18.6
Benzo(b)fluoranthene	12.9	15.2	118	22.5
Benzo(k)fluoranthene	12.9	12.9	100	14.0
Benzo(a)pyrene	11.6	10.7	92	21.6
Dibenzo(a,h)anthracene	9.8	9.1	93	24.5
Benzo(g,h,i)perylene	11.4	12.0	105	23.7

[1] A total of 6 amended sediments were analyzed at 2 spike levels. The average percent recovery of all spike levels is presented.
[2] Method detection limit was determined from the standard deviation of the analysis of the spikes, according to CFR (1991).

PCBs and pesticides

Chlorine-containing compounds (pesticides and PCBs) were analyzed using gas chromatography with electron capture detection (GC-ECD; Hewlett-Packard 5890 series II), equipped with 2 columns, a 30 m × 0.25 mm i.d. (0.25-µm film thickness) DB-5 (5% phenyl; J&W Scientific) and a column with equal dimensions and 50% phenyl (Rtx-50; Restek Corp.). At the head of each column, a 5-m guard column was used to protect the analytical column. The carrier gas was held at a constant average linear velocity of 33 cm/s by pressure programming the injector. The carrier and detector makeup gases were helium and argon:methane (95%:5%), respectively. The injector and detector temperatures were 250 °C and 320 °C, respectively. A 2-μL sample was injected using a splitless Grob technique (1-min split time). The sample was then split so that nearly equal portions were sent to each column. The initial oven temperature was 50 °C with a 1-min hold, followed by a ramp to 170 °C at 4 °C/min, then from 170 °C to 210 °C at 1 °C/min then from 210 °C to 310 °C at 4 °C/min with a 10-min hold. A Windows-based EZ Chrom software (Scientific Software Inc.) was used to digitize and process the detector signal.

A mixed standard of target analyte (chlorinated pesticides, NIST SRM 2261; and PCB congeners, NIST/NOAA intercalibration mixture) prepared with internal standards (DBOFBP, PCB congeners 103 and 198) was used to calibrate the instrument. There were 3 concentrations of the standards prepared that bracketed the sample concentrations. The slope of the response curve with respect to the internal standards was used to quantify the concentrations of the analytes. The calibration curve was verified at the beginning of each sample set by injection of a check standard, which was required to be within ±20% of the known value for each analyte or the instrument was recalibrated.

Retention data were simultaneously acquired from the 2 columns and were used to identify the analytes. On each column, unknown peaks were identified relative to standards. If the unknown analyte peak fell within ±0.05 min of the standard and was present on both columns, then the peak was determined to be authentic. The analyte amount was determined on each column, and the lower amount was reported.

Trace metals

Samples for metal analyses were microwave-digested (CEM Corporation 1988) in closed Teflon vessels with nitric acid. The digestate was analyzed on a Perkin-Elmer Inductively Coupled Plasma Sequential Spectrometer (USEPA 1982) for Cr, Cu, Ni, Pb, and Zn.

The metal Pb also was analyzed by graphite furnace atomic absorption (Perkin Elmer 5100 Atomic Absorption Spectrometer with a Zeeman HGA 600 Graphite Furnace). Prior to sample analysis, the instrument was calibrated with 5 separate concentrations of each metal, spanning approximately 1 order of magnitude. The modifier PO_4-$Mg(NO_3)_2$ was used for Pb. Samples were analyzed in duplicate and the results averaged.

Characterization of grass shrimp population

Palaemonetes pugio samples were collected monthly from April 1993 to March 1994. A dip net (31-cm length × 30-cm width × 4-mm mesh) was pushed 25 m along each bank at 3 different lateral stream locations (ebb, mid, and flood) per site. The contents of the 2 tows along each stream bank were combined to estimate population dynamics within each stream reach (n = 3/site). Grass shrimp were weighed wet to determine biomass (g/m stream) and density (#/m stream) was also enumerated. Samples were then fixed in 10% buffered formalin. Because of the large samples resulting from the pushnetting technique, random subsamples from each fixed collection (30 individuals/stream area) were selected and identified under a dissecting microscope as males, gravid females, or nongravid females to estimate population sex ratios. If gravid females were present, the clutch size (# eggs/female) and approximate egg stage were determined. The number of gravid females and clutch size data was then used to determine site-specific total egg production (product of the mean clutch size/site and the total number of gravid females found in an individual subsample). Site-specific water temperature (°C), dissolved oxygen (mg/L), and salinity (ppt) values were recorded at the time of each monthly collection, and the proportion of males, gravid females, and nongravid females for each site was calculated.

Statistical analysis

All physicochemical water-quality, chemical-contaminants, and grass-shrimp-population metrics data were statistically analyzed in the following manner. Initially, all data were analyzed for normality of their statistical distribution. If data were normally distributed, then parametric procedures were performed including analysis of variance (ANOVA) and both χ^2 and multiple sample comparisons (Scheffe and Bonferroni/Dunnett) to determine whether sites were significantly ($p \leq 0.05$) different from each other for a given parameter. Data that were not normally distributed were transformed and retested for normality. If transformed data were normally distributed, then the same parametric procedure outlined for normally distributed data (e.g., ANOVA and multiple comparison tests) were performed. If transformation still yielded data that were not normally distributed, then nonparametric procedures were followed for ANOVA (Kruskal Wallace (Zar 1974) and multiple comparison tests (Wilcoxon [Wilcoxon and Wilcox 1964] and Mann-Whitney [Zar 1974]). The objective of this phase of statistical analysis was to determine which sites were different from each other and, in particular, which urban and agricultural sites were different from the reference sites.

A second phase of statistical analysis involved multiple regression analysis of physicochemical parameters (salinity, temperature, and dissolved oxygen) and sediment chemical contaminant data (total PAHs) as independent variables and their correlation with the dependent variables, adult grass shrimp abundance and reproduction. Combined and individual correlation coefficients (R) were calculated, and the F statistic was used to determine whether the regression model itself was significant ($p \leq 0.05$) (Wirth et al. 1996).

Results

Water-quality parameters

Water temperature (°C) and dissolved oxygen (mg/L) were similar among sites, but salinity varied considerably (Figure 8-2). Water temperature ranged from 9.8 °C to 36 °C at all sites, and monthly temperatures at all sites were comparable. Similarly, dissolved oxygen concentrations were quite comparable at all sites, ranging from 3.4 mg/L to 9.9 mg/L. However, salinities were higher at MI sites, ranging from 28.5 ppt to 37.2 ppt. Salinities at the agricultural sites (KWA, TRT, and CTL) were much lower, varying from 2.3 ppt to 25.7 ppt. The widest salinity range was seen at NIOL with values spanning 7.0 ppt to 38.0 ppt. During periods of heavy rainfall (e.g., April, February, and March), salinities at NIOL were similar to the agricultural sites, usually less than 15 ppt.

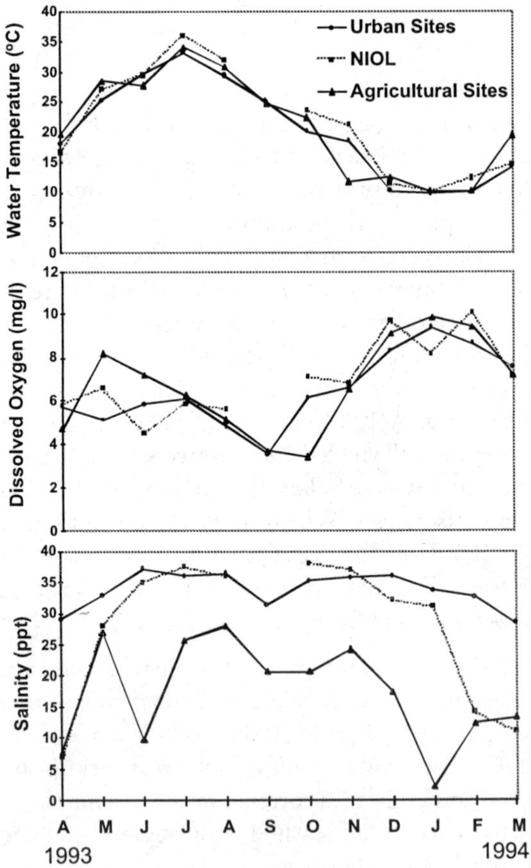

Figure 8-2 Monthly values for water temperature (°C), dissolved oxygen (mg/L), and salinity (ppt), during April 1993 to March 1994. Data from urban (OC-6, AC-1, AC-2, PS-3, MIF, and TP-1) and agricultural (CTL, TRT, and KWA) sites were averaged monthly and reported as means for each habitat type. Note the lower salinities observed at the agricultural sites.

Insecticides in agricultural estuaries

At KWA, high levels of azinphosmethyl (up to 21 μg/L) and endosulfan (up to 0.17 μg/L) in surface waters (Table 8-2) resulted in fish kills during 1988 and 1989 (Fulton et al. 1993) and again in 1993 (this study) and 1994 (G. I. Scott, unpublished data). During 1993, a fish kill was observed on 15 June at the KWA site, with azinphosmethyl concentrations of 1.42 μg/L detected. This was well above the azinphosmethyl 96-h LC50 value of 1.05 μg/L for *P. pugio* (Moore 1989). Similarly, high levels of endosulfan (e.g., 280 μg/kg), which are known to be toxic to benthic polychaetes and oysters (Chandler and Scott 1991), were detected in KWA sediment. At TRT, high concentrations (> 96-h LC50 values) of fenvalerate (0.89 μg/L) and deltamethrin (0.00131 μg/L) have been observed (Scott et al. 1992). During 1993, no toxicologically significant concentrations of fenvalerate, deltamethrin, azinphosmethyl, or endosulfan were observed. Sediment concentrations of fenvalerate have been observed at TRT and have inhibited reproduction in benthic copepods (Chandler and Scott 1991), but no acutely toxic concentrations were detected during this study. At the CTL site, only negligible (< 0.010 μg/L) concentrations of azinphosmethyl, endosulfan, and fenvalerate have been observed in surface waters, and only fenvalerate has been detected in sediments. The presence of these insecticides at the CTL site possibly was due to reflooding of the lower reaches of Leadenwah Creek, containing runoff from TRT. This runoff could have been diluted in the next flood tide and transported back up the western branch of Leadenwah Creek to the CTL area.

Table 8-2 Surfacewater and sediment insecticide concentrations measured in agricultural impacted estuaries (1986–1994)

Site	Insecticide	Media	Measured concentration[1]	*P. pugio* 96-h LC50 (mg/L) value[2]
KWA	Azinphosmethyl	Water	< dl[3]–21.0 mg/L	1.05
		Sediment	< dl	
	Endosulfan	Water	< dl–0.17 mg/L	1.10
		Sediment	< dl–280 mg/kg	
TRT	Fenvalerate	Water	0.0151–0.89 mg/L	0.052
		Sediment	< dl–90.0 mg/kg	
	Deltamethrin	Water	0.00131 mg/L	0.00051[4]
		Sediment	< dl	
CTL	Azinphosmethyl	Water	< dl	
		Sediment	< dl	
	Endosulfan	Water	< dl–0.014 mg/L	
		Sediment	< dl	
	Fenvalerate	Water	< dl–0.003 mg/L	

[1] Source: Scott et al. 1992
[2] Source: Baughmen 1986
[3] dl = detection limit, which varied with analyte and media sampled
[4] *Mysidopsis bahia* maximum allowable toxicant concentration

PAHs and trace metals in urbanized estuaries

Total PAH concentrations in MI sediment ranged from 284 ng/g (AC-2) to 708 (TP-1) ng/g dry weight (Figure 8-3). At NIOL, the total PAH concentration in sediments was 139 ng/g. There was a general trend in MI for PAH concentrations to increase from the southern end of MI at OC-6 (320 ng/g dry weight) to the northern end at TP-1 (708 ng/g dry weight).

While higher PAH concentrations were observed in sediments from MI, total and individual PAH concentrations did not exceed effects range low (ERL) sediment quality guidelines for toxicity as described by Long et al. (1995). ERL is the sediment concentration for a contaminant for which 10% of all published studies have found toxic effects. The expected % incidence for adverse effects (the number of data entries < ERL concentration in which biological effects were observed, divided by the total number of data entries in that range), based upon individual sediment PAH concentrations in MI and NIOL, were quite low, ranging from 10.3% (benzo(a)-pyrene) to 25% (anthracene) (Long et al. 1995).

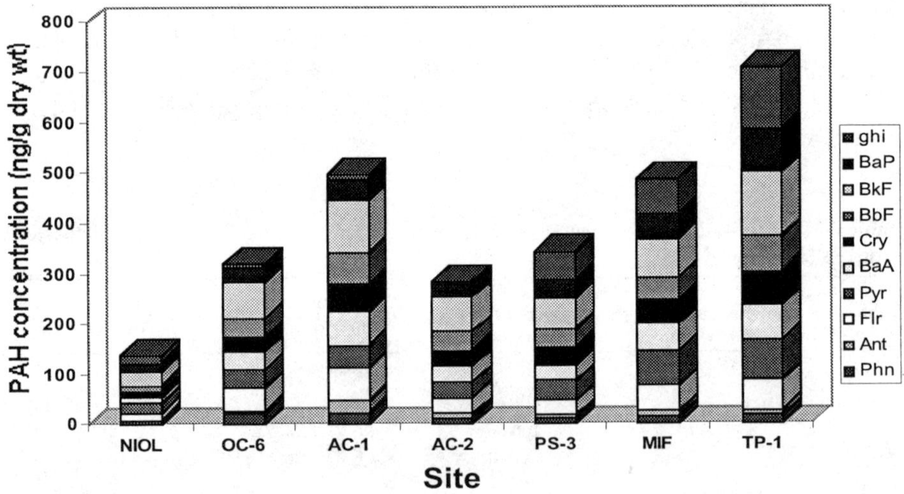

Figure 8-3 Concentrations of individual and total PAHs in sediments from NIOL and MI

Sediment concentrations of Cr, Cu, Ni, Pb, and Zn were similar in MI sites and NIOL, and no individual trace metal exceeded ERL sediment quality guidelines (Long et al. 1995). Figure 8-4 depicts sediment trace metal concentrations of these 5 most abundant trace metals. The % incidence of adverse effects based upon sediment quality guidelines, as described in Long et al. (1995), was low for both MI and NIOL, ranging from 1.9% to 9.4% for various metals.

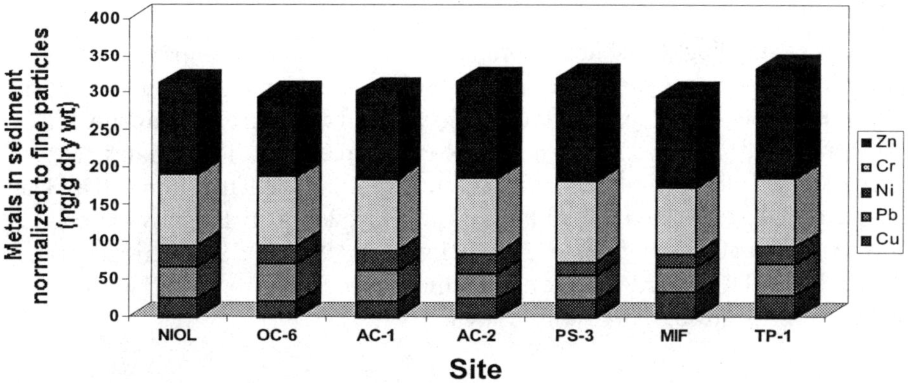

Figure 8-4 Concentrations of the 5 most abundant trace metals in sediment from NIOL and all MI sites

High sediment concentrations of DDT and α-chlordane were observed at MIF and TP-1, respectively (Table 8-3). At MIF, DDT concentrations (2.7 ng/g) exceeded the ERL sediment quality guidelines (Long et al. 1995). Similarly, at TP-1 the α-chlordane concentration (0.8 ng/g) exceeded the ERL sediment quality guidelines of 0.6 ng/g (Schantz et al. 1990). All other MI sites had nondetectible concentrations of these and other pesticides (t-nonachlor, DDE, and DDD) and PCBs. While T-nonachlor was detected at TP-1, concentrations were below those considered toxic to marine organisms (Long et al. 1995). Similarly, at NIOL no detectable levels of any insecticides or PCBs were observed in sediments.

Table 8-3 Summary of organochlorine pesticide concentrations (ng/g) in sediment at MI and NI

Estuary	Site	Total PCBs	α-chlordane	T-nonachlor	4-4'-DDE	4-4'-DDT
MI	0C	< dl	< dl	< dl	< dl	< dl
MI	AC-1	< dl	< dl	< dl	< dl	< dl
MI	AC-2	< dl	< dl	< dl	< dl	< dl
MI	PS-3	< dl	< dl	< dl	< dl	< dl
MI	MIF	< dl	< dl	< dl	< dl	2.7[2,3]
MI	TP-1	< dl	0.8[2,4]	0.7–2.1	< dl	< dl
NI	NIOL	< dl	< dl	< dl	< dl	< dl

[1] dl = detection limit
[2] Sediment concentrations exceeded ERL sediment quality guidelines for each analyte.
[3] ERL for 4-4'-DDT is 2.0 ng/g (Long et al. 1995).
[4] ERL for α-chlordane is 0.5 ng/g (Long et al. 1995).

Biomass

Analysis of standing stock biomass of male and female grass shrimp (Figure 8-5) indicated the reference site, NIOL, had the highest total biomass (1.90 ± 0.45 g/m). This was 4 times higher than the total biomass found at any urban study site. MI values ranged from 0.06 ± 0.03 g/m (MIF) to 0.43 ± 0.08 g/m (TP-1). Statistical analysis found all urban sites to be significantly ($p \leq 0.05$) different from NIOL. The KWA site had a total grass shrimp biomass of 0.63 ± 0.21 g/m. Biomass was only slightly greater at TRT and CTL (0.74 ± 0.21 g/m and 0.75 ± 0.19 g/m, respectively) than at KWA. TRT and KWA were not significantly different from CTL but were significantly ($p \leq 0.05$) different from NIOL.

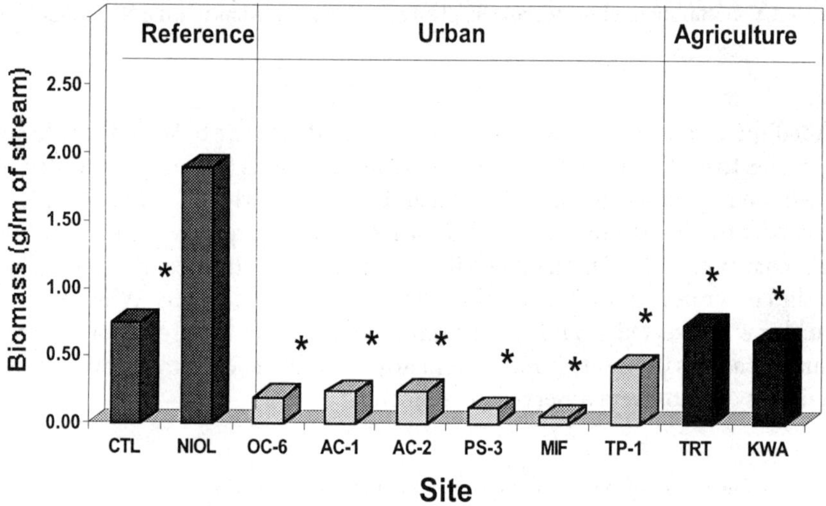

Figure 8-5 Total biomass of *P. pugio* from April 1993 to March 1994 in g/m of stream. Asterisks (*) indicate those sites with total biomass significantly different from NIOL ($p \leq 0.05$).

Abundance

The highest mean annual abundance of *P. pugio* (Figure 8-6), measured in #/m stream, was found at NIOL (13.7 ± 3.5/m). This was more than 4 times higher than any mean density found at MI, which ranged from 0.4 ± 0.2/m (MIF) to 3.3 ± 0.7/m (TP-1). Statistical analysis found all urban sites to be significantly ($p \leq 0.05$) different from NIOL. CTL had an overall mean abundance of 6.8 ± 1.8/m. Abundance was only slightly lower at TRT, with 6.3 ± 1.9/m. KWA had the lowest abundance for the agricultural sites, with 3.8 ± 1.1/m. KWA was the only agricultural site significantly ($p \leq 0.05$) different from NIOL. Neither TRT nor KWA was significantly ($p \leq 0.05$) different from CTL on an annual basis.

Comparisons of monthly grass shrimp abundance at NIOL (Figure 8-7) revealed decreased abundance (< 1.3/m) in the winter and early spring months (December to

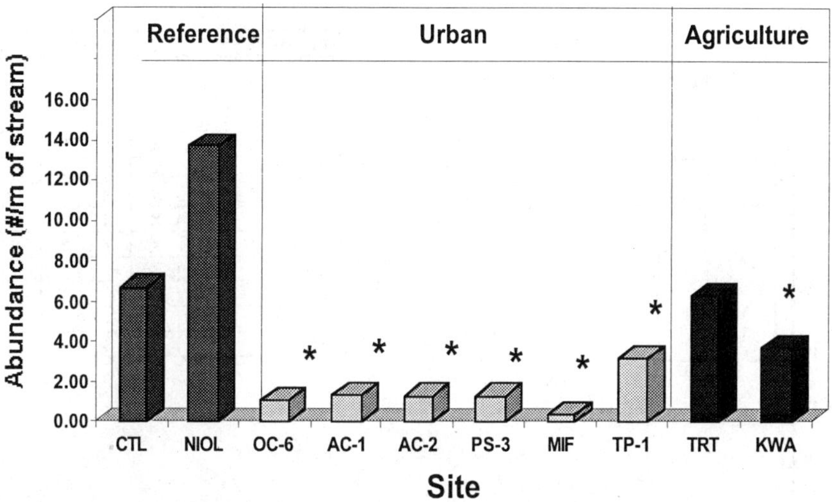

Figure 8-6 Abundance of grass shrimp from April 1993 to March 1994 in #/m stream. Asterisks (*) indicate those sites significantly different from NIOL ($p \leq 0.05$).

May). *Palaemonetes pugio* densities began to rise in NIOL during June and reached maximum abundance in August (39/m). NIOL grass shrimp density then fell rapidly until October (12/m) when *P. pugio* abundance remained steady through November (13/m) and finally reached its winter low (2/m) in December. Monthly grass shrimp abundance in the MI sites (Figure 8-7a) was similar to the low NIOL population densities from December to May. When the grass shrimp density at NIOL began to rise in June and July (4.1/m and 13.8/m, respectively), the populations at the urban sites continued to have very low densities, ranging from 0.08/m (PS-3) to 1.43/m (TP-1) in June and 0.05/m stream (MIF) to 2.9/m (AC-2) in July. All of the MI sites had significantly reduced abundance during July to November when compared to NIOL. The percentage of MI monthly samples that was significantly different from NIOL ranged from 41.7% (OC-6 and TP-1) to 83.3% (MIF). When the NIOL grass shrimp density peaked in August, the highest MI density (0.87/m), found at site AC-1, was 45 times lower. The population density in MI peaked in September with 8.6/m at the MIF site, which was less than one-fourth the peak population density reached at NIOL 1 month earlier. Significant ($p \leq 0.05$) abundance reductions were also seen in MI during the months of April (PS-3 and MIF), June (AC-1, PS-3 and MIF), January (AC-1, AC-2 and MIF), and March (AC-2 and MIF) when compared to NIOL.

Monthly grass shrimp densities at CTL (Figure 8-7b) revealed a peak in abundance during the month of August (19/m). Grass shrimp densities never peaked at levels as high as those seen in NIOL, but both populations were similar in their population growth, which can be seen by the similarity of their curves. The CTL population experienced its yearly low in November (0.06/m) and recovered densities above 4/m in the cold months of December and January. CTL abundance values were signifi-

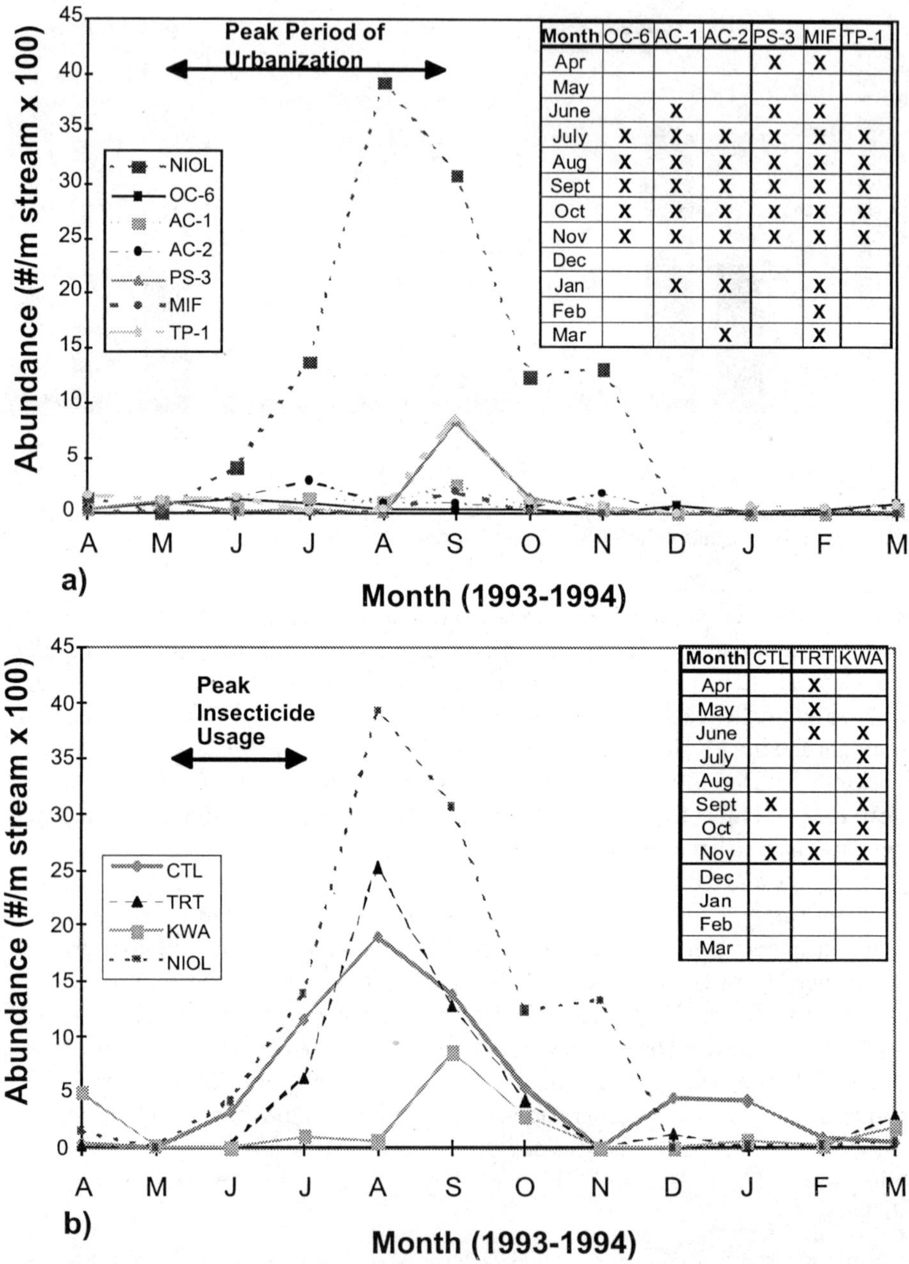

Figure 8-7 Monthly *P. pugio* abundance (#/m of stream) at all MI sites (a) and agricultural sites (b) as compared to NIOL. Peak periods of human activity were based upon demographic census/survey data (e.g., highway traffic counts and hotel/motel occupancy rates). Peak periods of insecticide usage were based upon farm logs of spray application in the region compiled by state regulatory agencies. Monthly statistical comparisons of urban and agricultural sites with the NIOL reference site that were significantly ($p \leq 0.05$) different are indicated in the box inset by an X.

cantly ($p \leq 0.05$) reduced when compared to NIOL during September and November only. This corresponds to a significant reduction in only 16.7% of the collections. The grass shrimp population at TRT also followed the same growth pattern as NIOL, even though the total abundance was reduced until December, when TRT densities became marginally higher than the grass shrimp population at NIOL (1.2/m and 0.02/m, respectively). The *P. pugio* population at TRT reached the greatest density of any agricultural site when it peaked in August with 25/m. Note the 89% reduction in grass shrimp abundance at KWA during June, which is attributed to an azinphos-methyl runoff event. Like the urban sites, KWA experienced a delayed peak in abundance during September (8.6/m), which was 1 month later than the peak abundances at NIOL, TRT, and CTL. This delay in recruitment at KWA may have been caused in part by mortality to larval grass shrimp during the June fish kill. These larval shrimp would have reached adult size (≥15 mm) and been sampled by our pushnetting technique 90 d later. By October, the population size at KWA had fallen (2.8/m), and by November, it had reached its winter low (0/m). Both TRT and KWA had significantly reduced abundance when compared to NIOL during 41.7% and 50.0% of the monthly collections, respectively. Significantly ($p \leq 0.05$) reduced population densities were found at KWA from June to November and at TRT from April to June and October to November.

Sex ratios

Variations in the distributions of male and female *P. pugio* during the NIOL reproductive period (April 1993 to September 1993) and for the entire 12-month sampling period (April 1993 to March 1994) are shown in Figure 8-8a and 8-8b, respectively. During the reproductive season, gravid females made up 13.8% of the population at NIOL. The largest portion of the population was male (65.6%), with the remaining 20.6% nongravid females. TP-1 was the only MI site with significantly ($p \leq 0.05$) different sex ratios from NIOL. At this northernmost site, 89.5% of the population was male and only 4.2% and 7.0% were gravid and nongravid females, respectively (Figure 8-8a).

The agricultural reference site and CTL had the lowest number of gravid females (2.8%). The majority of females were nongravid (40.1%), and more than half the population constituted males (57.1%). The TRT site was very similar to CTL with 3.6, 48.4, and 48.0% gravid females, nongravid females, and males, respectively. The KWA site had the highest percentage of gravid females found in the agricultural area (12.4%). At this site, nongravid females constituted 31.5% of the population, and the remaining 56.2% was male. Both CTL and TRT were significantly ($p \leq 0.05$) different from NIOL.

Analysis of the temporal population distributions revealed overall reductions in the percentage of gravid females at all sites due to a complete absence of gravid females in the colder winter months. Males constituted the greatest proportion of the population at NIOL (64.0%) (Figure 8-8b). Annually, 27.4% were nongravid females

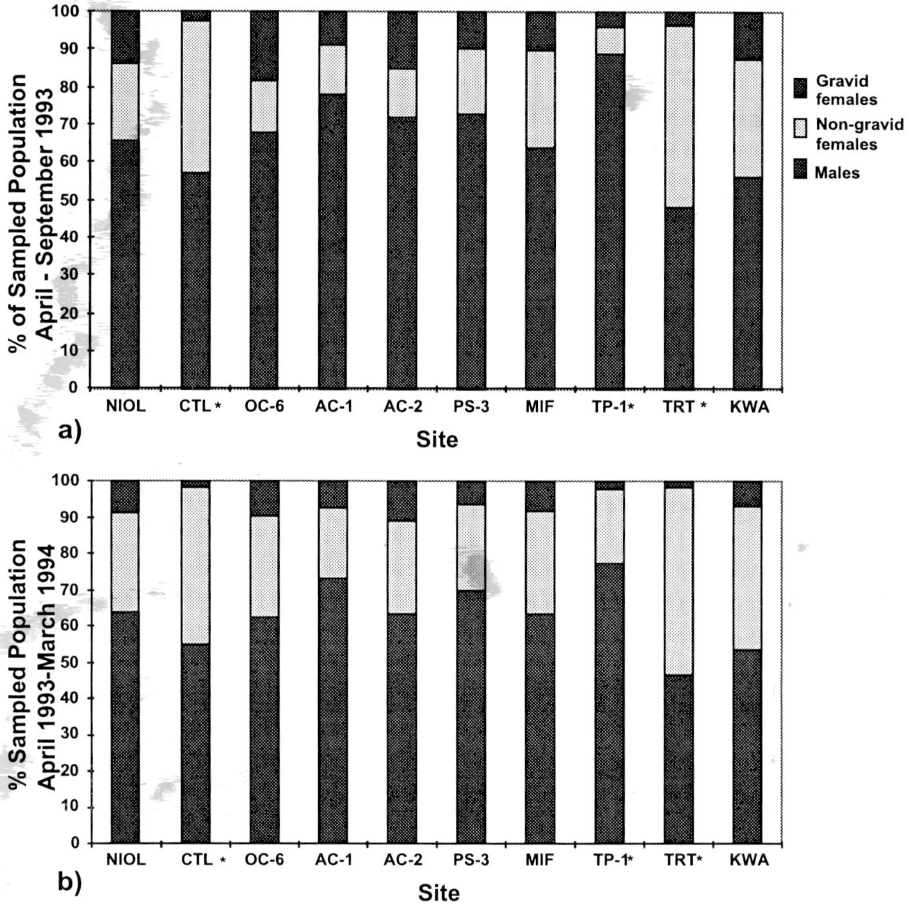

Figure 8-8 Percent gravid females, nongravid females, and males during the reproductive season (April 1993 to September 1993) (a) and the April 1993 to March 1994 12-month sampling season (b). Asterisks (*) indicates those sites with distributions significantly ($p \leq 0.05$) different from NIOL.

and 8.6% were gravid females. Males systematically made up > 50% of *P. pugio's* population at all MI sites. The greatest percentage of males was found at TP-1 (77.3%), with nongravid and gravid females constituting only 20.4% and 2.3% of the population, respectively. TP-1 was also the only MI site where population sex ratio distributions were significantly ($p \leq 0.05$) different from NIOL.

Yearly population distributions at the agricultural sites revealed marked similarity between the percentage of gravid females, nongravid females, and males at CTL and TRT (1.6%, 43.3%, and 55.1% versus 1.7%, 51.5%, and 46.8%, respectively) (Figure 8-8b). The only site studied with a female-dominated population structure was TRT. KWA had the greatest annual percentage of gravid females (7.0%) among all the agricultural sites. Both CTL and TRT had yearly population distributions significantly ($p \leq 0.05$) different from NIOL.

Clutch size and total egg production

Determination of the mean clutch size (Figure 8-9a) revealed NIOL to have an average female clutch size of 142 ± 10.7 eggs/female. All MI sites had mean clutch sizes larger than NIOL. MIF had the highest mean clutch size (248 eggs/female), while the lowest average clutch size was shared by OC-6 and AC-1 with 165 eggs/female. NIOL female grass shrimp produced significantly ($p \leq 0.05$) smaller clutches than did those at AC-2 or MIF.

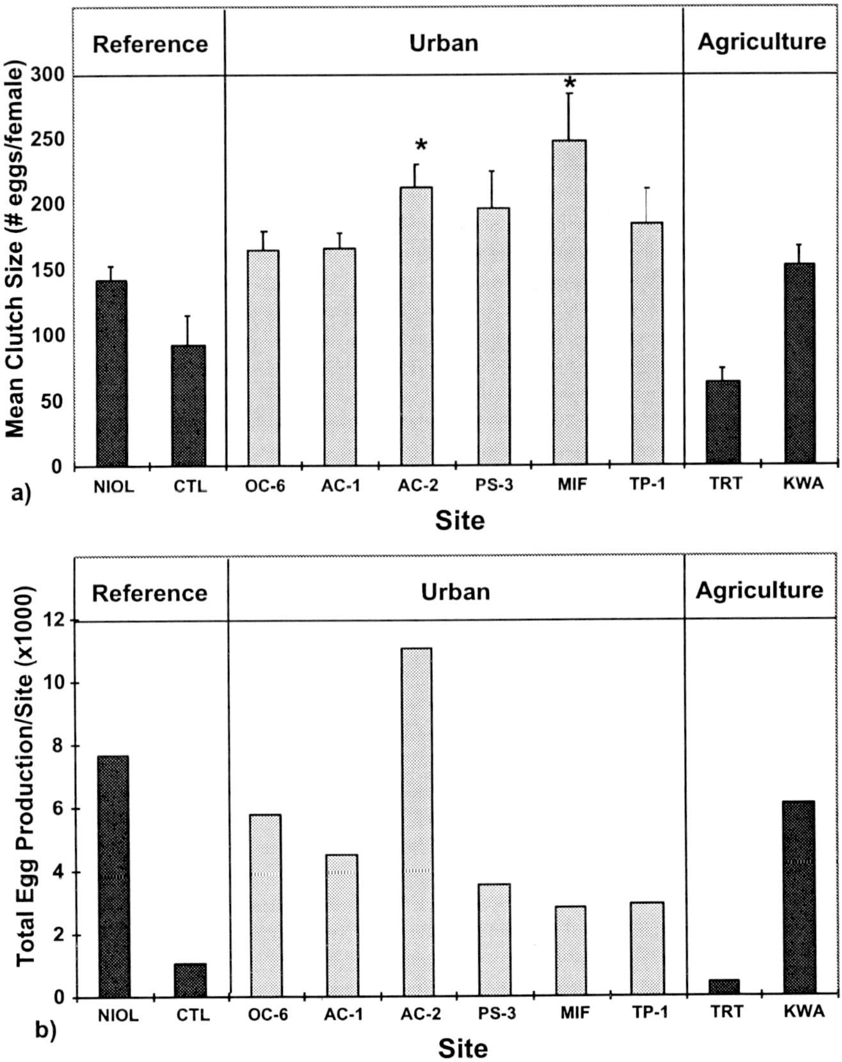

Figure 8-9 The mean clutch size of gravid *P. pugio* from each site (a) and the total egg production of collected females (mean clutch size/site × # of gravid females collected from each individual site) (b) during April 1993 to March 1994. Asterisks (*) indicate those sites found significantly different ($p \leq 0.05$) from NIOL.

The mean clutch size for CTL gravid females was 92 eggs/female ±22.0. KWA females had the highest average clutch size of 153 eggs/female ±10.5. The lowest mean clutch size was found at TRT (64 eggs/female ±14.8). Clutch size was not significantly ($p \leq 0.05$) different between CTL and the other agricultural sites or between NIOL and any agricultural site.

Total egg production/site (Figure 8-9b) reached almost 8.0×10^3 eggs/site at NIOL. The highest production level among the MI sites was found at AC-2 (11.0×10^3 eggs/site). Except for AC-2, production declined as sites moved northward in MI, reaching values only one-third that at NIOL. The lowest production found was at MIF, with only 2.8×10^3 eggs/site. Total egg production at CTL was low, reaching only 1.02×10^3 eggs/site. The lowest production in the agricultural area was found at TRT, with only 0.45×10^3 eggs/site. Surprisingly, KWA had the highest total egg production, with 6.1×10^3 eggs/site.

The contribution to the total egg production made by 2 different cohorts of females was also determined. In general, the overwintering females were older, larger, and carried larger clutches than the smaller, late season females. NIOL received equal contributions from both the overwintering (52%) and late season (48%) females (Figure 8-10). MI sites (Figure 8-11) varied widely in their dependence upon the 2 sets of females. The sites at the southern end of MI (OC-6, AC-1, and AC-2), where urbanization effects were minimized, remained roughly equal with overwintering females, contributing 58, 43, and 60%, respectively. At the northern end of MI, where urbanization effects were greatest, the largest egg contribution was made by the overwintering females with PS-3, MIF, and TP-1 populations having 84, 92, and 76% of their egg production dependent on the larger females, respectively. The CTL site (Figure 8-12) was very similar to NIOL, with roughly equal contributions coming from overwintering and late season females (46% and 54%, respectively). TRT had no observable overwintering females contributing to the egg production, which suggests high mortality in overwintering females and perhaps reliance entirely on the younger, late season females to maintain the population. KWA was similar to the highly urbanized sites in that most egg production was due to the overwintering (77%) and not the late season (23%) females.

Discussion

The discharge of NPS urban and agricultural runoff into estuarine ecosystems may have profound impacts on marsh and tidal creek fauna (Scott et al. 1992; Vernberg et al. 1992; Fulton et al. 1993). In addition to impacts from loading of chemical contaminants associated with NPS runoff, concerns about the effects of changes in the physicochemical water quality (e.g., salinity), reduced habitat availability or quality, and hydrographic regime (tidal flushing characteristics) have been reported (Scott et al. 1992; Vernberg et al. 1992) for urban and agricultural NPS runoff.

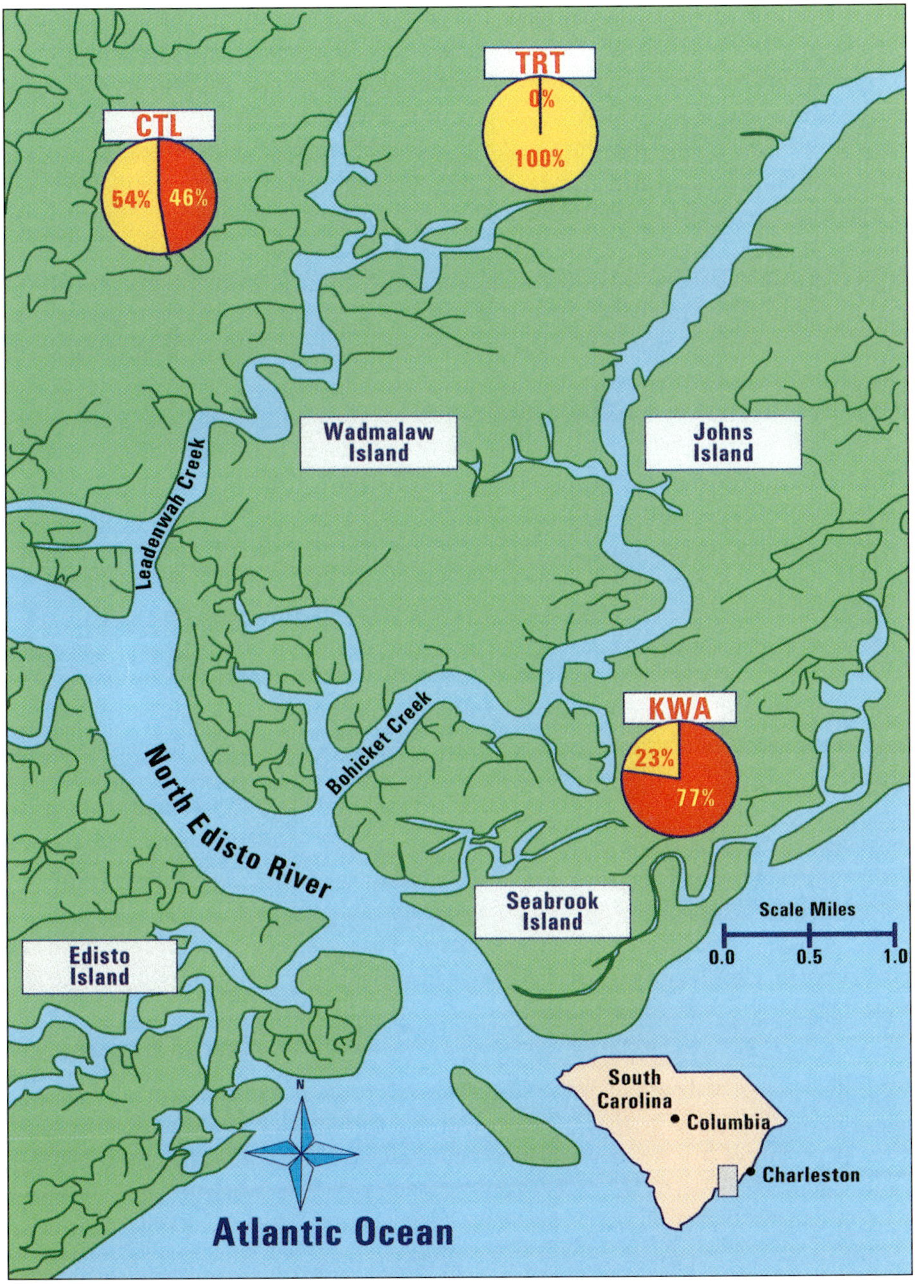

Figure 8-12 Agricultural sampling sites, CTL, TRT, and KWA, marked with pie charts representing late season total egg production (yellow), and overwintering female egg production (red). Note the complete loss of overwintering females at TRT and the increased proportion of overwintering female contribution at KWA.

In this study, differences in salinity were observed between the agricultural sites and NIOL and MI sites. Generally, lower salinities were observed at the agricultural sites, suggesting greater freshwater inputs into estuarine habitats adjacent to agricultural areas. Scott et al. (1992) have earlier reported that salinities declined from > 30 to < 5 ppt in 1 tidal cycle following a major runoff event at these agricultural sites. Additionally, the urban areas appeared to have higher salinities than NIOL or the agricultural sites during January and February, which is normally a wet weather period. It has been noted (Fulton et al. 1993, 1996) that salinities were much lower in NI than MI due to both the indirect effects of urbanization and salinity and the high fluctuation in salinity with the tidal cycle at NI. Highway drainage modifications and NPS urban runoff control measures have greatly reduced surfacewater flow and impounded surfacewater runoff, thereby affecting the hydrographic regime in MI. No notable differences were observed in other, measured physicochemical water-quality parameters (dissolved oxygen and water temperature). Fulton et al. (1993) earlier used continuous monitoring and found significantly higher dissolved oxygen concentrations at ebb tide in MI than in NI. This may enhance predator egress into tidal creek headwaters, which are nursery grounds, and potentially affect population abundance within these habitats. In this study, monthly (e.g., less rigorous) monitoring of dissolved oxygen did not discern this trend of reduced dissolved oxygen concentration. These findings suggest that urban and agricultural NPS runoff may potentially change freshwater flow into estuarine ecosystems and may alter the salinity regime of the environments affected. Salinity has been found to affect grass shrimp abundance in earlier studies of SC estuaries (Alon and Stancyk 1982), with reduced population abundances found in pristine areas with lower salinities (riverine versus nonriverine). The potential interactive effects of altered salinity and chemical contaminants on estuarine grass shrimp have not been well studied in the field. Scott et al. (1992) have reported that in laboratory studies using selected insecticides, low salinity only increased toxicity to grass shrimp by less than a factor of 2. Grass shrimp abundance is also known to increase at the CTL reference site after major rain events. These findings imply that contaminants in the runoff, rather than decreased salinity per se, may alter grass shrimp abundance (Scott et al. 1992).

Analysis of chemical contaminants in surfacewater runoff and sediments from agricultural areas (TRT and KWA) indicated that agricultural NPS runoff contained concentrations of insecticides that were potentially toxic to grass shrimp. Historically, significant concentrations of azinphosmethyl, endosulfan, and fenvalerate have been observed at both TRT and KWA (Scott et al. 1992). The development of pesticide NPS runoff controls has reduced pesticide concentrations at TRT by > 89% (Scott et al. 1992). This has greatly reduced ecotoxicological impacts at TRT, as indicated by comparisons of grass shrimp abundance during the peak of the agricultural growing season and the immediate period of subsequent adult recruitment in August (Figure 8-7). At KWA, no IPM, BMPs, or RPs were used; rather, a calendar application method (every 5 to 6 days during the growing season) was employed. During this study, the organophosphorus insecticide azinphosmethyl reached concentrations of 1.42 µg/L at KWA, causing a fish kill. Brain AChE levels in adult *Fundulus heteroclitus* were reduced by 93.7%, and peak azinphosmethyl concentrations in the water of 3.60 µg/L were predicted based upon brain AChE inhibition curves (M.H. Fulton, unpublished data). The 96-h laboratory LC50 for adult *P. pugio* was 1.05 µg/L, and the field-derived LC50 was 0.97 µg/L (Moore 1989). Predicted grass shrimp mortality based upon pushnet results in this study ranged from 89% (intrasite temporal comparisons at KWA) to 99.6% (intersite comparison with CTL).

This acute impact observed in the grass shrimp population at KWA during June 1993 may have resulted in > 55% reduction in mean annual grass shrimp abundance. Hampton (1987) observed delayed effects in grass shrimp populations exposed to endosulfan and azinphosmethyl. Delayed population abundance differences were observed at 90 and 180 d post pesticide exposure. Post initial acute toxicity most probably was due to reduced population densities of juvenile and larval grass shrimp, which require 90 and 180 d, respectively, to reach a 15-mm adult size that can be sampled by the pushnetting technique.

Reduced grass shrimp densities and biomass, compared to NIOL, were also observed at the urban sites in MI. This was especially interesting considering the increased egg production at all MI sites when compared to NIOL. These results were similar to whole life-cycle studies (Fulton et al. 1996) on a benthic copepod (*Amphiascus tenuiremis*) that found adult mortality and the percentage of females successfully producing clutches were not significantly ($p \leq 0.05$) different between NIOL and TP-1. However, the mean clutch size was significantly ($p \leq 0.05$) larger in gravid females from TP-1. In addition, even though no differences were found in the mean number of nauplii hatchings between NIOL and TP-1, larval survival or hatching success decreased at TP-1 when compared to the NIOL control population. This was determined from noting equal female survival and fertility rates between the 2 populations, even with significantly ($p \leq 0.05$) larger clutch sizes at TP-1. Because larval stages were not addressed in this study, we can only postulate that, as in the copepod study (Fulton et al. 1996), some constituent present in MI sediment inhibited proper development of one or more larval stages of *P. pugio* and thus prevented its development into a reproductively active adult. This helps explain the significantly ($p \leq 0.05$) reduced grass shrimp abundance and larger clutch sizes found in MI, compared to NIOL. In fact, Fulton et al. (1996) found a > 900% reduction in the mean number of copepod nauplii successfully metamorphosing and surviving at TP-1 when compared to the mean number at NIOL. Earlier studies (Vernberg et al. 1992; Fulton et al. 1993) have concluded that urban runoff containing PAH contamination was not acutely toxic to adult grass shrimp. Additionally, laboratory toxicity tests with larval grass shrimp have found that the total PAH concentration at MI did not exceed the mortality threshold (5913 ng/g) but did exceed the reproductive effect level (1164 ng/g) (Wirth et al. 1998). In addition to reduced grass shrimp abundance and biomass, alterations were observed in sex ratios, clutch size, total egg production, and the proportion of overwintering/late season gravid females. Statistical analysis of sex ratios indicated that those at TP-1, which had the highest total PAH concentration, were significantly different from those at NIOL. At TP-1, the proportion of gravid females was reduced by > 26.0%, compared to the proportion at NIOL. Additionally, on an annual basis, only TP-1 had significantly ($p \leq 0.05$) increased proportions of males (77.3%) in the population when compared to NIOL (64.0%).

Total egg production (egg production/site) was highly variable in urbanized MI. In the 3 southernmost stations (OC-6, AC-1, and AC-2), which are located in the least developed area of the estuary near a state park, total egg production (7.3×10^3 eggs/site, average) was comparable to NIOL (8.0×10^3). In the northernmost sites of MI (PS-3, MIF, and TP-1), egg production was reduced by 57.5%, compared to production at NIOL.

Perhaps the most striking difference between MI and NI grass shrimp populations was the alteration in the proportion of overwintering and late season gravid female egg contributions. In general, gravid females that first appear during March are from the large (> 25 mm) overwintering female population, which will produce the first of several egg clutches during the spring to mid summer (July). By July, smaller late season females, from the first spring clutch that have matured to adult size, begin to appear and dominate reproduction from July to October. At both reference sites, the proportion of overwintering to late season gravid females was approximately 50% (NIOL = 52:48; CTL = 46:54). At the southern, less urbanized region of MI (stations OC-6, AC-1, and AC-2), the proportion of overwintering to late season females was similar to that of NIOL (58:42, 43:57, and 60:40, respectively). At the northern, more urbanized regions of MI (stations PS-3, MIF and TP-1), the proportion of overwintering: late season females was greatly altered (84:16, 92:8 and 76:24, respectively). This profound difference suggests urbanization may cause delayed development of reproductively competent females at MI. This strategy results in the larger-sized females dominating reproduction. This life-history strategy is highly adaptive because the larger-sized females produce more eggs/female, resulting in increased reproductive output from depressed grass shrimp populations. Despite the > 89% reduction in the MI grass shrimp population density, overall egg production was reduced by only 20% estuarine wide.

Urbanization is a complex process involving both contaminant (trace metals, PAHs, and coliform bacteria) and noncontaminant (altered salinity, dissolved oxygen levels, and hydrographic regime) stressors that may impact living marine resources in a variety of ways (Vernberg et al. 1992; Fulton et al. 1993). The alterations in grass shrimp populations at MI observed in this study were profound, but trying to assign cause and effect to urbanization is a tenuous process at best. Two population metrics (adult grass shrimp abundance and the proportion of overwintering gravid females) were compared to independent variables (salinity, dissolved oxygen, temperature,

Table 8-4 Correlation of selected grass shrimp population metrics with independent environmental variables associated with urbanization

Independent variables associated with urbanization	Dependent variable: adult grass shrimp abundance	Dependent variable: proportion of overwintering females
Salinity	0.732[a]	< 0.022
Dissolved oxygen	< 0.068	0.134[a]
Temperature	< 0.068	0.247[a]
PAHs	0.200[a]	0.596[a]
Combined salinity and PAH	0.932[a]	
Combined PAH, temperature, and dissolved oxygen		0.977[a]

[a]Indicates that variable was significantly ($p \leq 0.05$) correlated.

and PAH concentration) using stepwise and backward regression procedures (Table 8-4). Results indicated that salinity was positively correlated ($R^2 = 0.73$) and sediment PAH concentrations were negatively correlated ($R^2 = 0.20$) with grass shrimp abundance variability. These findings suggest that the combination of lower salinity and elevated PAH concentrations, which would result from increased NPS runoff and loading in urban areas, could be causation factors affecting grass shrimp abundance. Together, salinity and sediment PAH concentration accounted for 93% of the abundance variability in MI. The proportion of overwintering to late season gravid females was positively correlated with sediment PAH concentration ($R^2 = 0.60$) and negatively correlated with temperature ($R^2 = 0.25$) and dissolved oxygen ($R^2 = 0.13$). Note that sediment PAH concentration accounted for almost 60% of the overwintering gravid female variability. Correlation with temperature was indicative of the seasonal nature of the reproductive cycle that declines as temperatures fall below 20 °C (Anderson 1985). These findings suggest that grass shrimp populations may be profoundly affected by NPS urban runoff containing PAHs, which may result in concomitant reduced salinities, altered dissolved oxygen levels, and increased sediment PAH concentrations. Thomas and Colborn (1992) have reported that PAHs may be endocrine-disrupting chemicals that may adversely affect reproduction. Our results are consistent with these findings, as reproduction in grass shrimp was significantly affected. Fulton et al. (1996) noted similar effects in copepods.

Conclusions

The need to characterize the health of estuaries and associated coastal wetlands after recent increases in runoff from urbanization and agricultural practices along our coastlines is necessary if proper management strategies are to be employed to minimize impacts. A comparison of the NIOL (high-salinity estuary) and CTL (riverine estuary) reference sites revealed differences in abundance, biomass, and sex ratio distributions. Much of the variability is likely due to physicochemical differences such as salinity. This clearly indicates the range of natural variability in grass shrimp populations that must be taken into account when reference sites are compared with potentially impacted sites. By focusing interest on the grass shrimp, *Palaemonetes pugio*, this study has revealed impacts such as populations with significantly decreased ($p \leq 0.05$) abundance and biomass in the highly urbanized MI area as well as in the areas subject to pulsed influxes of freshwater often contaminated with pesticides. Sediment analysis at MI sites revealed PAH concentrations up to 3 times that of the background concentration and pesticide concentrations (a-chlordane and 4,4'-DDT) that exceeded ERL sediment quality guidelines at 2 sites (TP-1 and MIF, respectively). As a result, PAH concentrations were significantly ($p \leq 0.05$) correlated with reduced adult grass shrimp abundance and altered proportion of overwintering females at MI sites. Water and sediment analyses at the agricultural sites have revealed azinphosmethyl and endosulfan concentrations well above the 96-h LC 50 values for *P. pugio* (1.05 and 1.10 mg/L, respectively) (Moore 1989). The result of increased contaminants from urban and agricultural NPS runoff may be a factor in the apparent restructuring of the grass shrimp life cycle based on results of the pushnet sampling method. In those areas highly impacted from NPS runoff, such as the northern stations of MI (PS-3, MIF, and TP-1), the female *P. pugio* appear to delay reproduction so that the larger, overwintering grass shrimp dominate the reproductive output, thus maximizing reproductive potential in sites with decreased population size.

Future research should be focused on the dynamics of urbanization effects in grass shrimp populations, particularly larval survival and developmental effects of PAH and other chemical contaminants or processes associated with urbanization. Additional study should also be undertaken to understand the interactions of changes that influence salinity in the hydrographic regime and changes in habitat availability in conjunction with chemical contaminant effects. This differentiation between contaminant versus noncontaminant stressors is essential in defining the cumulative impacts of urbanization on grass shrimp populations in estuarine environments.

References

Alon NC, Stancyk SE. 1982. Variation in life history patterns of the grass shrimp *Palaemonetes pugio* in 2 South Carolina estuarine systems. *Mar Biol* 68:265–276.

Anderson G. 1985. Species profiles: life histories and environmental requirements of coastal fishes and invertebrates (Gulf of Mexico) grass shrimp. 82(11.35). Biological Report. Slidell LA: U.S. Fish and Wildlife Service.

Baughmen DS. 1986. The acute toxicity of insecticides associated with agricultural runoff on the grass shrimp, *Palaemonetes pugio* [masters thesis]. Columbia SC: Univ South Carolina.

Buikema Jr AL, Niderlehner BR, Cairns Jr J. 1980. Use of grass shrimp in toxicity tests. In: Buikema Jr AL, Cairns Jr J, editors. Aquatic invertebrate bioassays. Philadelphia PA: America Society for Testing and Materials. STP 715. p 155–173.

Burkholder PR, Bornside GH. 1956. Decomposition of marsh grass by aerobic marine bacteria. *Bull Torrey Bot Club Bol* 84:366–383.

CEM Corporation. 1988. Microwave application note for acid digestion. Note a.m.-3. Matthews NC: CEM Corporation.

[CFR] Code of Federal Regulations. Definitions and procedure for the determination of the method detection limit. §40, Appendix B to part 136.

Chandler GT. 1990. Effects of sediment-bound residues of the pyrethroid insecticide fenvalerate on survival and reproduction of benthic copepods. *Mar Environ Res* 29:65–76.

Chandler GT, Scott GI. 1991. Effects of sediment-bound endosulfan on survival, reproduction and larval settlement of meiobenthic polychaetes and copepods. *Environ Toxicol Chem* 10:375–382.

Colborn T, Clement C. 1992. Chemically induced alterations in sexual and functional development: the wildlife/human connection. In: Mehlman MA, editor. Advances in modern environmental toxicology. Princeton NJ: Princeton Scientific. p 347–359.

[CEQ] Council on Environmental Quality. 1983. 14th Annual Report of the Council on Environmental Quality. Washington DC: CEQ.

Fisher WS, Foss SS. 1993. A simple test for toxicity of number 2 fuel oil and oil dispersants to embryos of grass shrimp, *Palaemonetes pugio*. *Mar Poll Bull* 26:385–391.

Fulton MH, Chandler GT, Scott GI. 1996. Urbanization effects on the fauna of a southeastern U.S.A. bar-built estuary. In: Vernberg FJ, Vernberg WB, Siewicki T, editors. Sustainable development in the southeastern coastal zone. Columbia SC: Univ South Carolina Pr. p 477–504.

Fulton MH, Scott GI. 1992. The effect of certain intrinsic and extrinsic variables on the acute toxicity of selected organophosphorous insecticides to the mummichog, *Fundulus heteroclitus*. *J Environ Sci Health* B26:459–478.

Fulton MH, Scott GI, Fortner A, Bidleman TF, Ngabe B. 1993. The effects of urbanization on small high salinity estuaries of the southeastern United States. *Arch Environ Contam Toxicol* 25:476–484.

Gardner WS, Lee RF, Tenore KR, Smith LW. 1979. Degradation on selected polycyclic aromatic hydrocarbons in coastal sediments: importance of microbes and polychaete worms. *Water Air Soil Pollut* 11:339–347.

Hampton TW. 1987. The use of ecotoxicology and biomonitoring to assess the effects of nonpoint source runoff from agricultural fields [masters thesis]. Columbia SC: Univ South Carolina.

Hoffman EJ, Latimer JS, Hunt CD, Mills GL, Quinn JG. 1985. Storm water runoff from highways. *Water Air Soil Pollut* 25:349–364.

Hoffman EJ, Mills GL, Latimer JS, Quinn JG. 1983. Annual input of petroleum hydrocarbons to the coastal environment via urban runoff. *Can J Fish Aquat Sci* 40:41–53.

Krahn MM, Wigren CA, Pearce RW, Moore LK, Boger RG, Macleod Jr WD, Chan SL, Brown DW. 1988. New HPLC cleanup and revised extraction procedures for organic contaminants. Technical Memorandum. Washington DC: National Oceanic and Atmospheric Administration. NMFS F/NWC-153.

Kucklick JR, Bidleman TF. 1994. Organic contaminants in Winyah Bay, South Carolina I: Pesticides and polycyclic aromatic hydrocarbons in subsurface and microlayer waters. *Mar Env Res* 37:63–78.

Kucklick JR, Sivertsen SK, Sanders M, Scott GI. 1997. Factors influencing polycyclic aromatic hydrocarbon distributions in South Carolina estuarine sediments. *J Exp Mar Bio Ecol* 213(1):13–29.

Lee RG, Gardner WF, Anderson JW, Blaylock JW, Barwell-Clarke J. 1978. Fate of polycyclic aromatic hydrocarbons in controlled ecosystem enclosures. *Environ Sci Technol* 123:832–838.

Long ER, MacDonald DD, Smith SL, Calder FD. 1995. Incidence of adverse biological effects within ranges of chemical concentrations in marine and estuarine sediments. *Environ Manag* 19:81–97.

Meehean OL. 1936. Notes on the freshwater shrimp *Palaemonetes paludosa* (Gibbes). In: Ackert JE, editor. Transactions of the American Microscopial Society. Menasha WI: Collegiate Pr. p 433–441.

Moore D. 1989. An integrated laboratory and field study of nonpoint source agricultural insecticide runoff and its effects on the grass shrimp, *Palaemonetes pugio* (Holthius) [Ph.D. dissertation]. Columbia SC: Univ South Carolina.

Murphy SD. 1986. Toxic effects of pesticides. In: Klaassen CD, Amdur MO, Doull J, editors. Toxicology: the basic science of poisons. 3rd ed. New York: Macmillan. p 519–581.

[NOAA] National Oceanic and Atmospheric Administration. 1994. Habitat protection accomplishments of the National Marine Fisheries Service. St. Petersburg FL: NOAA.

[NOAA] National Oceanic and Atmospheric Administration. 1995. Habitat conservation program synopsis. St. Petersburg FL: NOAA.

Neely WB, Blau GE. 1985. Environmental exposure from chemicals. Boca Raton FL: CRC Pr.

Pathirana S, Connell DW, Vowles PD. 1994. Distribution of polycyclic aromatic hydrocarbons (PAHs) in an urban roadway system. *Ecotoxicol Environm Safety* 28:256–269.

Sanders M. 1995. Distribution of polycyclic aromatic hydrocarbons in oyster (*Crassostrea virginica*) and surface sediment from 2 estuaries in South Carolina. *Arch Environ Contam Toxicol* 28:397–405.

Schantz MM, Benner BA, Chesler SN, Koster BJ, Hehn KE, Stone SF, Kelly WR, Zeisler R, Wise SA. 1990. Preparation and analysis of marine sediment reference material for the determination of trace organic constituents. *Fresenius J Anal Chem* 338:501–514.

Scott GI, Fulton MH, Crosby MC, Key PB, Daugomah JW, Waldren JT, Strozier ED, Louden CJ, Chandler GT, Bidleman TF, Jackson KL, Hampton TW, Hoffman T, Shultz A, Bradford M. 1992. Agricultural nonpoint runoff effects on estuarine organisms: correlation of laboratory and field bioassays and ecotoxicological biomonitoring. Final Report. Gulf Breeze FL: U.S. Environmental Protection Agency.

Scott GI, Fulton MH, Morre DW, Chandler GT, Key PB, Hampton TW, Marcus JM, Jackson KL, Baughman DS, Trim AH, Williams L, Louden CJ, Patterson ER. 1990. Agricultural insecticide runoff effects on estuarine organisms: correlating laboratory and field bioassays and ecotoxicological biomonitoring. Gulf Breeze FL: U.S. Environmental Protection Agency. EPA CR81338- 02-1.

Sikora WB. 1977. The ecology of *Palaemonetes pugio* in a southeastern saltmarsh ecosystem, with particular emphasis on production and trophic relationships [masters thesis]. Columbia SC: Univ South Carolina.

Sunda WG, Engel DW, Thoutte RM. 1978. Effect of chemical speciation on toxicity of cadmium to grass shrimp, *Palaemonetes pugio*: importance of free cadmium ion. *Environ Sci Technol* 12:409–413.

Thomas K, Colburn T. 1992. Organochlorine endocrine disruptors in human tissue. In: Colborn T, Clement C, editors. Chemically induced alterations in sexual and functional development: the wildlife/human connection. Princeton NJ: Princeton Scientific. p 365–394.

[USEPA] U.S. Environmental Protection Agency. 1979. Water related environmental fate of 129 priority pollutants. Volume II, Halogenated aliphatic hydrocarbons, halogenated ethers, monocyclic aromatics, phthalate esters, nitrosamines, and miscellaneous compounds. Washington DC: USEPA. EPA PB80-204381.

[USEPA] U.S. Environmental Protection Agency. 1980. Methods for the analysis of pesticides in tissue, sediment, and water. Washington DC: USEPA. EPA-600/8-80-038.

[USEPA] U.S. Environmental Protection Agency. 1982. Inductively coupled plasma-atomic emission spectrometric method for trace element analysis of water and wastes. Washington DC: USEPA. EPA 200.7.

van Dijk JJ, van der Meer C, Wijnans M. 1977. The toxicity of sodium pentachlorophenolate for three species of decapod crustaceans and their larvae. *Bull Environ Contam Toxicol* 17:622–630.

Vernberg FJ, Vernberg WB, Blood E, Fortner A, Fulton M, McKellar HN, Michener W, Scott GI, Siewecki T, El Figi K. 1992. Impact of urbanization of high salinity estuaries in the southeastern United States. *Netherlands J Sea Research* 30:239–248.

Welsh BL. 1975. The role of grass shrimp, *Palaemonetes pugio*, in a tidal marsh ecosystem. *Ecology* 56:513–530.

Williams AB, Wigley RL. 1977. Distribution of decapod crustacea off northeastern United States based on specimens at the northeast fisheries center. Technical Report. Woods Hole MS: National Oceanic and Atmospheric Administration. NOAA/407.

Wilcoxon F, Wilcox RA. 1964. Some rapid approximate statistical procedures. Pearl River NY: Lederle Laboratories. 53 p.

Wirth EF, Scott GI, Fulton MH, Van Dolah RF, Maier PP, Hadley N, Daugomah JW, Key PB. 1996. In situ monitoring of dredged material spoil sites using the oyster *Crassostrea virginica*. *Arch Environ Contam Toxicol* 30:340–348.

Wirth EF, Fulton MH, Chandler GT, Key PB and Scott GI. 1998. Toxicity of sediment-associated PAHs to the estuarine crustaceans, *Palaemonetes pugio* and *Amphiascus tenuiremis*. *Bull Environ Contam Toxicol* (In Press).

Wise SA, Benner BA, Byrd GD, Chesler SN, Rebbert RE, Schantz MM. 1988. Determination of polycyclic aromatic hydrocarbons in a coal tar standard reference material. *Anal Chem* 60:887–895.

Wood CE. 1967. Physioecology of the grass shrimp, *Palaemonetes pugio* in the Galveston Bay estuarine system. *Contrib Mar Sci* 12:54–79.

Zar JH. 1974. Biostatistical analysis. Englewood Cliffs NJ: Prentice-Hall. 620 p.

Zepp RG, Cline DM. 1977. Rates of direct photolysis in aquatic environment. *Environ Sci Technol* 11:359–366.

Chapter 9

Workgroup IV Synopsis: Regulatory Issues and Risk Assessment

Thomas Kelsch, chair
Rebecca L. Powell, co-chair
Kenneth R. Dixon, Anne Fairbrother, Judy C. Helgen, Stephen J. Klaine, Foster L. Mayer, Gary A. Pascoe, Jennifer L. Shaw, Russell F. Theriot

Greater public awareness of the importance of wetlands and the historical rate of their loss has given rise to several important federal, state, and local programs whose purpose is to stem the loss of these valuable ecological resources. Such programs have helped contribute to a significant reduction in the rate of wetlands loss, from 180,000 hectares/y in the mid-1970s to 120,000 hectares/y in the mid-1980s. Recent data from the U.S. Department of Agriculture's National Resources Inventory suggest that the net rate of loss is now below 40,000 hectares/y.

As the United States approaches its national goal for no overall net loss of its wetlands base, it is essential that greater attention be focused on restoring and maintaining the chemical, physical, and biological integrity of the remaining wetlands as is suggested in the goal of the Clean Water Act (CWA). No single protection or management program effectively addresses the multiple sources of chemical contamination to wetlands and the need for ecosystem rehabilitation.

Chapter Preview

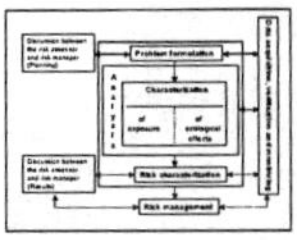

Ecotoxicology and Risk Assessment for Wetlands. Michael A. Lewis et al., editors.
 ISBN 1-880611-16-3

Rather, several programs based on federal and state legislation directly or indirectly affect the restoration and maintenance of the chemical integrity of wetland systems (Table 9-1). Many of these programs incorporate ecological risk assessment as a tool to evaluate scientific information about the adverse effects of physical and chemical stressors on the environment.

Table 9-1 Major federal environmental legislation

Legislation	Description
National Environmental Policy Act of 1969	Analysis of environmental impact of proposed actions and the alternatives; environmental impact assessments
Clean Air Act 1963; amended 1970, 1977, 1992	Protection and enhancement of the quality of the nation' s air resources; ambient air pollutant and emission standards
Federal Water Pollution Control Act 1972; amended 1977 (Clean Water Act)	Restoration and maintenance the chemical, physical, and biological integrity of the nation' s waters; regulation of point sources (Section 402) and discharges of dredged or fill material (Section 404); nonpoint source control (Section 319); water quality standards (Section 303)
Federal Insecticide, Fungicide, and Rodenticide Act 1972, 1975, 1978, 1988	Regulation of pesticides
Safe Drinking Water Act 1974	Establishment of drinking water regulations to protect public health in surface and ground water
Marine Protection Research and Sanctuaries Act of 1972 (Ocean Dumping Act)	Protection of human health, the marine environment, and ecological systems; regulates disposal of materials beyond territorial limits or 3 miles from shore and provides for designation and regulation of marine sactuaries
Coastal Zone Management Act of 1972	Development plans for coastal management
Resource Conservation and Recovery Act of 1976	Regulation of chemicals used in manufacturing; emphasis on the workplace and disposal
Toxic Substances Control Act of 1976	Regulation of new chemicals (other than pesticides)
Executive Orders 11990 and 11988 from 1977	Protection of wetlands and floodplain management
Comprehensive Environmental Response, Compensation, and Liability Act of 1980 (Superfund)	Assessment and cleanup of risks to human health and the environment at federally designated hazardous waste sites
Oil Pollution Act of 1990	Emergency response to oil spills in territorial waters

Source: Bartell et al. 1992

Risk can be defined in terms of the probability that a particular adverse effect will occur as the consequence of a specific action (Scala 1991). Risk by definition is probabilistic and is generally statistically derived from surrogate studies or subsamples of actual populations. A risk does not exist unless 2 criteria are met:

1) the stressor has the inherent ability to cause an adverse effect, and
2) the population of concern is in contact with the stressor for long enough, and at sufficient intensity, to elicit a response or is affected indirectly by the toxicity responses of closely associated species in the community (e.g., disruption of food resources).

An assessment of ecological risk, as modified from the U.S. Environmental Protection Agency's (USEPA) risk assessment framework (1992a, 1998), quantitatively or qualitatively evaluates the actual or potential adverse effects of stress on an ecosystem. Ecological risk assessments can help identify environmental problems, establish priorities, and provide a scientific basis for regulatory or management decisions. The risk assessment process has several advantages as applied to environmental decision-making and management of ecological hazards (Suter 1993):

1) It provides the quantitative bases for comparing and prioritizing risks.
2) By expressing results as probabilities, it acknowledges the inherent uncertainty in predicting future environmental states, thereby making the assessment more credible.
3) It requires the statement of clearly defined endpoints, thereby avoiding ambiguous goals that by their nature are unachievable.
4) It provides a scientific basis for cost–benefit analyses.
5) It clearly separates the scientific process of estimating the magnitude and probability of effects from the process of choosing among alternatives and determining the acceptability of risks.

The 2 general categories of risk assessments are predictive (or prospective) and retrospective. Predictive risk assessments generally are used to predict the consequences of a future action, such as the registration of a new pesticide or regulation of new effluents. They predominate in regulatory agencies and often lead to dichotomous decisions (i.e., permit issuance, pesticide registration). Retrospective risk assessments may be used to assess the existing damages of a particular site or action (e.g., evaluating the ecological effects at a hazardous waste site) or to reassess the effectiveness or appropriateness of a previous action or decision (e.g., evaluating new data on the risks of a previously registered pesticide). Whereas predictive risk assessments are primarily source-driven, retrospective assessments may be driven by information on sources, effects, or exposure (Suter 1993). Differences in the information driving the assessment will also change the flow of inference about contaminant sources, exposure, and effects (Table 9-2).

Table 9-2 Types of retrospective risk assessments and the associated flow of inference about sources, exposure, and effects

Retrospective risk assessment	Associated flow of inference
Source-driven assessments	Known source → Unknown exposure → Unknown effects
Effects-driven assessments	Observed effects → Unknown exposure → Unknown source
Exposure-driven assessments	Unknown source ← Observed exposure → Unknown effects

Source: Suter 1993

Various levels of complexity in the approach to performing an ecological risk assessment are possible. These range from simplistic and relatively inexpensive tests to sophisticated and expensive field- and laboratory-based assessments. Each successive increase in complexity generally increases the specificity of the assessment and refines the quantitative understanding of risk. A tiered approach to risk assessment is often recommended. Tiers may be similar to those described below.

1) Screening consists of a relatively simple comparison of stressor parameters, such as chemical concentrations in environmental media, with available standards and criteria on other ecological effect benchmarks such as proposed sediment quality guidelines.
2) Literature comparison consists of comparisons of chemical parameters, such as concentrations in environmental media or doses to organisms, with ecotoxicological data from the scientific literature. Ecotoxicological data, modeling of chemical fate and transport, food web trophic transfer, etc., are necessary information.
3) Field- and/or laboratory-based potential impacts are measured, or risks are estimated, by integrating empirical information from laboratory and in situ toxicity bioassays and ecological surveys. This approach provides very specific information on the 3 components of the risk assessment triad (i.e., identification, characterization, and assessment) and thereby minimizes uncertainty in the risk estimates.

The first 2 tiers, which should be done before Tier 3, can be limited by their dependence on predicted concentrations in environmental media, if measured concentrations are unavailable, and on the use of surrogate species for derivation of criteria or literature values. This is particularly a problem with wetland assessments because toxicity data on unique wetland species, such as obligate wetland vegetation or semiaquatic mammals, are underdeveloped in comparison to those for more typical aquatic or terrestrial organisms. The first 2 tiers minimize the specificity of the risk assessment and subsequently limit the usefulness of the analysis; however, they are appropriate under a variety of conditions as screening-level tools. The literature comparison can incorporate ecosystem-specific information on toxicology and bioavailability of chemical contaminants if that information is available in the literature. Should an indication from the comparisons in the first 2 tiers suggest a possible ecological risk, further data gathering in the form of field- and/or laboratory-based tests would be necessary to refine the likelihood of the risk for a specific wetland.

Risk management is the process of evaluating alternative options and selecting among them (NRC 1983). Design of a risk assessment and the consequential risk management decisions are made based on considerations of stakeholders in the project or issue. Stakeholders can include a diversity of groups or individuals, such as regulators, affected or interested citizens, and the regulated community or industry. While conducting a risk assessment may not be the solution for addressing all environmental problems, nor is it a prerequisite for effective environmental management, use of the overall risk assessment thought process should increase the efficiency and quality of management decisions.

Risk Assessment Procedures

Several agencies or organizations have developed procedures for performing ecological risk assessments. Most of the procedures are directly applicable to a particular program of the sponsoring organization. However, many are applicable to assessing risks to wetlands from ecological stressors.

USEPA Superfund Program

A risk assessment approach similar to that of the Risk Assessment Forum (see USEPA Risk Assessment Forum Section) is provided in guidance by USEPA's Office of Solid Waste and Emergency Response for Superfund-type hazardous waste sites. The Superfund guidance is outlined in several newsletters and documents (USEPA 1991, 1992d, 1997) and supersedes earlier guidance on conducting environmental evaluations under the Comprehensive Environmental Response, Compensation, and Liability Act (CERCLA) (USEPA 1989).

As part of an effort to develop a cooperative guidance among various offices to address wetlands contamination, USEPA has formed the Core Working Group Considering Wetlands at Hazardous Waste Sites (USEPA 1992e). Such concerns as the ecological significance of wetlands and how remedial processes may affect wetlands have been published as a result of this group's work (USEPA 1994).

U.S. Army Corps of Engineers Hydrogeomorphic Classification

The U.S. Army Corps of Engineers (USACOE), in cooperation with USEPA, administers the CWA Section 404 Regulatory Program for permitting the discharge of dredged or fill material in waters of the U.S., which include wetlands. The USACOE has released guidance on assessing wetland functions to satisfy technical and programmatic requirements of Section 404 such as determination of minimal effects (USACOE 1991). The approach described in the guidance, frequently referred to as the "hydrogeomorphic (HGM) classification approach," is very similar to the approach to assessing ecological risks described in USEPA's framework document discussed in the next section (Brinson 1993; Smith 1993). However, the terminology differs substantially. For example, the development and characterization phases of HGM are equivalent to USEPA's problem formulation phase, the HGM assessment phase is similar to USEPA's analysis phase, and the analysis phase of the USACOE guidance is similar to the risk characterization phase of USEPA's framework document.

USEPA Risk Assessment Forum

USEPA's Risk Assessment Forum has suggested an approach (Figure 9-1) and methodology for assessing stressor (i.e., chemical and nonchemical) risks to the environment in its Framework for Ecological Risk Assessment (USEPA 1992a, 1992b, 1992c, 1998). The framework has several advantages that make it useful for assessing wetland ecological risks:

1) Comprehensive: The procedures outline a process for evaluating a variety of scientific information used in assessing risks of stressors to ecological systems. Stressors may be physical, chemical, or biological entities that can adversely affect the environment, although the focus of the framework document is on physical and chemical stressors.
2) Flexible: The procedures can be applied to risk assessment questions considering one or more stressors at any spatial or temporal scale.
3) Iterative: Although the framework document defines each component of the process for completing an assessment, a strength of the process is its iterative nature, allowing a return to earlier phases of the assessment to reexamine previous analyses in light of new data or refined priorities.
4) Identifies the risk management role: The procedures clearly describe the role of risk management and its relationship with risk assessment.
5) Establishes terminology: The procedure was designed to be applicable across regulatory bodies for multiple types of stressors and provides consistent terminology to satisfy this goal.

The approach outlined in the framework documents was adapted from the 4-step methodology developed by the National Academy of Sciences for assessing human health risks (NRC 1983). The Risk Assessment Forum has developed further recommendations on implementing the framework (USEPA 1998). The Risk Assessment Forum's framework approach consists of 3 primary phases:

1) Problem formulation—Defines the objectives and scope. Focus is on collecting information to design exposure and ecological effects assessments. The ecosystem or type of ecosystem to be protected is defined, and appropriate assessment and measures of exposure are identified. The end product is a conceptual model of the situation, in which contaminants and receptors of concern and potential pathways of exposure are outlined.

2) Analysis—Consists of 2 steps, the first of which is characterization of exposures, which quantifies the magnitude, duration, and type of actual or potential exposures of ecological receptors to site contaminants. The focus is on characterizing receptors and quantifying contaminant exposure point concentrations. The second step is characterization of ecological effects, which links concentrations of contaminants to adverse biological or ecological effects.
3) Risk characterization—Compares the exposure assessment with the ecological effects assessment. Risk characterization is usually not a probabilistic risk estimate, due to a lack of probability distributions for input parameters. Uncertainties in the assessment are described, and the ecological significance of the results is interpreted.

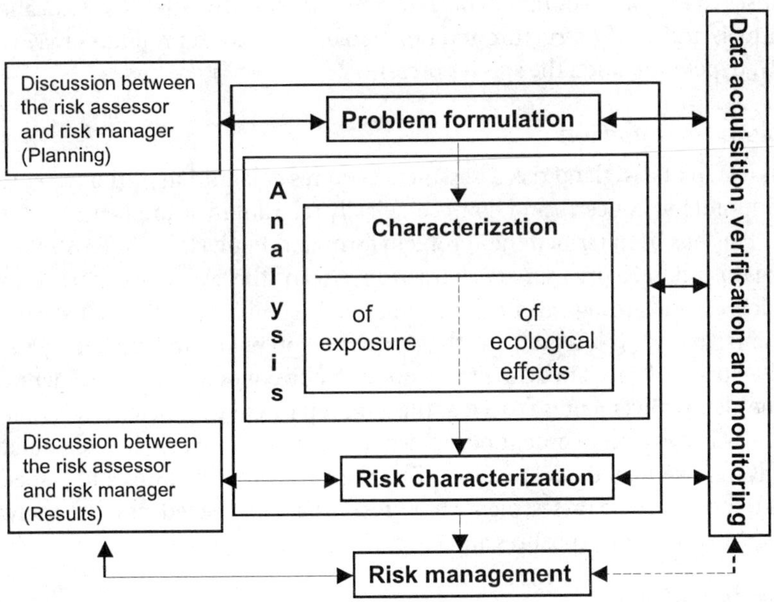

Figure 9-1 USEPA's framework for ecological risk assessment

The Risk Assessment Forum framework is useful for performing and reporting risk assessments for a wide variety of environmental conditions and program objectives and under a wide breadth of complexity, from simple criteria comparisons to complex field- and laboratory-based assessments. The remainder of this chapter illustrates the applicability of these recommendations for a variety of wetland risk assessments under the existing management programs. Additional information on how to conduct a risk assessment is available in several publications. In particular, readers are encouraged to read USEPA's Framework for Ecological Risk Assessment (USEPA 1992a) and the related guidelines (USEPA 1998).

Application of the Risk Assessment Framework to Wetlands

Wetlands represent complex environments for assessing ecological risks. Habitats may vary from estuarine to riverine to basin type. They include such diverse media as surface water, ground water, sediments, and upland and saturated soils. Given the diversity of wetland habitats, it is not surprising that a number of species are unique to these ecosystems. Wetland biota include wholly aquatic organisms such as fish, semiaquatic or upland organisms that feed on aquatic biota (e.g., waterfowl and shorebirds), and animals such as amphibians that utilize both environments. Plants also have adapted to the semiaquatic wetland environment and include aquatic phytoplankton, floating plants, and rooted macrophytes that require continual or periodic inundation of the root zone. All of these organisms may be affected by environmental stresses, particularly chemical contamination. Because ecosystem responses to chemical contaminants tend to be specific, the effects of toxicants on individuals and on the structure and function of wetland communities may vary greatly, depending upon the species present.

Problem formulation

The first step in a wetland risk assessment requires a definition of the system at risk, the endpoints of concern, and how ecologically relevant measurements will be taken. This has been termed the "problem formulation phase" (USEPA 1992a, 1998). During this phase, a preliminary characterization of the available exposure and toxicological and ecological effects information is combined with other scientific data. This, in turn, is integrated with information on policy and regulatory issues and site-specific factors to define the scope and objectives for the assessment. Stakeholder involvement is crucial at this point, particularly for wetlands that frequently involve very contentious issues. The result of the problem formulation phase is a conceptual model that identifies the ecological functions and associated values to be protected (assessment endpoints), the data needed, and the analyses to be used (measures of exposures and effects).

Assessment endpoints

The identification of assessment endpoints appropriate for wetlands is dependent on the ecological functions and values of the wetland. Key ecological functions have been grouped into categories such as habitat for characteristic communities and wildlife, hydrologic flux, and biogeochemical processes such as nutrient cycling (Richardson 1994). Values ascribed to wetlands, on the other hand, include such things as providing habitat for fishing, hunting or wildlife viewing, timber harvesting, and flood control. The introduction of stressors such as chemical contaminants can alter the wetland functions and, in turn, the wetland values that are derived from these functions.

Taken together, ecosystem functions and values comprise a set of assessment endpoints for wetlands. Although not inclusive, wetland functions and values have been compiled and grouped into categories for purposes of developing assessment endpoints (Table 9-3). Selection of functions and values as assessment endpoints for wetlands helps to ensure that the ecological risk assessment will address the full extent of possible concerns about risks to wetlands.

Table 9-3 List of potential assessment and measurement endpoints for wetlands

Assessment endpoints	Measurement endpoints
Hydrologic flux and storage	Suborganismal level
Flood control and storage	Biomarkers
Open space	
Water supply	
Shoreline stabilization	
Saltwater intrusion control	
Groundwater recharge and discharge	
Biological productivity	Individual level
Timber production	Bioassays
Shrub crop production	Body burdens
Food production (fish, ducks)	Reproductive success
Historical, cultural, archaeological resources	Reduced photosynthesis
	Growth rate
	Time to sexual maturity
	Number of young produced
	Number of reproductive cycles/y
	Viability of young
	Cell division rate
Biogeochemical cycling and storage	Population level
Sediment control	Growth
Wastewater treatment	Lifespan
Nutrient removal	Distribution
Water quality	Recruitment
	Age structure (size distribution)
	Altered gene pool
	Percent deformities
	Mark/recapture study
	Fitness
Decomposition	Community or ecosystem level
Community energetics	Change in abundance or biomass
Carbon and energy flow	Shifts in interspecific competitive advantage
CO_2 sink	Change in species dominance
	Change in diversity
	Change in species richness
	Change in structure
Community or wildlife habitat	Change in net productivity
Recreation	Change in stability of fluctuation patterns
Visual and cultural	Loss of a population
Hunting and fishing	Indices of biotic integrity
Preservation of flora and fauna	Microbial respiration
Medical	Presence or absence of specific populations
Education	Decomposition rates
Threatened, rare, endangered species habitat	Net loss of essential elements
	Nutrient cycling
	Microbial index

Measurement endpoints

While assessment endpoints are explicit expressions of the actual environmental value that is to be protected, measurement endpoints are measurable responses to a stressor that are related to the valued characteristics (Suter 1993). Measurement endpoints link the assessment endpoints to the risk management process. For each assessment endpoint listed in Table 9-3, a number of measurement endpoints may be appropriate.

Measurement endpoints are either single numbers (e.g., LC50s) or, preferably, multidimensional descriptive models (Suter 1993). Selection of measurement endpoints must be carefully thought out before an ecological risk assessment is undertaken.

The conceptual model

Wetland ecosystems may be affected by adjacent land use or by any stressor imported from an upstream system. The major focus of the conceptual model is the development of working hypotheses regarding how stressors might affect ecological components of the natural environment. The conceptual model may become increasingly detailed during the various iterations that refine the risk assessment process. From a conceptual standpoint, the wetland can begin to appear as a series of compartments that represent various land uses and aquatic ecosystems, each connected by potential contaminant transport arrows. While this may seem simplistic, it facilitates the formulation of hypotheses concerning spatial and temporal exposure scenarios and the impact of stressors on the ecosystem.

For example, it is critical to understand hydrology within the watershed, as this ultimately dictates exposure for many wetland receptors. The incorporation of different land-use hydrology into exposure scenarios can be a significant aid to visualizing spatial and temporal relationships between stressors and ecological components within the wetland watershed. In addition, visualizing these relationships in a diagram can help develop and prioritize hypotheses for the conceptual model.

Analysis phase

The analysis phase consists of 2 activities: characterization of exposure and characterization of ecological effects. The purpose of the exposure characterization is to estimate or measure the distribution and magnitude of a stressor spatially and temporally and to determine its potential for contact with the ecological components of concern. The purpose of the characterization of ecological effects is to identify and quantify the adverse effects resulting from exposure to a stressor and, to the extent possible, to describe the cause-and-effect relationships. Indirect effects of the stressor on the receptors of concern also need to be identified, when possible.

Characterization of exposure

Exposure characterization evaluates the co-occurrence or contact of the stressor with ecological components. Exposure generally is expressed in terms of concentration of the chemicals of concern in environmental media. For organisms in aquatic habitats (e.g., fish, macroinvertebrates, amphibians), this is the concentration of the chemical in the water column or sediments. For wetland plants, water, sediment, or soil concentrations also are important determinants of exposure. Terrestrial animal (e.g., birds, mammals, amphibians) exposure generally is measured by concentration of chemicals in food items, such as aquatic invertebrates, plants, or fish.

Exposure profiles need to be developed for each scenario identified in the problem formulation phase. Questions to be addressed include

1) which media are significantly contaminated and how is the contamination transferred between media,
2) which contaminated media are the organisms of concern in contact with and for how long,
3) what are the routes by which the organisms are exposed, and
4) can and will the exposed organisms modify their behavior to reduce exposure (Suter 1993).

Furthermore, physicochemical parameters such as temperature, pH, and water hardness may influence the amount of contaminant that is available for uptake by biota. This information must be taken into account when the relationship between the chemical in the abiotic and biotic components of the environment is being established.

Most chemical stressors are transported into a wetland through water flow. Point source discharges, nonpoint source entry, groundwater seepage during base flow, simple downhill water flow from one aquatic ecosystem to another, and dry and wet fallout should all be considered as potential transport pathways. Except for ephemeral wetlands caused by heavy rainfall or flooding, most wetlands are intimately connected with ground water in freshwater systems or tidal waters in estuarine and coastal marsh systems. This connection allows for the development of pathways of contaminant transport and modification that may be of greater concern than in other ecosystems. For example, riverine wetlands may be affected by surface waters transporting contaminants onto the site and by surface currents releasing contaminants from underlying sediments. In an estuarine wetland, storm action and unusually high tides can alter contaminant loading, groundwater seeps, or dilution mechanisms. Surfacewater infiltration to ground water may transport contaminants from sediments into ground water, particularly if the geochemistry of the contaminated sediments is modified by changes in surfacewater pH or redox status. Contaminants also can be transferred between environmental media through partitioning, sorption, solubilization, volatilization, etc.

Transformation of stressors through abiotic factors such as oxidation/reduction, hydrolysis, and photolysis or biotic factors such as metabolism and primary production also is important in evaluating exposure (Suter et al. 1994). As a result of these processes, the parent chemical may be activated to more toxic forms, broken down, or simply detoxified by minor structural alterations. Secondary toxic products may also be formed. Chemical transformation occurs more readily in wetlands than in other ecosystems. Flooding creates a highly reduced oxidation state in soils. This results in pH shifts, thereby increasing mobilization of many nutrients as well as contaminants. Biotic transformation of chemicals in wetlands by the microbial community is well documented and supports the use of constructed wetlands for treating contaminated water. Both mineralization and metabolism can occur, depending on the contaminant and the microorganisms. Anoxic conditions will significantly alter the type of biota available for transformation.

Exposure potential

Exposure requires the presence of a stressor and receptor in the same place at the same time for a certain length of time. Several characteristics are used to describe the exposure potential, including spatial and temporal relationships between the stressor and the receptor and frequency and duration of the contact. All these factors must be considered to develop an accurate exposure profile.

In wetland systems, fluctuating hydrological cycles can have a major influence on frequency of exposure by altering chemical fate. Regulated wetting and drying cycles, such as tidal fluxes and seasonal fluxes, or unregulated events, such as heavy rainfall or flooding, can bring contaminants in contact with critical components of the wetland. Such alterations have the potential for releasing chemicals adsorbed to soils or sediments and may result in periodic pulses of contaminants. For example, in the western United States, the dissolution and release of Cu salts from the banks of rivers in mining areas during spring snowmelt and flooding can result in an influx of dissolved Cu downstream. In addition, lowered pH caused by snowmelt can increase the availability of soil-bound metals for transport (Brooks and Moore 1989).

It is critical to understand hydrology within the watershed, as this ultimately dictates exposure for many scenarios. Different land uses have different stormwater hydrographs, resulting in different exposure durations. In addition, runoff from different land uses may vary in intensity, resulting in physical stresses (e.g., hydrology, erosion, sedimentation) on the receiving stream ecosystem. Alterations of the hydrological conduit exacerbate or ameliorate some of these physical stresses (e.g., channelization increases the velocity of the water; impoundments decrease the water velocity). These alterations may significantly change exposure scenarios as well as critical ecological components potentially at risk. The incorporation of different land-use hydrology into exposure scenarios can be a significant aid to visualizing spatial and temporal relationships between stressors and ecological components within the wetland watershed. In addition, visualizing these relationships in a diagram can help develop and prioritize hypotheses for the conceptual model.

Route of exposure

There are numerous routes in which organisms can be exposed to chemical stressors in wetlands, including plant and animal uptake or sorption, inhalation or respiration both from air and water, ingestion of soil or sediment, ingestion of water, and food-chain transfer.

Organisms also may be exposed to a contaminant by several routes simultaneously and/or during different life stages. For instance, the primary route of exposure for a fish may be through respiratory transfer; however, dietary intake and dermal exposure also can occur (Suter et al. 1994). Amphibians spend portions of their life cycle in both the terrestrial and aquatic environment and could be exposed in numerous ways. While tadpoles could accumulate toxicants through several routes in the aquatic environment, adult frogs are susceptible to exposure through both aquatic and terrestrial routes. Emergent macrophytes that are in contact with contaminants through both the sediment and water columns have shown a significant ability to adsorb chemicals through both their roots and shoots.

Food-chain interactions and the potential for biomagnification, in which certain chemicals can increase in concentration with each trophic level, should also be addressed in the exposure assessment. Plants, as the primary producers, play an important role in food web interactions. Insects, tadpoles, and snails that graze over plant and sediment surfaces will ingest deposited contaminants. Filter-feeding zooplankton will ingest planktonic algae and suspended organic detritus. As organisms such as birds and mammals feed on the contaminated species, toxicants may be transferred up the food chain.

Exposure modeling

Numerous wetland ecosystem models have been developed, beginning in the early 1970s. Types of wetlands modeled include coastal salt marshes, mangrove wetlands, freshwater marshes, swamps, and riparian wetlands. Most of these models were simple compartment models designed primarily to simulate biomass or nutrient dynamics. They were developed by systems ecologists and did not consider the transport and effects of contaminants. At the same time that these ecosystem models were being developed, process models that did include contaminant mobility and bioaccumulation also were being constructed. These models were designed by civil, hydraulic, and chemical engineers and attempted to describe hydrodynamics, sediment transport, or food-chain accumulation. There has been little interaction between the different modeling efforts, and as a result, few environmental transport models that emphasize physical and chemical aspects of contaminants have been developed for wetland ecosystems (Dixon and Florian 1993).

Surface hydrologic models, such as Hydrological Simulation Program Fortran (Donigian et al. 1983) and groundwater loading effects of agricultural management systems (GLEAMS) (Leonard et al. 1987), predict the runoff of toxicants from the land surface. Wetland models can obtain input from surface runoff models and predict the change in toxicant concentration within the wetland. Modeling for wetlands usually entails separate considerations of terrestrial root-zone transport modeling (e.g., for pesticides) and sediment transport modeling in aquatic systems.

Hydrodynamics of wetlands include precipitation, freshwater inflow, circulation, and turbulence. Flow dynamics in tidal marshes are complicated by tidal processes and saline density and mixing. Circulation and flow models have been developed for the Chesapeake Bay (Ward 1980), Gulf Coast estuaries (Hauck and Ward 1980) and estuaries of Puget Sound (PSWQA 1994). The effects of draining wetlands in eastern North Carolina were modeled by Philips (1985).

Sediment transport depends on the underlying hydrodynamics. A hydrodynamics model, therefore, must be verified before a sediment transport model can be developed. Transport mechanisms include convection, turbulent diffusion, gravitational settling, and resuspension at the sediment–water interface. A model of contaminant flux, together with hydrodynamic and wave models, was used to simulate sediment dispersion in the western basin of Lake Erie (Sheng 1980) and contaminated sediment transport through wetlands of the Clark Fork River, Montana (Pascoe 1994). Models of contaminant uptake have been developed for algae (Seip 1979; Thomann 1981), zooplankton (Dixon 1975), and fish (Barber et al. 1988, 1991; Clark et al. 1990).

Characterization of effects

An effect is a change in the state or dynamics of an organism resulting from exposure to a chemical, physical, or biological stressor (USEPA 1992a). It can be a direct effect when the stressor acts on the organism. Alternatively, a stressor can indirectly affect an organism by changing the state of another part of the ecosystem that is important to the maintenance of the organism of concern.

In ecotoxicological risk assessment, direct effects are the result of a stressor such as a contaminant causing adverse changes in an individual organism. However, it must be remembered that toxic effects are not manifested unless the chemical concentration is high enough to overcome the physiological detoxification, elimination, or sequestration processes in the organism. In other words, the dose makes the poison.

Although chemicals act on and cause adverse changes to individuals, in an ecological assessment, concern generally centers on ecological attributes such as maintenance of viable populations or communities. However, effects on individuals may be important for protected species such as endangered species or migratory birds. The effects on individuals involve an assessment of the indirect effects of the contaminants of concern on associated organisms in the food web. Contaminants also can indirectly alter the relationship of the affected organisms to the abiotic cycling of nutrients and other factors in the environment. This expands the toxicological effects on individual organisms to the entire population of the target species and the community in which it is embedded. Population effects occur when sufficiently large numbers of individuals are affected by the toxicant to change the mortality, reproductive, and recruitment rates of the population. Intraspecific competition can be altered as well as dominance roles; eventually, the gene pool can be changed, resulting in the emergence of more tolerant strains and/or less genetic diversity, with increased susceptibility to other environmental stressors. Community associations are altered as individual and population fitness traits affect interspecific competition and predator–prey relationships. Shifts in community structure may result in a reversion to an earlier successional stage or a change in the rate at which succession is occurring. Composition of the vascular plant community is important in defining the type of wetland environment that is experienced by the benthic organisms as well as the wildlife that are attracted to the area. Therefore, simple changes in vegetative structure may profoundly influence the habitat quality for wetland-associated animals.

Ecosystems are, however, more than just a collection of different species in one place. They provide important biogeochemical cycles that integrate living organisms with their abiotic environments. Wetlands are recognized for their role in the maintenance of hydrological regimes, nutrient cycling, and carbon sequestration. Contaminants can interfere with many of these functions, by either directly or indirectly affecting organisms that are responsible for the maintenance of cycles (including bacteria). For example, destroying vegetation through the use of herbicides or other phytotoxic chemicals would allow water to move through a wetland at a faster rate, thereby increasing the amount of oxygen in the system which, in turn, may increase the rate of decomposition, liberating increased amounts of phosphorous. Changes in vegetative structure may also influence sedimentation rates, thereby changing the value of the wetlands in sediment trapping and flood control. Therefore, it is important to assess ecosystem functions as well as attributes in ecotoxicological risk assessments.

When dealing with ecosystem processes, it is important to remember that all systems have functional redundancies and some degree of resiliency that allow them to absorb environmental and anthropogenic stresses up to a certain point. Determining how much assimilative capacity is available, and when it is likely to be exceeded, obviously is not a trivial task. In addition, stochastic environmental factors contribute a great deal of uncertainty to any prediction efforts. Moreover, ecosystems are constantly changing through time as successional influences change the composition of the community. Therefore, what really is being assessed during the risk assessment process is how a proposed action would change the trajectory along which an ecosystem is moving, not how far a system deviates from a static state. Because wetlands are boundary systems (between aquatic and upland ecosystems or between inland and marine systems), they tend to be very dynamic in nature. Short-term changes are influenced by attributes such as tidal regimes, flood and drought cycles, and seasonal temperature fluctuations. Long-term cycles are driven by climatic changes, sediment accretion and depletion, natural successional processes, and large-scale landscape or hydrological alterations. Assessments of the risks of anthropogenic activities to wetland structure and function must be placed within this context of continual change. Preference should be given to approaches that use response and exposure distributions in a probabilistic framework for risk perceptions. This will capture the system variability during the selected temporal scale and allow comparisons to the range of variability within the selected reference systems. If long time frames are used in the assessment, the predicted magnitude of change of the system and/or its components should be compared with predicted changes in reference systems. Ecosystem attributes should be included in wetland risk assessments whenever possible.

Risk characterization phase

The final step in the ecological risk assessment, the characterization of risks, usually is the most difficult part of the process. Its purpose is to provide an estimate of current and potential risks to receptors and ecological components (which may be individual organisms, populations, communities, or ecosystems). The risk characterization phase integrates the results of the exposure and ecological effects analysis to evaluate the likelihood of adverse ecological effects associated with exposure to a stressor. The resulting risk characterization forms the basis for further discussions with risk managers prior to the use of the risk assessment information in decision-making.

One approach to risk characterization is the development of a matrix of the results of the exposure and effects analysis and the assignment of weighing factors to each of the measured endpoints (Pascoe 1993). Values of plus or minus are assigned to the variables of chemistry, toxicity, and ecology for each bioassessment area, based on statistical differences from control samples, reference area surveys, or trends analysis. A positive chemistry value is defined as an elevation above a reference area concentration, or it may be related to the lowest concentration above which an effect is observed in a sensitive bioassay. A positive toxicity value is defined as a statistically significant response in a bioassay, compared to control responses. A positive ecology value is a significant difference in community structure, compared to a reference area, or in a trends analysis, as exceeding a percentage change in a community parameter from that observed at areas with lower contamination levels.

Where comparison to reference areas is not possible, or for multiple variables within each triad category, a ranking scheme described by Kreis (1988) may be useful to fit the measured variables into the 3 categories. The ranking scheme essentially ranks the results of measurements of various subcategories, then calculates an average ranking within each of the 3 variables. For example, the chemistry category may include rankings of chemical concentrations and measures of bioavailability, such as cation exchange capacity or sulfide concentrations. The toxicology category may rank results of a number of toxicity tests. From these rankings, an average ranking of chemistry and toxicity can be generated. Final rankings are then used to generate the valuation matrix.

Ecological significance

Risk managers depend on an adequate description of the ecological significance of the risk findings in making decisions about managing a contaminated wetland during permitting actions. The difficulty in defining ecological significance becomes apparent when one evaluates sublethal effects observed in toxicity bioassays, or imbalances in community parameters when actual effects on species diversity or abundance are lacking (Barnthouse et al. 1989; Adams et al. 1992; Birge et al. 1992; Dickson et al. 1992; Krantzberg and Boyd 1992; Suter 1993). The USEPA working group on contamination will address ecologically significant issues with respect to characterizing risks and making remedial decisions (USEPA 1992c).

The definition of ecological significance can be addressed by a relative ranking of impacts, as outlined by Duinker and Beanlands (1986):

1) Major impact—Affects an entire population or species in sufficient magnitude to cause a decline in abundance and/or change in distribution beyond which natural recruitment (reproduction, immigration from unaffected areas) would not return that population or species, or any population or species dependent on it, to its natural level.
2) Moderate impact—Affects a portion of a population and may bring about a change in abundance and/or distribution over one or more generations but does not threaten the integrity of that population or any population dependent upon it.
3) Minor impact—Affects a specific group of localized individuals within a population over a short time period but does not affect other trophic levels or the population itself.
4) Negligible impact—Any impacts below the minor category are considered negligible.

A more recent development in describing the significance of ecological risk assessment findings is to place the results in one of several categories based on consequence (Suter et al. 1995). In this approach, risk thresholds for a variety of parameters are calculated, with a statistical basis, and the risks grouped into categories according to a selective threshold or cutoff criterion:

1) *De manifestis* risk: Risks that exceed a defined threshold, such as percentage change in abundance, production, number of species, or area loss, and have legal protection or extraordinary local value. Indicates management (e.g., remediation) is needed.
2) Intermediate risk: Risks that exceed the defined threshold but the species or population has no special status.

3) *De minimus* risk: Risks less than the threshold in a unit area, or the population is of negligible ecological value, or only short-term impacts are expected.

Although none of the above approaches to describing the ecological significance of the risk assessment may be appropriate for a given wetland or condition, they nonetheless provide a conceptual starting point for risk managers to consider in their management of wetlands.

Nontoxicant Stressors

Types of nontoxicant stressors

Although the focus of this document is on anthropogenically released chemical stressors, there are many nonchemical stressors that may affect wetland ecosystems. Nontoxicant stressors may impact wetlands independently or may act in conjunction with toxicants. Chemical stressors usually are associated with increases in concentration, availability, and/or toxicity of metals and synthetic organic compounds (Adamus and Brandt 1990). For instance, toxicity of metals and metalloids may be significantly influenced by changes in nonchemical attributes such as pH, dissolved oxygen, water hardness, and sediment loading.

Because of the interaction of chemicals with changes in the physical attributes, wetland risk assessments should always include an evaluation of the magnitude, duration, and frequency of all potential stressors. Otherwise, accurate cause-and-effect relationships cannot be established. The following nonchemical stressors warrant consideration, as described by Adamus and Brandt (1990):

1) Nutrient enrichment and eutrophication: Enrichment and eutrophication are caused by increases in concentration or availability of N and P. These stressors usually are associated with fertilizer application, cattle feedlots, ineffective wastewater systems, fossil fuel combustion, and agricultural or urban runoff.
2) Organic C loading and reduced dissolved oxygen (DO): Organic C loading results from wastewater effluent, feedlot drainage, and nutrient enrichment. Reduced DO results from increases in C loading. The organic matter (OM) causes an increase in respiration or biological oxygen demand, which reduces DO in sediments and the water column. Lower DO leads to increases in toxic gases such as hydrogen sulfide and ammonia. These stressors usually are a result of ineffective wastewater systems.
3) Acidification: Acidification may result from mining or atmospheric deposition from fossil fuel combustion and is expressed as an increase in acidity (decrease in pH). Changes in pH can alter the bioavailability and toxicity of some compounds.

4) Salinization: Salinization results in an increase in dissolved salts (especially chloride), conductivity, and alkalinity. This stressor usually is associated with the use of road salt for winter ice control, recycled irrigation water, seawater intrusion, and domestic and industrial waste.
5) Sedimentation: Sedimentation results in partial or complete burial of organisms and alteration of substrate. This stressor usually is a result of agricultural practices, urban runoff, ineffective wastewater treatment systems, deposition of dredged or other fill material, and erosion from mining and construction sites.
6) Turbidity or shading: Increased turbidity is caused by a suspended sediment, whereas shading is caused by overstory vegetation, algal blooms, or other physical obstructions. Both stressors result, however, in a reduction or blockage of solar radiation. Turbidity may increase as a result of agricultural practices, urban runoff, ineffective wastewater treatment systems, erosion from mining and construction sites, and resuspension by wind or aquatic organisms.
7) Vegetation removal: Removal of vegetation in wetlands, by defoliation or timber harvesting, can result in increasing solar radiation. Vegetation removal may result from aquatic weed control, agricultural or silvicultural practices, channelization, bank stabilization, urban development, defoliation by aerial spraying of defoliants, disease, fire, and grazing by aquatic herbivores such as muskrat, nutria, grass carp, and waterfowl.
8) Temperature alteration: Changes in temperature regime may be caused by power plants, other industrial facilities, removal of riparian vegetation, and global climate warming.
9) Dehydration: Dehydration results from a reduction in water levels and/or increase in the frequency, duration, or extent of desiccation of wetland sediments. This stressor is usually associated with ditching, channelization of nearby streams, invasion by highly transpirative plant species, outlet widening, subsurface drainage, and ground- or surfacewater withdrawals for agricultural, industrial, or residential use.
10) Inundation: Inundation results from increases in water levels and/or frequency, duration, or extent of saturation of wetland sediments. This stressor is associated with impoundment (e.g., for cranberry or rice cultivation, flood control, water supply, waterfowl management). It also is associated with subsidence and changes in watershed land use that result in more runoff water being provided to wetlands. Permanent inundation can alter the wetland ecology.
11) Habitat fragmentation: Fragmentation of habitat is characterized by reduction in the size of habitat patches and increases in the distance between patches. This stressor is associated with urbanization and other land-use changes. A minimum distance between wetlands in the landscape

must be maintained to ensure movement and sustainable populations of biota.

12) Exotic species: Exotic plant and animal species can alter the structure of wetlands and eliminate native species. Nutria can be destructive to vegetation and may displace native muskrats. Melaleuca and Brazilian pepper have affected the Everglades. The European purple loosestrife threatens wetlands across the United States. Cordgrass and common reed are other undesirable plant species in some areas.

Differentiation between toxicant and nontoxicant stressors

It is not always possible to differentiate between the effects of anthropogenic and natural chemicals or between chemical and nonchemical stressors. For example, surface runoff from agricultural fields contains both suspended sediment and pesticides, and it may be difficult to differentiate the effects resulting from each stressor. An example of co-occurring chemical and nonchemical stressors is the runoff of the herbicide atrazine and suspended sediment into streams, rivers, and wetlands of North America (Solomon et al. 1996). The most susceptible organisms in these systems are plankton, periphyton, and macrophytes. Exposure to atrazine is in the form of pulses from runoff from agricultural fields recently treated with atrazine. The runoff also may contain heavy loadings of suspended sediment. It is not clear from previous work what the relative or combined effects of atrazine and suspended sediment would be on plant growth. The mode of action of atrazine is inhibition of photosynthesis through blockage of electron transport in Photosystem II. In the absence of light, atrazine does not affect plants. Confounding stresses, such as sediment loading, that co-occur with atrazine concentrations associated with runoff events also inhibit photosynthesis. Because both stressors inhibit photosynthesis, it is not clear which stressor (chemical or nonchemical) has the greater effect. This makes the assignment of risk and selecting the appropriate risk management options difficult.

External stressors to wetlands

Wetland risk assessments must consider external stressors to the system. Two examples of this would be changes in land use and atmospheric deposition. Land use in the watershed that drains into the wetland significantly affects the hydrologic conduits upstream from the wetland. Whether these conduits are small or large, land use dictates both hydrograph and chemograph of rainfall runoff events; these, in turn, significantly affect exposure regimes within the wetland. Turning forested land into row crop agriculture steepens the hydrograph, resulting in higher peak flows. In addition, many contaminants migrate into the receiving streams faster than from forested land. Urbanization significantly compresses the hydrograph, resulting in the highest peak flows (with the greatest amount of scouring energy) and the most rapid export of contaminants. In addition, if land use changes, both intensity and duration of runoff may change, particularly if the soils in the watershed are highly impervious. Widely fluctuating stream flow, erosion, and sedimentation are severe stresses on wetlands. These stresses, even in the absence of contaminant stressors, can result in significant loss of wetland function.

Atmospheric particles and gases can be transported from sources hundreds of miles away from the wetland where they are deposited. These substances can be both toxicants and nontoxicants. Sources include nuclear and coal-fired power plants, municipal and hazardous waste incinerators, and gases or resuspended particles from hazardous waste sites or landfills.

Case Studies

The following sections are case study examples of how the risk assessment approach described in the preceding sections can be implemented within current regulatory programs.

Superfund assessments

Legislative basis

CERCLA (1980) was envisioned as a cleanup effort that would use existing knowledge to assess and clean up the nation's abandoned hazardous waste sites. The amendments to this statute, known as the Superfund Amendments and Reauthorization Act (SARA) of 1986, made major changes to CERCLA by clarifying and expanding its role for protection of human health and the environment with respect to releases (or potential releases) of contaminants from abandoned hazardous waste sites. CERCLA is made up of 4 major parts. The first, consisting of Sections 102 and 103, outline USEPA responsibilities for the identification and reporting of hazardous substances. The USEPA is required to define what constitutes hazardous substances, while operators and owners of hazardous waste facilities are required to notify USEPA of the presence and potential release of hazardous substances at their facilities. The second part, Section 104, authorizes the federal government to remove and remediate the effects of hazardous waste releases. These actions are to be in compliance with the National Contingency Plan (NCP) developed by USEPA (Section 105). The final 2 parts of CERCLA involve the establishment of a Hazardous Waste Trust Fund (or Superfund) for remedial and removal activities. Section 107 also makes any party that was responsible for the release of hazardous substances financially liable for all the costs of removal or remediation action, other necessary response actions, and damage to natural resources. This provision offers guidance for responsibilities for the cleanup, either voluntarily or through enforcement.

In order to meet its requirement to promulgate regulations to implement the cleanup of hazardous waste sites, USEPA developed the NCP, which calls for identification and mitigation of the environmental impacts of these sites and the selection of remedial actions that are "protective of environmental organisms and ecosystems." CERCLA requires USEPA to ensure the protection of the environment through the selection of remedial alternatives for particular hazardous waste sites and the assessment of the degree of cleanup necessary. In addition, numerous federal and state statutes and regulations concerning environmental protection are potentially "applicable or relevant and appropriate requirements" (ARARs). An ARARs manual (USEPA 1988a) should be used to assist in determining potential legislative requirements on a case-by-case basis. Some federal environmental statutes that may be ARARs for a particular site include the

1) Resource Conservation and Recovery Act (RCRA) of 1976, as amended;
2) Federal Water Pollution Control Act, as Amended (also known as the Clean Water Act);
3) Clean Air Act of 1970, as amended;
4) Toxic Substances Control Act (TSCA);
5) Federal Insecticide, Fungicide, Rodenticide Act (FIFRA);
6) Endangered Species Act of 1973, as reauthorized in 1988;
7) Fish and Wildlife Conservation Act of 1980;
8) Marine Protection, Research and Sanctuaries Act of 1972;
9) Coastal Zone Management Act of 1972;
10) Wild and Scenic Rivers Act of 1972;
11) Fish and Wildlife Coordination Act, as amended in 1965;
12) Migratory Bird Treaty Act of 1972; and
13) Marine Mammal Protection Act of 1972.

Compliance with these laws and regulations may require evaluation of a site's ecological effects and the measurements needed to mitigate those effects.

Remedial Investigation and Feasibility Study

Once it has been determined that an ecological assessment is required at a site under CERCLA or other ARARs, the remedial project managers are responsible for all phases of the remedial process, including, but not limited to, the remedial investigation and feasibility study (RI/FS) (USEPA 1988b). An ecological assessment of appropriate detail may be conducted during either the RI or FS following the process described in the Framework for Ecological Risk Assessment (USEPA 1992a, 1998), Risk Assessment Guidance for Superfund, Volume II, Environmental Evaluation Manuals (USEPA 1989), *Eco Updates* (USEPA 1991, 1992d) and Ecological Assessment of Hazardous Waste Sites: A Field and Laboratory Reference (Warren-Hicks et al. 1989).

The baseline risk assessment component of the RI is intended to "provide an evaluation of the potential threat to human health and the environment in the absence of any remedial action." This process involves the identification and characterization of levels of contamination in relevant media, including biota, and potential human and environmental receptors. The effects characterization considers the types of adverse health and environmental effects associated with single and multiple chemical exposures. The risk characterization phase evaluates the potential exposures to surrounding ecological receptors and potential effects associated with such exposures. Assessment endpoints to consider include adverse effects to populations of plants and animals and the extent of perturbations to ecological communities from direct and indirect effects.

The FS involves reviewing remediation alternatives for effectiveness, including potential impacts to the environment during the construction and implementation phase. Alternatives should be evaluated to ensure protection to the environment from potential exposure pathways of concern.

Natural Resource Damage Assessments

CERCLA, and its amendments under SARA, goes beyond the cleanup of hazardous waste sites. Section 107(f)(1) of the act contains provisions for the payment for damages to natural resources caused by the release of hazardous substances, known as the Natural Resource Damage Assessment (NRDA) process. However, this requirement is restricted to the residual damages that exist after an USEPA-approved remedial action. These damages are defined as injury to, destruction of, or loss of a natural resource, but these terms (i.e., injury, destruction, and loss) are not defined in CERCLA. Subsequent case law has provided extremely broad definitions of the terms, such that physical alteration or chemical contamination of a habitat may be considered to cause damage if a biological community can no longer exist in a pre-release condition. Also, natural resources requiring restoration under CERCLA are not restricted to those at the site under consideration. The damage caused to off-site resources, by transport in air, surface or ground water, or soil, must also be restored. Under CERCLA, natural resources are defined as land, fish and wildlife, biota, air, surface and ground water, drinking water supplies, and other resources belonging to, managed by, held in trust by, appertaining to, or otherwise controlled by the government.

Case study example

Four co-located Superfund sites near Tampa, FL are surrounded by 3 freshwater wetlands, designated North, Central, and South Wetlands. The Bay Drums, Peak Oil, and Reeves Southeastern area-wide wetland impact study (AWIS) was initiated in 1988 and later rewritten as an ecological risk assessment (Stober and Auwarter 1993). The purpose was to assess the cumulative impact of the 4 Superfund sites on the viability of the wetland habitats. In particular, assessment endpoints included quantity and quality of surfacewater; contribution to groundwater recharge; and habitat for birds, fish, macroinvertebrates, and several species of endangered plants and animals. Wetland attributes were further analyzed with the Wetland Evaluation Technique (WET) (Adamus et al. 1987) and ranked as high, moderate, or low. Overall, the wetlands rated as moderate to high in ecological values and functions.

Stressors included multiple contaminants and physical alterations. Contaminants consisted of an array of volatile organic compounds, semivolatile organic compounds, organochlorine pesticides, polychlorinated biphenyls, and metals (Fe and Zn). Alteration of wetland habitat resulted from drum storage and recycling processes, deposition of 53,200 cubic meters of shingles, and construction of drainage control berms and wastewater holding ponds, as well as backfilling of wetland areas.

Because this study was initiated as an impact assessment, not as a risk assessment, the problem formulation phase was incomplete. No conceptual model was developed to describe potential exposure pathways from the sources of contamination to the wetlands and their biological receptors. Hypotheses regarding cause-and-effect relationships between contaminants or physical alterations and wetland integrity were poorly developed. Finally, the possible synergism of the various receptors was not addressed.

The exposure analysis phase included a characterization of the transport of chemicals into and through the wetlands and a hydrological assessment. Because the bottom elevations of the wetlands were at approximately the same level as the groundwater table, the potential for interaction of shallow ground and surface waters was pronounced. There was no significant confining layer to reduce vertical migration of the site contaminants; therefore, the wetlands represented a direct pathway to groundwater. A ditch from 2 of the Superfund sites connected directly to the North Wetland. The other 2 sites had surface runoff into an unnamed creek, which also drained the North Wetland. The South Wetland received runoff from a spray irrigation site at a central sewage treatment facility. Two nearby wetlands served as reference sites.

Surfacewater and sediment samples were collected from all the wetlands and from the unnamed creek. Spatial distributions of the metals and organics were characterized in a general manner (e.g., the surface water from the South Wetland and unnamed creek were the most contaminated with metals, but no spatial isopleths or geographic information systems (GIS) mapping was done to characterize the distribution within each wetland). Whole-body contaminant levels in aquatic organisms were also measured to provide an indication of exposure and to develop site-specific bioaccumulation factors. Mosquitofish (*Gambusia affinis*) were collected by seine or dip net and crayfish were collected from all sampling stations. Most of the tissue residue measurements were not above reference levels, except for high concentrations of Fe and Zn found in fish and crayfish from the unnamed creek. Al, Ba, Cu, Fe, Mn, Ti, and Zn were slightly elevated above reference. None of the organics were found in tissue samples.

Biological effects studies were based on toxicity bioassays. More than 400 samples of surface water, sediment, soil, and ground water were taken from the industrial sites and wetlands for chemical analyses. Of these, 100 samples were split for toxicity testing, with the exception that no groundwater samples were tested. Water samples were tested with the Microtox bacterial assay (*Photobacterium* nr. *phosphoreum*), a freshwater alga (*Selenastrum capricornutum*), a freshwater cladoceran (*Ceriodaphnia dubia*), a freshwater fish (*Pimephales promelas*), and a terrestrial plant (lettuce, *Lactuca sativa*). Soils and sediments were eluted, and the eluates were tested with the same suite of organisms.

The toxicity test results demonstrated toxic media at all 4 of the Superfund sites. At the Bay Drum site, water was highly toxic to daphnids but not to the other species. Sediments were also toxic to daphnids as well as to algae and lettuce seed germination. At the Peak Oil site, water, soil, and sediments were toxic to all species tested. Pond water and sediments at the Reeves sites were highly toxic, except for the inactive ponds at the southeastern galvanizing portion. Soils from the extreme eastern edge of the site were nontoxic, while the remaining areas were toxic to all organisms tested. *Daphnia* were the most sensitive of all the species tested at any of the sites.

The major weakness in the analysis phase of this risk assessment was the lack of study of ecological effects. While toxicological effects to laboratory indicator species were evident, uncertainty associated with laboratory-to-field extrapolations and interspecific toxicity differences weakened the conclusions that could be drawn. Furthermore, the 2 reference wetlands were not well chosen, as they apparently received runoff from the land application of treated domestic wastewater. The sediment of one of the reference ponds had extremely low DO and was found to be highly toxic to the test organisms. Furthermore, extrapolation from effects in laboratory bioassays to the chemical residues in tissues from wild-caught organisms was not possible because tissue residues from the laboratory organisms were not measured. No attention was given to measurement of any wetland functions. Finally, no attempt was made to look for impacts on higher-trophic-level organisms (e.g., waterfowl) that may have been using the marsh.

The risk characterization phase of the assessment simply compared the concentrations of chemicals of concern in the various media to available criteria or toxicity threshold concentrations. Water samples were compared to USEPA freshwater ambient water quality criteria. Sediment and soil concentrations were compared with biologically effective sediment concentrations derived from a National Oceanic and Atmospheric Administration technical memo (Long and Morgan 1990). Effects range-low criteria for sediments were used as the soil criteria. The risk quotients derived from dividing the environmental concentration at each sampling site by the various benchmark values were examined to find areas with the highest ratio. This was used as an estimate of the spatial distribution of risk. The highest ratio (194) was found for chlordane in the North Wetland area. Most risk quotients were less than 100, and many were less than 10.

Field observations of the number of benthic macroinvertebrate taxa at each sampling site provided a weight-of-evidence for ecological effects. A total of 53 taxa were collected from the 5 wetlands, with similar species richness at all wetland sites, except for 1 sampling station in the South Wetland and in the unnamed creek.

This was an extremely limited Risk Characterization. It would be adequate for an initial screening study, but more in-depth descriptions of the ecological effects of the contamination were missing. Furthermore, better spatial characterization of the contaminant distributions relative to areas where toxicity and/or ecological responses were seen is needed to identify where cleanup decisions should be made. Finally, the benchmark reference values used for the Risk Quotients, particularly for soils, have a large amount of uncertainty associated with them, and a quantitative analysis of uncertainty, such as a probabilistic statement of risk, was not performed.

Clean Water Act Section 404 Program

Legislative basis

Section 404 of the CWA establishes a permit program to regulate the discharge of dredged or fill material into waters of the United States, including wetlands. Activities in wetlands that are typically regulated under this program include fills for development, water resource projects (such as dams and levees), infrastructure development (such as highways and airports), dredging activities, and the conversion of wetlands for agriculture and forestry. The basic premise of the program is that no discharge of dredged or fill material can be permitted if a practicable alternative exists that is less damaging to the environment or if the project would significantly degrade the nation's aquatic ecosystems.

Specifically, project proponents must demonstrate

1) that they have avoided wetland impacts to the extent practicable (i.e., through the analysis of project alternatives);
2) that impacts are minimized to the extent appropriate and practicable, e.g., by downsizing the project or avoiding highly valuable wetlands; and
3) that remaining unavoidable impacts are offset through the provision of compensatory mitigation (e.g., through the restoration or creation of similar wetlands). Finally, no permit can be issued if the project would otherwise violate other applicable environmental laws or regulations, including the Endangered Species Act and state water quality and toxic effluent standards.

The Section 404 program provides an important regulatory framework for protecting the ecological integrity of the nation's wetlands and other aquatic resources. In ensuring compliance with requirements established under USEPA's Section 404(b)(1) guidelines, the USACOE routinely considers the relative ecological risk of necessary development activities in wetlands. For the majority of activities that would only cause minimal adverse effect, either individually or cumulatively, and therefore pose little or no ecological risk, authorization may occur under a "general" permit. General permits may be issued on a nationwide, regional, or state basis and may be conditioned, as appropriate (e.g., by requiring mitigation), to ensure that activities are only minimal in effect. For activities that pose more significant ecological risk, an "individual" permit is typically required. The level of review for individual permits is commensurate with the relative severity of the proposed impact (i.e., its ecological risk).

It can be concluded from the program requirements discussed above that the Section 404 regulatory program, in fact, operates in a manner consistent with USEPA's risk assessment framework. Based on a more explicit use or consideration of the framework, however, there is an opportunity for program decision-makers to ensure that the intent of the Section 404 of the CWA and its implementing regulations are met with respect to minimizing the ecological risk of proposed discharges.

Moreover, use of the framework may be particularly important when one is considering the direct or indirect effect of chemical stressors associated with proposed discharges. Such impacts do not typically receive the attention they merit, in part because the focus of the Section 404 program historically has been on the physical loss of habitat (i.e., acreage) and not necessarily on the chemical degradation of the aquatic system posed by discharge activities. There are several ways USEPA's risk assessment framework may be utilized to improve decision-making within the Section 404 program with respect to the maintenance and potentially the restoration of the chemical integrity of wetlands and other aquatic resources. First, a detailed risk assessment, consistent with the process identified in USEPA's Framework for Ecological Risk Assessment (1992a), may be used to evaluate the potential impact of an individual project that has the potential to contaminate wetlands or to evaluate the cumulative effect of multiple authorizations. The risk assessment framework also lays out a sound decision-making process, which can be used in the review of routine permit applications to ensure that adequate consideration is given to the potential adverse effects of all chemical and nonchemical stressors associated with proposed discharges. Finally, this approach may be adapted to address the ecological risk of particular policy decisions.

Application of risk assessment framework in review of individual permits

Certain activities regulated under Section 404 have the potential to adversely affect the chemical integrity of the nation's wetlands and other aquatic resources and thereby pose a significant ecological risk. Examples of such projects include dredging projects involving contaminated sediment or soil; the proposed location of a potential contaminant source in or adjacent to wetlands (e.g., municipal landfill, oil or gas pipeline installation); projects that would significantly alter wetland hydrology, thereby altering the chemical equilibrium and leading to, e.g., saltwater intrusion; and coastal development projects with the potential to contribute disproportionate quantities of impaired runoff into receiving wetlands or other waterbodies.

These are examples of the types of projects that typically involve a thorough review of project alternatives and actions to minimize and mitigate proposed impacts as part of the individual permit review process. However, as indicated above, the focus of the analysis is typically on the physical loss of habitat. It is not clear, in such cases, whether the potential chemical effects are adequately and objectively considered.

Given the potential for significant direct or indirect adverse effects in such cases, it may be appropriate that a detailed ecological risk assessment be conducted using the procedures established within the USEPA framework document to ensure that permit decisions are based upon a sound scientific assessment of all ecological risks. An ecological risk assessment can assist permit reviewers in identifying the least damaging project alternative, in identifying possible steps to minimize potential adverse effects, and in evaluating the effectiveness of mitigation options. Moreover, such an analysis can provide a scientific basis for deciding whether a proposed activity would cause or contribute to the significant degradation of the aquatic ecosystem. It is important to note that this level of analysis is consistent with the intent of the regulations (i.e., Section 404(b)(1) guidelines) and agency guidance, which clarifies that the level of analysis should be commensurate with the severity of the proposed impact.

Adaptation of decision-making process for routine permit actions

For minor discharges or those activities that may be authorized under a general permit, the evaluation steps and protocol of the assessment framework provide a logical decision-making process to ensure that all appropriate and practical steps have been taken to reduce the ecological risk associated with a proposed activity. A thorough identification of all stressors, and subsequent analysis, is critical for conducting an accurate assessment of the ecological risk of a proposed activity. The framework can be interpreted or adapted accordingly.

Problem formulation

1) Stressors: Identify chemical, physical, and biological stressors associated with the proposed activity (e.g., partial fill, draining, dredging, impoundment, storm water, nature of fill material).
2) Ecosystems at risk: Identify the individual wetlands and other aquatic resources that may be directly or indirectly affected. Specifically consider the scope of any landscape effects of the proposed activity.
3) Ecological components: Identify the ecological components at risk (e.g., plant and animal communities, receiving surface and ground waters, threatened and endangered species).
4) Endpoints: Identify assessment endpoints (i.e., wetland functions and/or values) of concern and the endpoints (e.g., measures of exposure, measures of effects, measures of ecosystem characteristics) that can be used to assess the effect on assessment endpoints.

Exposure and effect assessment

As appropriate, given the severity of the proposed impact, permit reviewers should characterize the exposure (i.e., the magnitude and duration of stressors) and the ecological effects. The latter step can be accomplished through the use of an appropriate functional assessment methodology (e.g., HGM) that incorporates the necessary measurement endpoints to permit a detailed description or quantification of ecological effects on the functions or values of concern (i.e., assessment endpoints).

Risk characterization

Considering the results of the assessment phase, the landscape context of a proposed activity, and alternatives for minimizing and mitigating impacts, permit reviewers should characterize the relative ecological risk of the activity and of potential alternatives.

Risk management

The risk characterization analysis may subsequently guide the permit decision, e.g., less scrutiny for projects that truly pose little ecological risk, appropriate mitigation decisions, permit conditioning or denial, as necessary. Consideration of risk to guide decisions, in addition to other considerations (e.g., practicality of alternatives), is consistent with the program requirements.

The chemical degradation of aquatic systems may often be the result of the cumulative effect of multiple stressors within the particular watershed in question. Many of these activities (e.g., fills for development) may be regulated under Section 404. Conducting a detailed risk assessment on a watershed basis may assist in determining the individual and cumulative contribution of these activities on the chemical integrity of the aquatic system. This analysis may be conducted as part of the assessment phase of a comprehensive wetland or watershed management planning effort.

Case study example

The USEPA's Office of Research and Development applied the ecological risk assessment framework to evaluate the risk to water quality of wetlands and adjacent surface waters based on the frequency, type, and intensity of physical disturbances (deposition of fill, dredging, impoundment, sedimentation, and stormwater or pumped groundwater inputs) (USEPA 1992). Stressor intensities were quantified as to wetland fill area, percentage wetland filled, change in water depth due to dredging or impoundment, changes in the ratio of watershed to wetland area, changes in the ratio of impervious surface area (urban or residential land use) to wetland area, and the ratio of construction area (bare earth) in the watershed to wetland area. Assessment endpoints were potential water quality effects relative to wetland biota (reduced transparency, altered ionic strength, low DO/high ammonia stress, and Pb toxicity) and potential water quality impacts on downstream surface waters (eutrophication, reduced transparency, nitrate/nitrite toxicity, and Pb toxicity). Measurement endpoints were changes between pre- and postdisturbance conditions in temperature, DO, conductivity, turbidity, N, P, organic C, suspended solids, and total extractable Pb. Thirty-three sites were identified and sampled for up to 1 year prior to disturbance, during the peak distribution, and over a 1- to 2-year postdisturbance or recovery period. A multiple regression approach was used to quantify stressor–response relationships.

Risk characterization required integrating cause–effect relationships identified through site-specific investigations with information on regional distributions of stressor type and intensity. A major uncertainty in the study area was in estimating the true incidence or intensity of unregulated or incompletely regulated physical or hydrologic disturbances, especially with respect to small, isolated headwater wetlands. In addition, estimates of ecological risk to aquatic biota in wetlands were difficult to determine because of the uncertainty in extrapolating to wetlands water quality standards that were derived for different classes of surface waters.

Federal Insecticide, Fungicide, and Rodenticide Act

Legislative basis

FIFRA is the basis for regulations governing the use of pesticides in the United States and is managed by the Office of Pesticide Programs (OPP) within the USEPA. Within OPP, the Environmental Fate and Effects Division is responsible for environmental risk assessment, and the Biological Evaluation and Analysis Division conducts agricultural benefits assessments. Risk management divisions include the Registration Division and Special Review and Reregistration Division. Risk assessment tends to be prospective, prior to registration or reregistration of a pesticide. Ecological risk assessment integrates the estimated environmental concentration (EEC) and effects estimates (acute and chronic toxicity of various organisms) into a risk quotient. This output is compared to a level of concern (LOC). Regulatory decisions, and triggering of the next tier to refine the assessment, are based on exceedance of the LOC. Levels of concern differ for acute and chronic effects and for endangered species. Many endangered and threatened species occupy wetland habitat. In the past, where LOCs have been exceeded, biological consultations with the U.S. Fish and Wildlife Service have occurred. Recently, endangered species location information relative to specific crops has been requested in order to determine risk and appropriate mitigation.

The current pesticide risk assessment process is such that wetlands are not normally considered as a separate ecosystem. Management of ecosystems tends to be conducted in programs other than FIFRA. Due to methodological limitations, FIFRA is aimed at protecting individual component resources of an ecosystem, while the overall structural and functional aspects of an ecosystem are intended to be protected by the conservative nature of the ecological risk assessment process.

Recently, an Aquatic Risk Assessment and Mitigation Dialogue Group (ARAMDG) was formed to review pesticide risk assessment and mitigation (risk reduction) for aquatic ecosystems within OPP's integrated risk-assessment paradigm and to offer recommendations for technical implementation and use of risk mitigation measures in regulatory risk assessment scenarios. They recommend a deterministic first tier based on point estimate data. In later tiers, an overlay of probabilistic distributions of exposure and effects data is conducted. Effects are based on laboratory toxicological data, and the approach does not account for secondary, tertiary, indirect, and sublethal effects associated with the structural and functional integrity of ecosystems. Mitigation options for exposure reduction are presented, the outcomes of which are modeled. Field study data are used to validate exposure simulation models.

Lower-tier risk assessments for aquatic and terrestrial organisms represent a conservative screen and are considered protective of organisms occupying wetlands. However, wetlands are considered only in relation to specific types of nontarget organisms. Wetland-specific environmental-exposure estimates are used for semiaquatic, nontarget plants. Exposure estimations are calculated using a channelized runoff scenario, similar to that used for aquatic exposure estimates (i.e., farm pond), except that depth is set at zero and therefore a concentration was not considered. This approach may yield unusually high EECs. The ARAMDG questions the adequacy of surrogate species currently used in toxicity tests; current plant toxicity tests do not incorporate semiaquatic species, and the mallard duck is the only wetland avian species targeted.

Endpoints pertaining to structural and functional aspects of the wetland ecosystem are not considered by ARAMDG. Nonetheless, the approach fits well within USEPA's Risk Assessment Framework and allows flexibility to account for wetland specific characteristics. An example of how the ecological risk assessment framework could be applied to wetlands exposed to pesticides is illustrated in Figure 9-2.

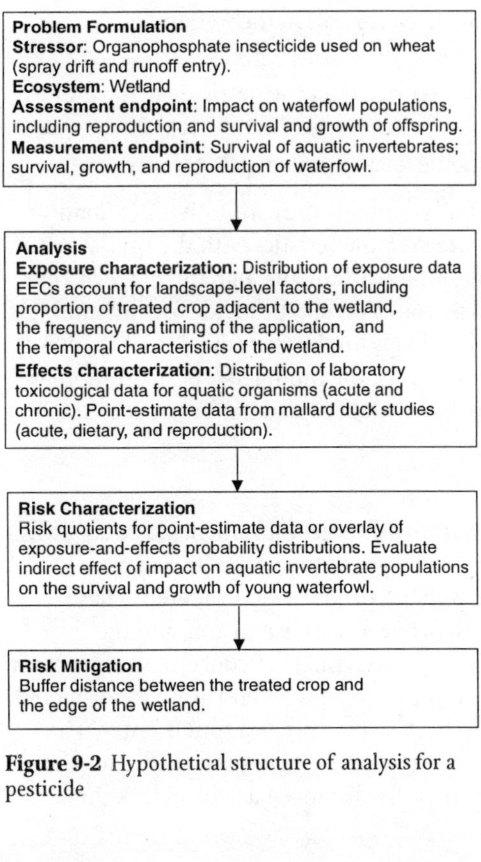

Figure 9-2 Hypothetical structure of analysis for a pesticide

Case study example

Problem formulation

The development of a conceptual model for assessing risks of a pesticide-exposed wetland under FIFRA should consider the following types of information.

1) Geographic aspects include
   - the presence of wetlands in pesticide use area,
   - the types of wetland in the area of concern and its seasonal characteristics, and
   - the compartments of the wetland at potential risk of exposure.
2) Pesticide use pattern includes
   - the specific crop to be treated;
   - the timing and frequency of application in relation to the presence of the potential routes of entry to the wetland (entry will be dependent on the properties of the chemical, type of application, formulation, and how these interact with the soil, water, and vegetation); and
   - the matrix between the treated or contaminated area and the wetland of concern.
3) Other stressors (chemical, physical, or biological) in the wetland of concern require answers to these questions:
   - Do these stressors present a greater risk than the pesticide being evaluated?
   - Do they interact with the pesticide to change its risk?

Geographic information systems are useful for obtaining quantitative information on the scale and the integration of use-pattern characteristics with the spatial factors of the ecosystem of concern. It is possible, after working through this stage of the assessment process, that the ecological risk from a certain pesticide use does not exist. For example, where the concern is for effects on the reproduction of dabbling duck populations that utilize ephemeral wetlands, the timing of a pesticide application (e.g., late in the season) may not coincide with occupied habitat or even the presence of ephemeral wetlands.

Analysis - exposure

Exposure from pesticides typically results from off-target movement via spray drift or runoff (overland, or drainage channels flowing into the wetland). Factors affecting the entry of the pesticide to the wetland need to be considered. These include the distance and nature of the area between the treated area and the wetland. Depending on what component of the wetland is of concern, the characteristics of the margins of the wetlands and the aquatic area should also be considered. Distance and vegetation act as a barrier to both spray drift and runoff entry. The Spray Drift Task Force has recently generated comprehensive spray drift data and models for pesticide exposures. However, they are distance-based and lack the necessary consideration of the mitigative effects of the physical and biological structure of the wetland. For example, emergent vegetation may be important in mitigating the effects of insecticide spray drift on aquatic invertebrates. Another consideration regarding the entry and impact of a pesticide is the specific location or compartment of the wetland that is exposed. An extreme example would be a direct overspray of a wetland; however, more likely, only a portion of the wetland would be affected. Wetland compartmentation is important in characterizing the extent of exposure because uncontaminated areas may act as refuges for organisms from exposed areas and also provide a source of inoculum to allow impacted areas to eventually recover.

Models to characterize exposure in wetlands are poorly developed (Dixon and Florian 1993). This represents a major gap in our ability to adequately conduct refined risk assessments for pesticide-contaminated wetlands. Existing models, e.g., the PRZM2/EXAMS model used for aquatic (farm pond) risk assessment, could be modified to better represent the conditions in a wetland (e.g., increased organic material, surface area, etc.) (Burns 1997). In many respects, because of the rapid adsorptive capacity of newer pesticide chemistries, the organic-rich nature of wetlands represents a high potential for decreased bioavailability in comparison to a standard aquatic scenario (such as a pond or stream) and should be considered in the exposure analysis.

Analysis - effects

Limitations in testing parameters (e.g., the selection of toxicity thresholds and the use of surrogate species) can present limitations to nontarget plant testing for pesticide exposures. Further data acquisition to refine the effects estimate should be generated from laboratory studies with more realistic exposure, as recommended by ARAMDG (Baker et al. 1994), or should be based on in situ bioassays or micro/mesocosm field studies carefully designed to provide data on primary, secondary, and tertiary effects and on recovery. An understanding of trophic-level effects and indirect effects of pesticides will require an understanding of the interface between ecosystem compartments, including the integration of effects estimates from one compartment with that of others. For example, a pesticide may impact aquatic invertebrates that are an essential component of the diet of waterfowl young occupying the wetland.

Risk management

Risk management and mitigation is used to reduce unacceptable risk and, in the case of pesticide applications, requires the careful consideration of use-pattern information pertaining to the pesticide of concern. Mitigation can be defined as the actions necessary to reduce or eliminate concentrations of pesticides or byproducts that may affect wetland habitats and their components. Several methods for mitigating pesticide runoff and drift have been suggested by ARAMDG (Baker et al. 1994). These include elimination of aerial application, lower use rates, soil incorporation, and buffers such as vegetative buffer strips. Implementation of risk mitigation for pesticides is by product label instructions. The ARAMDG (Baker et al. 1994) recommends a 3-phase process to quantify effects of pesticide risk mitigation:

1) simulation modeling,
2) field or laboratory study data to validate model estimates, and
3) field investigations of the actual performance of mitigation in reducing exposure and effects.

Other wetland-specific mitigation options for pesticide applications would include the use of a constructed wetland to "treat" the pesticide. This approach can be useful for managing and mitigating pesticide residues in a channel draining into a wetland. Other practices important in pesticide exposure mitigation are integrated pest management, best management practices, and the construction of retention ponds. Where retention ponds and/or constructed wetlands are utilized, it is important that the exposure analysis phase be based on the outflow to receiving wetlands from these systems. As a final consideration, FIFRA legislation mandates that management decisions be based on a risk-benefit analysis, and agricultural benefits are to be considered in any risk-related decisions.

Water quality standards

The protection of water quality is one of the more established cases in which ecological risk assessment can be applied to wetlands. The primary components of water quality standards include

1) assigning designated uses or use classes to waters,
2) establishing the criteria to protect the designated uses, and
3) applying the nondegradation policy.

Wetlands, which are considered "waters of the U.S." (40 CFR S. 232.2(q)), should be considered when establishing water quality standards.

Water quality standards are established to protect waters according to use classes. An understanding of the use classes for wetlands is critical to applying the principles of risk assessment. For example, wetlands such as fens and bogs can be designated by the CWA as Outstanding National Resource Waters and therefore receive the highest level of protection under water quality standards. Other wetlands may be placed within the designated use of "aquatic life and recreation." Under this designation, water quality is to be maintained to permit the propagation and maintenance of a healthy community of aquatic and terrestrial species indigenous to the wetland. The waters shall be suitable for boating and other forms of aquatic recreation for which the wetland is usable.

To meet the water quality standards, USEPA is required under the CWA of 1977 (Section 304[a][1]) to review and publish national water quality criteria to protect public water supplies. The criteria should also be protective of the plant and animal species that occupy various trophic levels in the aquatic community.

Water quality standards have been proposed for wetlands (USEPA 1990). Through legislation and regulation, USEPA has asked the states to improve their water quality standards, including those for wetlands. Because national criteria may be either underprotective or overprotective, states may adapt national water quality criteria to local conditions. Although no states are yet using biological criteria specific to wetlands, some states such as Ohio apply existing water quality standards to wetlands.

The process of ecological risk assessment could be used to benefit the development and use of water quality standards for wetlands. National water quality standards serve as benchmarks with general applicability, and risk assessment could be used to make them more site-specific (Spehar and Carlson 1993). Quality standards based on criteria for water should be considered in conjunction with criteria for sediment and biota. Substantial modification, however, may be necessary to develop standards that are appropriate for wetlands. Ecological risk assessment could be used to identify key parameters that are "sensitive indicators," and critical to the wetlands of interest, and therefore highly appropriate factors for full consideration in the development of quality standards. The standards must also be appropriate for the specific wetland type and associated ecological function, in addition to the socioeconomic value of the wetland.

Ecological risk assessment could be used to quantify the detrimental effect of not maintaining established quality standards and to identify the limiting factors in achieving the required standards. For example, where wetlands could potentially be exposed, standards for National Pollution Discharge Elimination Systems that are supported by ecological risk assessment could provide improved risk management decisions that afford greater protection of wetlands.

Finally, where wetlands have already been degraded, a retrospective risk assessment could prevent further degradation. Further, standards may be used as a goal for restoration of quality. In this situation, risk assessment could be the underlying basis for risk management that is necessary to meet these goals.

Gaps in Information, Methodologies, and Tools for Utilizing the Risk Assessment Framework

In order to conduct a wetlands ecological risk assessment, it is necessary to characterize hydrological, biogeochemical, and biological functions. This is critical to both the exposure and effects assessments. A review of the literature suggests that our understanding of how these functions affect contaminant bioavailability is inadequate, and the effects of stressors on many wetland organisms are not known. Moreover, how one stressed species impacts the rest of the wetland ecosystem has not been addressed. Research is needed in this area in order to effectively address ecological risk assessment in wetlands.

Facilitating exposure assessment in wetland ecosystems could be improved by better understanding of contaminant fate in these organic-rich, alternatingly aerobic and anaerobic systems. Knowing the impact of these biologically rich ecosystems on chemical assimilation is also critical. These processes may ultimately dictate a very different exposure scenario than would be expected in other aquatic systems. Effort is also indicated to develop new contaminant transport and fate models that accurately predict movement within a wetland. These models should be able to accept water and chemical input from upstream watersheds as hydrographs and chemographs. This would facilitate both spatial and temporal characterization of contaminant exposure.

Effects assessment in wetland ecosystems requires more definitive toxicity information dealing with trophic levels not typically studied in aquatic ecosystems but integral to wetland function (e.g., mosses and fungi). The extrapolation of the results of these laboratory bioassays to field situations is a major research need. Integrative biochemical endpoints, biomarkers, are also needed to better understand the influence of stressors on wetland functions, not just on an individual or species. The water:land interface that is peculiar to wetlands has not been well studied to characterize either its response to contaminants or its role in wetland functions. Evaluation of biotic indices and community profiles and their relationship to wetland function is also needed. While the development of these indices is straightforward, the significance of the index in terms of ecosystem fitness has not been clearly defined.

The entire issue of reference sites for wetland ecological risk assessment must be investigated. Is it realistic to think that one wetland should behave like another? Can we find adequate reference sites? Do we produce a range of function values that encompass the variability inherent in each wetland type?

Finally, there is a need for specific research involving the sociological aspects of ecological risk assessments in wetlands. Stakeholder dynamics, hidden or redefined agendas, and "turf battles" all enter into the problem formulation phase. If not solved, problems in this phase ultimately lead to a poor or incomplete characterization of risk.

Summary of Regulatory Issues and Risk Assessment Workgroup Discussions

The discussions in this workgroup started with an identification and brief explanation of U.S. regulations pertaining to wetlands. The Framework for Ecological Risk Assessment developed by the USEPA Ecological Risk Assessment Forum was then reviewed in relation to the unique aspects of conducting a wetland assessment. Assessment and measurement endpoints as well as the development of conceptual models for conducting ecological risk assessment were discussed. Issues surrounding exposure and effects characterization, including spatial and temporal relationships, frequency and duration of contact, direct and indirect effects, and modeling of systems, were covered. The ecological significance of the data and their interpretation were also talked about. The importance of nontoxicant stressors to wetlands and the difficulty of separating them from chemical stressors were recognized. Finally, the workgroup finished with a review of 4 regulatory programs and how the ecological risk assessment thought process can and is being used to assist in management decisions.

It was concluded that the ecological risk assessment approach is data-driven and that the proper assessment depends on our ability to characterize wetland specific hydrological, biogeochemical, and biological functions as they relate to the exposure and effects of toxicants. Our limited understanding of how wetlands function and the effects of stressors on many wetland organisms make it necessary to improve and refine existing ecological risk assessment methods for use in these unique environments. Various recommendations were developed to identify and fill technical data gaps and to develop methods and models to process the data at various spatial and temporal scales.

References

Adams SM, Crumby WD, Greeley MS, Ryon MG, Schilling EM. 1992. Relationships between physiological and fish population responses in a contaminated stream. *Environ Toxicol Chem* 11:1549–1557.

Adamus PR, Clairain Jr EJ, Smith RD, Young RE. 1987. Wetland evaluations technique (WET). Volume II, Methodology. Vicksburg MS: U.S. Army Corps of Engineers Waterways Experiment Station. Operational Draft Technical Report Y-87-10.

Adamus P, Brandt K. 1990. Impacts on quality of inland wetlands of the United States: a survey of indicators, techniques, and applications of community-level biomonitoring data. Washington DC: U.S. Environmental Protection Agency. EPA/600/3-90/073.

Baker JL, Barefoot AC, Beasley LE, Burns LA, Caulkins PP, Clarke JE, Feulner RL, Giesy JP, Graney RL, Griggs RH, Jacoby HM, Laskowski DA, Maciorowski AF, Mihaich EM, Nelson Jr HP, Parrish PR, Siefert RE, Solomon KR, van der Schalie WH. 1994. Aquatic dialogue group: pesticide risk assessment and mitigation. Pensacola FL: SETAC. 227 p.

Barber MC, Suarez LA, Lassiter RR. 1988. Modeling bioconcentration of nonpolar organic pollutants by fish. *Environ Toxicol Chem* 7:545–558.

Barber MC, Suarez LA, Lassiter RR. 1991. Modeling bioaccumulation of organic pollutants in fish with an application to PCBs in Great Lakes salmonids. *Can J Fish Aquat Sci* 48:318–337.

Bartell SM, Gardner RH, O'Neill RV. 1992. Ecological risk estimation. Chelsea MI: Lewis. 252 p.

Barnthouse LW, Suter GW, Rosen AE. 1989. Inferring population-level significance from individual-level effects: an extrapolation from fisheries science to ecotoxicology. In: Suter GW, Lewis MA, editors. Aquatic toxicology and environmental fate. 11th volume. Philadelphia PA: American Society for Testing and Materials. ASTM STP 1007.

Birge WJ, Keogh DP, Price DJ, Gray BR. 1992. Integrating community ecology and aquatic toxicology in assessing effects of chemical stresses on freshwater biota. Proceedings, 13th Annual Meeting, Society of Environmental Toxicology and Chemistry, Cincinnati OH, 14–18 Nov 1992. 37 p.

Brinson MM. 1993. A hydrogeomorphic classification for wetlands. Vicksburg MS: U.S. Army Corps of Engineers Waterways Experiment Station. Technical Report WRP-DE-4.

Brooks R, Moore JN. 1989. Sediment-water interactions in the metal-contaminated floodplain of the Clark Fork River, Montana, USA. *Geo Journal* 19.1:27–36.

Burns LA. 1997. Exposure analysis modeling system (EXAMS): users guide for version 2.97.5. Athens GA: USEPA. EPA-600/R-97/047.

Clark KE, Gobas FAPC, Mackay D. 1990. Model of organic chemical uptake and clearance by fish from food and water. *Environ Sci Technol* 24:1203–1213.

Dickson KL, Waller WT, Kennedy JH, Ammann LP. 1992. Assessing the relationship between ambient toxicity and instream biological response. *Environ Toxicol Chem* 11:1307–1322.

Dixon KR. 1975. Thermal plumes and mercury dynamics in zooplankton. Proceedings, International Conference on Heavy Metals in the Environment. Toronto, Ontario, 27–31 Oct 1975. p 875–886.

Dixon KR, Florian Jr JD. 1993. Modeling mobility and effects of contaminants in wetlands. *Environ Toxicol Chem* 12:2281–2292.

Donigian Jr AS, Imhoff JC, Bichnell BR. 1983. Predicting water quality resulting from agricultural nonpoint source pollution via simulation—HSPF. In: Schaller FW, Bailey GW, editors. Agricultural Management and Water Quality. Ames IA: Iowa State Univ Pr. p 200–249.

Duinker PN, Beanlands GE. 1986. The significance of environmental impacts: an exploration of the concept. *Environ Manage* 10:1–10.

Hauck LM, Ward GH. 1980. Hydro-dynamic model of deltaic systems. In: Hamilton P, Macdonald KB, editors. Estuarine and wetland processes with emphasis on modeling. New York: Plenum. p 247–268.

Krantzberg G, Boyd D. 1992. The biological significance of contaminants in sediment from Hamilton Harbour, Lake Ontario. *Environ Toxicol Chem* 11:1527–1540.

Kreis RG. 1998. Integrated study of exposure and biological effects of in-place sediment pollutants in the Detroit River, Michigan: an upper Great Lakes connecting channel. Final Report. Duluth MN and Grosse Isle MI: Office of Research and Development, U.S. Environmental Protection Agency.

Leonard RA, Knisel EG, Still DA. 1987. GLEAMS: groundwater loading effects of agricultural management systems. *Trans ASAE* 30:1403–1418.

Long ER, Morgan LG. 1990. The potential for biological effects of sediment-sorbed contaminants tested in the National Status and Trends Program. National Oceanic and Atmospheric Administration (NOAA) Technical Memorandum NOS OMA 52. Office of Oceanography and Marine Assessment. Seattle WA: NOAA.

[NRC] National Research Council. 1983. Risk assessment in the federal government: managing the process. National Research Council, National Academy of Sciences. Washington DC: National Academy Pr.

Pascoe GA. 1993. Wetland risk assessment. *Environ Toxicol Chem* 12:2293–2307.

Pascoe GA. 1994. Human health and ecological risk assessment of sediment releases (continued releases). Milltown Reservoir operable unit, Milltown Reservoir Sediments Site. Prepared for U.S. Environmental Protection Agency Region 8, Helena, MT.

Philips JD. 1985. Stability of artificially drained lowlands: a theoretical treatment. *Ecol Model* 27:69–79.

[PSWQA] Puget Sound Water Quality Authorities. 1994. Fifth annual report of the Puget Sound ambient monitoring program. Olympia WA: Puget Sound Water Quality Authorities, Washington Department of Ecology.

Richardson CJ. 1994. Ecological functions and human values in wetlands: A framework for assessing impacts. *Wetlands* 14:1–9.

Scala RA. 1991. Risk assessment. In: Amdur MO, Doull J, Klaassen CD, editors. Casarett and Doull's toxicology: the basic science of poisons. 4th ed. New York: Pergamon Pr. p 985–996.

Seip KL. 1979. A mathematical model for the uptake of heavy metals in benthic algae. *Ecol Model* 6:183–197.

Sheng YP. 1980. Modeling sediment transport in a shallow lake. In: Hamilton P, Macdonald KB, editors. Estuarine and wetland processes with emphasis on modeling. New York: Plenum. p 299–337.

Smith RD. 1993. A conceptual framework for assessing the functions of wetlands. Vicksburg MS: U.S. Army Corps of Engineers, Waterways Experiment Station. Technical Report WRP-DE-3.

Solomon KR, Baker DB, Richards RP, Dixon KR, Klaine SJ, La Point TW, Kendall RJ, Weisskopf CP, Giddings JM, Giesy JP, Hall Jr LW, Williams WM. 1996. Ecological risk assessment of atrazine in North American surface waters. *Environ Toxicol Chem* 15:31–76.

Spehar RL, Carlson AR. 1993. Ecological risk assessment case study. Toxic discharges to surface waters: assessing the risk to aquatic life using national and site-specific water quality criteria. In: A review of ecological assessment case studies from a risk assessment perspective. Washington DC: U.S. Environmental Protection Agency. EPA/630/R-92/005.

Stober QJ, Auwarter AG. 1993. Ecological risk assessment case study: the Bay Drums, Peak Oil, and Reeves Southeastern area wide wetland impact study. In: A review of ecological assessment case studies from a risk assessment perspective. Washington DC: U.S. Environmental Protection Agency. EPA/630/R-92/005.

Suter II GW. 1993. Ecological risk assessment. Chelsea MI: Lewis. 538 p.

Suter II GW, Cornaby BW, Haddeng CT, Hull RN, Stack M, Zafran FA. 1995. An approach for balancing health and ecological risk at hazardous waste sites. *J Risk Anal* 15:221–231.

Suter II GW, Gillett JW, Norton S. 1994. Issue paper on characterization of exposure. Ecological risk assessment issue papers. Washington DC: U.S. Environmental Protection Agency, Office of Research and Development. EPA/630/R-94/009.

Thomann RV. 1981. Equilibrium model of fate of microcontaminants in diverse aquatic food chains. *Can J Fish Aquat Sci* 38:280–296.

[USACOE] U.S. Army Corps of Engineers. 1991. Environmental effects of dredging, technical notes. U.S. Army Corps of Engineers Technical Note EEDP-06-15. Vicksburg MS: Waterways Experiment Station.

[USEPA] U.S. Environmental Protection Agency. 1988a. CERCLA compliance with other laws manual: interim final. Washington DC: USEPA. EPA/540/G-89/006.

[USEPA] U.S. Environmental Protection Agency. 1988b. Guidance for conducting remedial investigations and feasibility studies under CERCLA. Washington DC: USEPA. EPA/540/G-89/004.

[USEPA] U.S. Environmental Protection Agency. 1989. Risk assessment guidance for Superfund. Volume 2, Environmental evaluation manual. Interim final report. Washington DC: Office of Emergency and Remedial Response, U.S. Environmental Protection Agency. EPA/540/1-89-001.

[USEPA] U.S. Environmental Protection Agency. 1990. Water quality standards for wetlands. Washington DC: Office of Water. EPA/440/5-90/011.

[USEPA] U.S. Environmental Protection Agency. 1991. Ecological assessment of Superfund sites: an overview. In: Eco update, Volume 1, Number 2. Washington DC: Office of Solid Waste and Emergency Response. Publication 9345.0-05I.

[USEPA] U.S. Environmental Protection Agency. 1992a. Framework for ecological risk assessment. Washington DC: Risk Assessment Forum, USEPA. EPA/630/R-92/001.

[USEPA] U.S. Environmental Protection Agency. 1992b. Report on the ecological risk assessment guidelines strategic planning workshop. Washington DC: Risk Assessment Forum, USEPA. EPA/630/R-92/002.

[USEPA] U.S. Environmental Protection Agency. 1992c. Peer review workshop report on a framework for ecological risk assessment. Washington DC: Risk Assessment Forum, USEPA. EPA/625/3-91/022.

[USEPA] U.S. Environmental Protection Agency. 1992d. Developing a work scope for ecological assessments. In: Eco update, Volume 1, Number 4. Washington DC: Office of Solid Waste and Emergency Response, USEPA. Publication 9345.0-05I.

[USEPA] U.S. Environmental Protection Agency. 1992e. BTAG forum, Volume 2, Number 2. Washington DC: Office of Solid Waste and Emergency Response, USEPA. Publication 9200.5-325I.

[USEPA] U.S. Environmental Protection Agency. 1994. Considering wetlands at CERCLA sites. Washington DC: Office of Emergency and Remedial Response. EPA/540/R-94/019.

[USEPA] U.S. Environmental Protection Agency. 1997. Ecological risk assessment guidance for Superfund: process for designing and conducting ecological risk assessments. Washington DC: Office of Solid Waste and Emergency Response. EPA/540/R-97/006.

[USEPA] U.S. Environmental Protection Agency. 1998. Guidelines for ecological risk assessment. Washington DC: Risk Assessment Forum. EPA/630/R-95/002F.

Ward Jr GH. 1980. Hydrography and circulation processes of Gulf estuaries. In: Hamilton P, Macdonald KB, editors. Estuarine and wetland processes with emphasis on modeling. New York: Plenum. p 183–215.

Warren-Hicks W, Parkhurst BR, Baker SS. 1989. Ecological assessment of hazardous waste sites: a field and laboratory reference. Corvallis OR: U.S. Environmental Protection Agency, Environmental Research Laboratory. EPA/600-3-89-013.

Chapter 10

Workgroup V Synopsis: Constructed Wetlands as a Risk Mitigation Alternative

John H. Rodgers, Jr., chair
Gary W. Dickson, Tom Dillon, Philip B. Dorn, Janis E. Farmer, Robert A. Gearheart, Jerry F. Hall, Beverly McFarland, Marcia K. Nelson, Peter Nix, Curtis J. Richardson, Dennis P. Tierney

Constructed and natural wetlands have been used to treat a variety of point and nonpoint sources (Table 10-1) (Bastian et al. 1989; Baker 1992). Wetlands have the ability to transform, sequester, and transfer materials in wastewater streams. For that reason, the resulting aqueous discharge from a wetland decreases the impact of physical and chemical stressors on receiving waters. Constructed wetlands can improve the quality of point and nonpoint source (NPS) discharges, and they can also be used to mitigate damaged wetland areas. This chapter results from the Constructed Wetlands Workgroup's discussion on the use of constructed wetlands for treatment of point and nonpoint sources, which is the focus of this chapter.

Chapter Preview

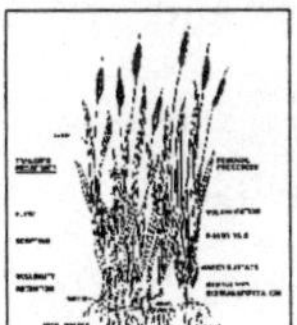

 ISBN 1-880611-16-3

Table 10-1 Applicability of constructed wetlands for treatment of point and nonpoint source materials

Materials	Parameters
Point source	
Domestic effluent, 2% treated	Biochemical oxygen demand (BOD), suspended solids (SS)
Domestic effluent	N, P
Domestic effluent	Trace elements (e.g., Cu, Zn)
Industrial effluent	Organics
Industrial effluent	Inorganics
Industrial effluent	BOD, etc.
Nonpoint source	
Agriculture/Forestry	Sediments
Agriculture/Forestry	Pesticides
Agriculture/Forestry	Animal waste
Urban runoff	Organics, metals
Acid mine drainage	Metals

Chapter Objectives

The 3 principal areas discussed in this chapter are

1) the application of constructed wetlands for point and NPS treatment,
2) a decision-support system as the basis for the design and implementation of constructed wetlands and for dealing with risk management issues, and
3) some guidance regarding research and development needs.

The application of constructed wetlands for rehabilitation and restoration is valuable but beyond the scope of this workgroup.

Background

Some history is needed regarding the use of wetlands for wastewater treatment: why have we moved from using natural to constructed wetlands? Where did the often-accepted ecological concept that wetlands function as efficient nutrient sinks (e.g., nutrient retention areas) come from? We know that wetlands can function as both nutrient sources or sinks, depending on the nutrient in question or the season of the year, but often we do not realize that the most important role for wetlands in the landscape may be as nutrient or material transformers (Richardson 1989). Is the sink concept for nutrients, xenobiotics, or trace metal retention flawed by being based simply on empirical input/output studies for systems that have not yet reached saturation? Do we understand the mechanisms controlling retention capacity in both natural and constructed wetlands to the degree that we can predict recycling rates and storage capacity for materials once we know loading rates? Can we use process information from natural wetlands to design constructed wetland systems that will optimize treatment for a specific chemical?

A brief historical review and an analysis of the work from pioneer research groups over the past 2 decades provide some insight into many of the above questions. It is not our intent to discuss these studies in detail but rather to highlight some of their generic findings as they led to a change from the use of natural wetlands to constructed wetlands. Numerous reports describe specific design criteria for wastewater treatment in wetlands (Godfrey et al. 1985; Richardson and Nichols 1985; Reddy and Smith 1987; Hammer 1989; Cooper and Findlater 1990). These sources also provide wetland design criteria for nutrient storage and processing for both point and nonpoint runoff. Understanding and quantification of the mechanisms responsible for retention and processing of chemicals in wetland ecosystems are also essential for predicting the efficiency of chemical storage or transformation by wetlands. Information on many of these processes can also be found in the above citations.

Historical View

Nearly 20 years ago, a research team was formed by the Kadlec brothers at the University of Michigan to investigate using wetlands to remove nutrients (primarily N and P) from wastewater. The concept that wetlands were "Mother Nature's kidneys" had led a number of scientists (e.g., Tourbier and Pierson 1976) to hypothesize that wetlands were efficient nutrient sinks. It was an exciting area of research during the 1970s because data on nutrient cycling and retention in wetlands in the U.S. were almost nonexistent, and the National Science Foundation was willing to fund applied research through a program known as Research Applied to National Needs.

Researchers at the Houghton Lake peatlands, along with a number of scientists in Florida (H. T. Odum group), Wisconsin (Spangler group), Maryland (Good and Whigham team), Germany (Siedel group), and North Carolina (Richardson team), were studying the effects of adding nutrients to natural and constructed wetlands. Results from these studies were presented at a national symposium in Ann Arbor, Michigan during May 1976 (Tilton et al. 1976). Review of those unpublished proceedings reveals 2 opposing views of the capacity of wetlands to store and remove nutrients as well as 2 different criteria for determining success, e.g., black box input/output analysis versus process studies on controlling mechanisms. Not surprisingly, these perspectives and methods still exist today.

First, most engineers, hydrologists, and biological researchers at the symposium who presented simple input/output studies were quite optimistic about the potential for using wetlands for wastewater treatment. This was based in part on the general findings that consistently indicated biochemical oxygen demand (BOD) removal ranging from 77 to 91%, high potential for N removal through denitrification, and P removal of over 99% (over a 3-year period). In fact, Dr. Maxwell Small at Brookhaven National Laboratory even stated "today there is operating a 10,000 gallon per day (37.8 m^3 day) sewage treatment system that consists only of a marsh and a pond ... the influent is raw sewage ... the effluent is potable water."

At this time, the mechanistic approach was in its infancy. Many of the studies concluded by reporting that they were not sure why, how, or for what time period their system could store or process nutrients or metals, or in other cases why they unpredictably exported nutrients. Almost all of the papers ended with a statement that more research was needed. However, the euphoria that a simple, cost-effective nutrient retention system could be created using wetlands spread like wildfire through the consulting world as well as the United States Environmental Protection Agency (USEPA). Without understanding whether or how these systems worked, some governmental agencies were pushing in the late 1970s for a policy to utilize natural wetlands for wastewater treatment.

However, the Clean Water Act (CWA) as amended in 1977 considers wetlands to be surface waters of the United States and therefore under the jurisdiction of the CWA (see "Classes of chemicals for constructed wetlands treatment" section). A primary objective of the act is to ensure that designated instream uses and natural processes are maintained and protected. Natural wetlands in the U.S. under current law cannot be degraded by a wastewater discharge. They must be considered as receiving systems and not as treatment systems (Kadlec and Knight 1996). This change in the CWA has resulted in a switch from natural to constructed wetlands for treatment systems. It should be noted that wastewater continues to be placed in thousands of wetlands nationwide, but the distinction is that they are being considered as polishing systems downstream of a permitted treatment system. Alternatively, they are being used as buffer systems on the landscape for nonpoint runoff treatment by agriculture and forestry, industries not as tightly regulated by the CWA. The CWA also requires all states to develop a system of classifications and standards to protect the best use of surface waters. Each discharger of wastes to surface waters is required to obtain a U.S. National Pollutant Discharge Elimination System (NPDES) permit that specifies the allowable pollutant load. Effluent limitations contained in NPDES permits are either technically and economically achievable or water quality-based, reflecting treatment levels required to meet water quality standards. Many states have set technology-based limits (e.g., secondary treatment for municipal wastewater) for wetland dischargers because there is no proven method for predicting wastewater assimilation in wetlands. This approach is currently changing with new information on predicting assimilative capacity for wetlands based on an analysis of the North American database for wastewater in wetlands (Kadlec and Knight 1996; Richardson et al. 1997).

There was no doubt early on that many natural wetlands were processing and storing some nutrients, metals, and organics. However, early studies were based on preliminary data from a variety of natural and constructed systems, some of which were not even constructed to function as wetlands, and most important, the mechanisms controlling ion removal and storage for these systems were for the most part unknown. In addition, few researchers realized that the transformation and nutrient retention often were carried out in the substrata (microbial processing and sorption by soils) of the system and not by the plants. For example, Spangler et al. (1976) had reported that only 5% of P went into harvestable plant tissue in their artificial marshes, and in fact, the unvegetated gravel controls often removed as much P as the vegetated systems. Other studies also reported that macrophytes showed no significant uptake of N or P in the field under increased nutrient loading conditions, as most of the added P accumulated in the litter and soils (Richardson and Craft 1993). These and additional studies have noted that outputs of nutrients increased significantly during the winter when the plants and other biotic components died back. It was clear from these early studies that wetland chemical retention and processing differed greatly among wetland types and for each element, that the processes were biologically controlled to a great degree, and that output concentrations varied seasonally. Additionally, output concentrations and retention efficiency often showed no consistent pattern among different wetlands, and the controlling mechanisms for many ions were not known. However, if one reviewed the limnology and soils literature available at the time, along with several studies in European peatlands, it would be clear that information emanating from other systems would be very helpful. For example, it was known that Al, Fe, and Ca controlled phosphate chemistry and that anaerobic conditions resulted in the release of P in acid lake waters due to the conversion of insoluble ferrous phosphate to phosphate (Wetzel 1975). Unfortunately, little of this process information was used in wetland design criteria, with the result that a large number of natural and constructed wetlands failed, especially in terms of P retention. The same fate was true for many other materials, but there were also many success stories.

The good news is that many of the preliminary findings of that 1976 Michigan symposium have since been reconfirmed many times in wetland systems, and recent symposia have now summarized key information on wetland processes as well as provided suggestions for wetland design (Godfrey et al. 1985; Richardson and Nichols 1985; Reddy and Smith 1987; Hammer 1989; Cooper and Findlater 1990). In general, these studies have shown that N outputs are generally not a problem because of high denitrification rates and storage in wetland systems. Sediment retention and BOD reductions are highly efficient in most wetlands (Richardson and Nichols 1985; Richardson 1989; Kadlec and Knight 1996). However, the problem with inconsistencies in P nutrient release data from wetlands continued into the

1980s but was ignored, misunderstood, or of little interest to wastewater engineers and many scientists. The problems related to removal of organics or trace metals have received much less attention, but it is known that wetlands are great sinks for many trace metals (Giblin 1985; Eger et al. 1993; Kadlec and Knight 1996). Much more work is needed on these materials as well as on the use of constructed wetlands to treat organics, oil processing wastes, or specific chemicals from point sources and nonpoint sources.

Classes of Chemicals for Constructed Wetlands Treatment

The decision to develop a constructed wetland for chemical removal is contingent upon many criteria, one of which is an understanding of the specific chemicals to be treated and the desired final discharge concentration. For example, understanding the transfer and transformation factors for pesticides (Figure 10-1) would aid in the development of wetlands that maximize their removal. Knowledge of the specific chemicals to be treated aids in estimating the potential for their removal in the constructed wetland. Several of these analyte-specific removal efficiencies are shown in Table 10-2. The decision to develop a constructed wetland treatment system should be contingent on prior knowledge of its successful application, on the fate of the targeted chemical or materials, or on data from laboratory microcosm-scale pilot experiments.

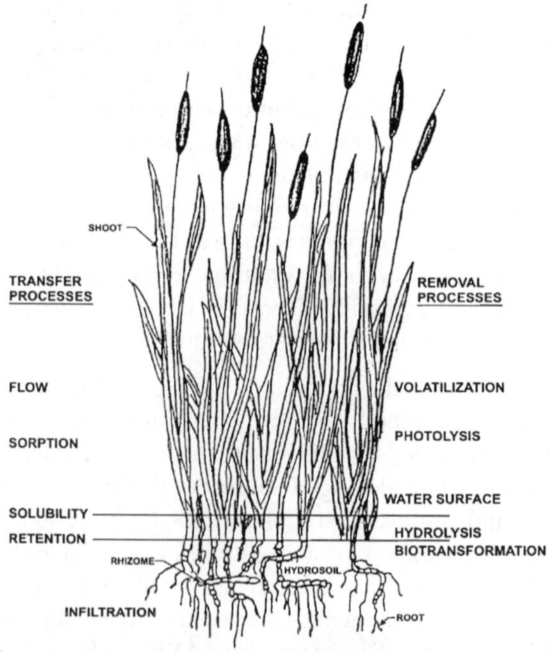

Figure 10-1 Transfer and removal processes in wetlands that are important in mitigation of nonpoint source pesticide runoff

Table 10-2 Contaminant retention efficiencies reported for constructed wetlands in North America

Contaminant	Retention efficiency	Reference
Cations	Low–high	Dunbabin and Browner 1992
Al	>35–>98.1	Morea et al. 1989; Sanford et al. 1990
Cd	50–>99.7	Daukas et al. 1988; Morea et al. 1989
Cr	50–>98.2	Daukas et al. 1988; Morea et al. 1989
Cu	50–100	Eger and Lapakko 1988; Daukas et al. 1988; Machemer et al.1990; Morea et al. 1989; Wildeman et al. 1990
Fe	84.6–100	Morea et al. 1989; Machemer et al. 1990; Sanford et al. 1990
Pb	80–95	Daukas et al. 1988; Morea et al. 1989
Mn	16.4–90	Morea et al. 1989; Sanford et al. 1990; Shea-Albin 1992
Hg	50–90	Daukas et al. 1988
Ni	>84.3–80	Eger and Lapakko 1988; Morea et al. 1989
Zn	27–100	Daukas et al. 1988; Machemer et al. 1990; Morea et al. 1989; Sanford et al. 1990; Wildeman et al. 1990
Organic N	95	Watson and Danzig 1993
Ammonia-N	62–98	CH2M Hill 1986, 1987; Girts 1988; Kadlec 1988; Watson 1990; Watson and Danzig 1993
Nitrate-N	57–94	Girts 1988; Watson 1990; Watson and Danzig 1993
Total N	51–98	CH2M Hill 1986, 1987; Girts 1988; Watson 1990; Watson and Danzig 1993
Chemical oxygen demand	54–95	Batcherer et al. 1990; Birkbeck et al. 1990; Brix and Schierup 1990; Litchfield 1993
BOD	71–97	Brix and Schierup 1990; Batcherer et al. 1990; Litchfield 1993; Birkbeck et al. 1990
Total suspended solids	80–100	Batcherer et al. 1990; Litchfield 1993
Phosphate	51–94	Batcherer et al. 1990; Birkbeck et al. 1990; Brix and Schierup 1990
Benzene	97	Wolverton 1987
Toluene	98	Wolverton 1987
p-Xylene	92	Wolverton 1987
Chloroform	68	Wolverton 1987
Tetrachloroethylene	75	Wolverton 1987

Metals

Metals removal in constructed wetlands is largely based upon biogeochemistry (Sinicrope et al. 1992), which is presented in Chapter 3. Metal removal may be contingent upon water quality and sediment factors such as reduction-oxidation potential (Eh), pH, hardness, alkalinity, acid volatile sulfides, cation exchange capacity (CEC), and sediment texture (sediment sand/silt/clay, with emphasis on fine particles). As an example, a reducing sediment with overlying water with basic pH would be better for sorbing Zn and Cu than would an oxidizing environment with an effluent pH of less than 7.0.

Organic chemicals

Organics may be amenable to treatment in constructed wetlands. The environmental compartment within which organic chemicals partition may be indicated by their water solubility, volatility, and sorption. The fate of the chemical is also determined by its ability to be moderated by environmental processes such as hydrolysis, photolysis, and biodegradation. In addition, partitioning into lipid-like mimics such as octanol indicates potential for uptake into biota.

Water solubility

Water solubility of a chemical indicates its likelihood of remaining in solution and being transferred through the aqueous phase with low probability of contacting sediments and high probability to biologically degrade. Chemicals that are highly water soluble are benzene, toluene, xylene, and phenols, for example. Those that are poorly water soluble are high-molecular-weight polynuclear aromatic hydrocarbons (e.g., fluoranthene) and chlorinated pesticides. Solubility as a property alone does not adequately indicate treatability in a constructed wetland.

Vapor pressure

The movement of chemicals between water and air can be estimated by the vapor pressure or by Henry's law constant (HLC). The higher the HLC, the more chemicals will move from water into air. Chemicals with high atmospheric partitioning (affinity for air) may be poor candidates for surfacewater constructed wetland treatment. Chemicals with high atmospheric partitioning coefficients are ethers, low mole alcohols, and trichloroethylene.

Sorption to soil

Sorption is an important chemical property that determines the ability of a material to attach to solids or surfaces. The partitioning of chemicals to soils may reduce biological availability and may allow removal by precipitation. The higher the partitioning coefficient, Kp, the less likely a chemical will remain in solution through a treatment system. Chemicals sorbing extensively to wetland surfaces become available for microbial activity or uptake, or sequestration onto soil surface may be highly amenable to treatment. Chemicals with high sorption properties would include those that are poorly water-soluble (e.g., polycyclic aromatic hydrocarbons [PAHs] and long-chain hydrocarbons). Many metals, such as Cu, Zn, and Pb, as well as many cations (e.g., Ca^{++}, Mg^4, Mn^{++}), are tightly sorbed depending upon prevailing water-column conditions, solids concentrations, and characteristics such as organic carbon content, CEC, and clay/solids content.

Octanol/water partitioning

The octanol/water partitioning coefficient (K_{ow}) is an indication of the potential for a chemical to bioconcentrate into tissue and is also related to partitioning and sorption onto solids. Chemicals with high K_{ow} would be expected to sorb onto wetland surfaces. These chemicals would not be expected to have high water solubility. Many pesticides, high-molecular-weight hydrocarbons, and polychlorinated biphenyls (PCBs) have a high K_{ow}.

Hydrolysis rate

The rate or ability to hydrolyze a chemical indicates whether a specific pH condition in a wetland would be amenable to degrading the chemical and thus removing it. Those chemicals possessing a high rate of either acid or base hydrolysis will be degraded in conditions that approximate those values. Textile dyes, fluridone, and chlorpyrifos are examples of chemicals with high hydrolysis rates. Atrazine and lindane are examples of chemicals that are poorly affected by hydrolysis.

Photolysis

Some chemicals are sensitive to light and may be degraded in the presence of ultraviolet (UV) or sunlight. Chemicals possessing this property may be treated in constructed wetlands with no surface vegetation cover and considerable open space in shallow areas. Chemicals with high photolysis rates may be better treated in open shallow lagoons with ample opportunity for interaction with sunlight.

Biodegradability: BOD/COD

Biodegradability is often measured by the biochemical oxygen demand (BOD) of a chemical. The ratio between BOD and chemical oxygen demand (COD) is an estimate of a chemical's biodegradability. If these tests are conducted in acclimated systems simulating treatment system conditions, the degradability may be higher than under actual conditions. Organic chemicals with high biodegradability are alcohols, phenols, and low-molecular-weight acids. Those that are not easily biodegraded include chlorinated hydrocarbons and high-molecular-weight PAHs. Estimates of the chemical half-life are very important to include in the design of constructed wetlands in order to ensure that sufficient chemical degradation is achieved in the system.

Toxicity

The inherent toxicity of the chemical should be identified to ensure that it is not introduced at toxic concentrations to microbial communities that may degrade the chemical and that it is not phytotoxic to plants that are growing in the wetland. Toxicity to indigenous flora and fauna may be of interest, but it may not be significant if the objective of the wetland excludes its use as wildlife habitat. The wetland discharge should reduce aqueous toxicity to a specifically targeted level. The measurement or test for satisfactory demonstration is a site-specific issue and may include *Daphnia,* fish, or other appropriate test organisms, as suggested by USEPA requirements.

Chemicals Incompatible with Constructed Wetlands

Some chemicals may not be compatible with constructed wetland treatment either because they are recalcitrant in the system or because another treatment would be a better candidate. If, e.g., volatile chemicals are of interest, biological treatment with activated sludge and air stripping may be more appropriate than constructed wetlands. Chemicals with high photolysis rates would be better treated in open shallow lagoons. Highly phytotoxic chemicals such as nonspecific herbicides may also be poor candidates. Highly refractory chemicals that bioaccumulate, such as PCBs, may also be better handled in other treatment systems or subsurface flow wetlands.

Integrated Design of Constructed Wetlands

Wetlands have unique abilities to transfer, sequester, and transform materials, including many chemicals (Greeson et al. 1978; Mitsch and Gosselink 1993). They may act as processing systems for sediments and contaminants, and they may remove nutrients along with other materials by enhancing filtration, degradation, and partitioning of chemical stressors into plants and sediments (Kusler and Brooks 1988). Several contaminant removal mechanisms are shown in Table 10-3. Constructed wetlands have been built for a variety of purposes and have been effective in removing a variety of chemicals (metals, organics, etc.) from wastewater derived from municipal and industrial sites (Wolverton et al. 1983; USEPA 1988; Sinicrope et al. 1992; Kadlec and Knight 1996). Other wetlands are constructed for rehabilitation or replacement of damaged wetlands for remediation purposes.

When wetlands are constructed to accomplish diverse objectives, it is apparent that their design must integrate our understanding of their primary components (hydroperiod, hydrosoil, and vegetation). These are the primary components of a constructed wetland that influence the potential functions and enhance or constrain the functions attained.

Table 10-3 Contaminant removal mechanisms in constructed wetland systems

Removal mechanism	Description
Sedimentation	Gravity settling of contaminants to cell substrates. Principal process for the removal of settleable and colloidal solids. This process is incidental to the removal of BOD, nutrients, heavy metals, organics, and pathogens.
Filtration	Solids and organic matter filtered mechanically as water passes through the system. Important in retention of chemical precipitates formed by wetland metabolism.
Adsorption	Particulate organic matter, media substrates, and root surfaces can have a high affinity for nutrients and refractory organics. Process possibly short-lived with removal potential high during the wetland maturation period and lower thereafter. Principal removal processes include adsorption, chelation, and cation exchange.
Plant metabolism	Wetland macrophytes will actively take up and store contaminants in the root zone. They may also sorb materials and become involved in co-metabolic processes.
Carbonate precipitation	Alkalinity and its interaction with available cations thought to be highly significant in the control of metals in constructed wetland systems. Typically occurs at relatively high pH, with importance probably greater during initial maturation phase. Long-term effectiveness most probably dependent upon the composition of cell media materials, interstitial chemistry, and influent water quality.
Co-precipitation	Co-precipitation of trace metals or toxic nonmetallic elements such as As typically with Fe, or Mn oxyhydroxides can be quantitatively significant in constructed wetland systems. Generally insoluble precipitates retained with the wetland matrix.
Dissimilatory sulfate reduction	The principal metals removal mechanisms in constructed wetlands. Microbiologically mediated process resulting in the formation of metabolic sulfides. Driven by the decomposition of labile organic matter under reducing conditions. Bacteria driving processes are ubiquitous and resistant to high concentrations of heavy metals. Process occurs in the subsurface anaerobic environment of the wetland.
Metal oxidation and hydrolysis	Microbiology mediated process in which ferric and manganic oxyhyroxides scavenge other metabolic cations in solution. Bacterially-oxidized states are thermodynamically stable and thus resistant to remobilization. It is an important process for metal removal in a constructed wetland. In a subsurface flow system, it occurs in the aerobic rhizosphere surrounding marsh plant root hairs and in the surficial oxic aerobic layer of the treatment media.
Decomposition	Decomposition or alteration of less stable compounds (e.g., refractory organics) by processes such as UV irradiation, oxidation, and reduction.
Microbial metabolism	Removal of colloidal solids and soluble organics by suspended, benthic, and plant-supported bacteria. Specific examples include nitrification/dentrification and the microbially mediated oxidation/reduction of metals. Important constructed wetlands process for the removal of colloidal solids, BOD, N species, refractory organics, and metals. Thought to be the most dominant contaminant removal pathway in a constructed wetland system for many materials.

Table 10-3 *continued*

Removal mechanism	Description
Plant absorption	Can be an important removal pathway for N, P, metals, and refractory organics. Under proper conditions, significant quantities of these contaminants can be taken up by plants. However, they recycle to the constructed wetland litter/soil layer upon plant death.
Peat accretion	Long-term process of organic matter buildup (1 to 2 mm) from partial decay of dead organic matter. Important long-term sink for most compounds, metals, and organics.
Natural dieoff	Removal of pathogenic organisms (e.g., bacteria and viruses) through natural decay or introduction to an unfavorable environment. With proper design, constructed wetlands can be very effective for removal of pathogens.

Hydrology in Design of Constructed Wetlands

Hydraulic regime

Hydrology in constructed wetlands is probably the controlling component that largely determines whether a constructed wetland meets its design objective. Facets of hydrology that should be considered in design of a constructed wetland are those related to loading, including flows as well as concentrations of solids and chemical constituents. Components of flow include both volume and periodicity. Constructed wetlands are typically designed to accommodate both average or typical flows and extreme flows (both minimum and maximum). For some constructed wetlands, flow is carefully maintained within a narrow range. However, constructed wetlands must occasionally be able to tolerate drought conditions as well as flooding. In many cases, hydraulic retention time (HRT), which is linked to flow, is a critical design consideration. The HRT can be changed by expanding area or altering water flow or depth in the wetland. These are not trivial considerations because the HRT can influence transfers and transformations of chemicals. Water depth within the wetlands can influence hydrosoils in wetlands (sediment reduction or oxidation). The hydraulic regime should be compatible with chosen vegetation as well as contribute to attaining the desired functions (e.g., negative hydrosoil redox to assist in sequestering metals). Often the selected hydraulic regime is a compromise.

Variance in the concentration of chemicals in the inflow to constructed wetlands may also influence the selected design. Both mass loading and concentration must be considered to arrive at a design that will accommodate the anticipated range in treatment rate.

Hydrosoil selection

Constructed wetlands often are built on sites where wetlands did not previously exist. In that case, selection of an appropriate hydrosoil can contribute to attainment of the desired functions. In some cases, wetlands previously existed and the hydrosoil is suitable.

Typical hydrosoil selection criteria for constructed wetlands include

1) appropriate chemical and physical characteristics
2) ability to contribute to desired functions,
3) minimal background chemical concentrations,
4) compatibility with the selected wetland plant species,
5) availability of nutrients for growth of the selected plant species,
6) location and availability, and
7) transportation costs.

Candidate hydrosoils can be evaluated by chemical, physical, and biological analyses (Faulkner and Richardson 1989). Chemical analyses may include measurements of background metals, organics, pesticides, pH, redox, acid volatile sulfides, and nutrients. Physical analyses may include particle size distribution, organic matter (OM) content, percent water, percent solids, bulk density, and pore space. Biological analyses could include evaluation of background toxicity using sediment toxicity tests (e.g., *Hyalella azteca*, *Chironomus tentans*, etc.).

Vegetation Selection

Vegetation selection is an important component in constructed wetlands design. Plants can be screened for use in constructed wetlands based upon previous knowledge, experience, and scientific literature (e.g., Armstrong 1978; Armstrong et al. 1990). Selection criteria might include

1) influence on hydrosoil characteristics such as redox and pH (Brix 1990),
2) influence on water characteristics such as suspended solids and BOD,
3) compatibility with selected hydrosoil,
4) compatibility with the local climate,
5) ability to withstand hydroperiod fluctuation or changes in HRT,
6) resistance to herbivory,
7) cost/availability, and
8) endemism.

Preliminary screening experiments can provide useful information to arrive at a final decision regarding appropriate vegetation for the constructed wetlands (Brix and Schierup 1990; Brix 1993).

Site Selection and Constraints

Once the land requirements are established, through the design process, then potential sites are assessed for compatibility, constructability, and constraints. The design process establishes the characteristics in the wetland to support the values selected for a particular project. The first filter in the site selection process should consider sites with the closest hydrological, vegetation, and soil or geomorphological conditions required to support the wetland values for the proposed constructed wetland. Landscape and watershed issues are among the essential considerations in siting a constructed wetland, if ecological functions are being considered. Land use designations, ownerships, parcel sizes, and proximity to the source of the wasteload are also critical considerations in choosing a site. Connectivity to other existing wetlands, riverine and riparian zones, migration pathways, critical habitats, buffer zones, etc., can enhance (or detract from) the value of the constructed wetland.

Scaling in Designing Constructed Wetlands

At least 2 aspects of scaling are important considerations in developing design criteria for constructed wetlands. First, there are spatial considerations or spatial scaling factors that may be nonlinear. Second, there are temporal considerations or temporal scaling factors that may not be directly applicable as the design moves from bench to pilot-scale and subsequently to full-scale construction. Spatial scaling in constructed wetland design may involve laboratory studies to provide transformation and fate-and-effects information. These laboratory studies, or bench-scale studies, may also provide information on hydrosoil–water interactions (e.g., pH, redox development), compatibility of the selected vegetation with the candidate hydrosoil, and other screening-level experiments that contribute to reducing uncertainty in the design phase. Caution must be exercised as these data are extrapolated to intermediate-scale testing or as the project moves to full-scale construction. If the project is relatively large or involves critical processes, then pilot-scale studies might be appropriate to minimize the extrapolation distance and uncertainties. Pilot-scale studies can address questions about hydrodynamics and other factors that may influence success in accomplishing the objectives, thus minimizing uncertainties in extrapolation to full-scale construction. Again, the nonlinearities in scaling factors should be incorporated. For example, if the transformation or transfer process required to accomplish the objectives of the constructed wetland is linked to plant density (density-dependent), then differences in plant density must be accounted for in scaling from laboratory or bench-scale to pilot-scale and subsequently to the full-scale constructed wetland. Another example is spatial scaling when transport is considered. There can be considerable nonlinearities in large- versus small-scale movement of water in constructed wetlands. Other considerations regarding spatial scaling may include issues such as the ultimate size of the constructed wetland within the watershed or landscape. The size issue is usually resolved based upon process design kinetics (processing rate versus HRT) or area- or volume-linked processing rates. Positioning within the landscape depends upon such factors as adjacent land use and availability or the role that position may play in accomplishing the desired objective.

Temporal scaling in wetland construction involves additional considerations. If the spatial scaling is sufficient to include the function and values of interest (see Chapter 1) then that implies that the rate kinetics and HRT have been coupled such that these functions can be realized within the wetland boundaries. One issue of concern in developing constructed wetlands is longevity, or design life. Currently, we do not have sufficient information to accurately assess the design life or useful life of constructed wetlands. However, management or maintenance practices can help maintain the desired functions and values for as long as possible. Other temporal considerations might include changes in function as a wetland "matures" or undergoes succession. Again, maintenance may be required to achieve desired function by "resetting" the wetland to the appropriate successional immature state.

Feedback

Feedback in the design and operation of constructed wetlands may occur at any step of the process. Negative feedback would indicate that using a constructed wetland may not be suitable for accomplishing the stated objective, but some adjustments may be possible. These may include

1) altering the objective,
2) adjusting components of the constructed wetland (hydrology, hydrosoil, vegetation),
3) increasing or decreasing scaling factors (temporal, spatial), and
4) redesigning the system (e.g., with pretreatment or settling).

With development of this relatively new technology, it is important that both successes and failures be reported in the published literature. Usually, failures and analyses of reasons why systems failed to achieve stated objectives are difficult to publish. Progress or improvement of designs can be accomplished most rapidly if communication is efficient. Thus positive and negative feedback in the design and operation of constructed wetlands is crucial in the process for both course correction and progress.

Management and Maintenance Issues

Management and maintenance issues for the design of constructed wetlands revolve around treatment performance optimization (e.g., maximum contaminant reduction) and support for system sustainability (e.g., operational stability). In some instances, these 2 issues are so interrelated as to be indistinguishable; e.g., the removal of contaminated sediment/sludge would likely impact both treatment performance and operational stability. In other instances, there might be a difference, at least in the short term, in the impact of management versus maintenance issues; for example, the removal of mosquito larvae would not have an impact on treatment but might be a valued aspect of any maintenance program in terms of public acceptability.

Treatment performance

The design of a managed system should result in better treatment performance and/or in a decrease of the HRT required for a given level of performance. A more managed constructed wetland implies an active treatment approach such as the addition of nutrients, flow controls, and/or aeration to enhance microbial degradation of contaminants. Just as with engineered waste treatment systems, limitations of oxygen supply and diffusion gradients into the bacterial biofilm on plant surfaces may limit the performance of treatment wetlands. More innovative measures can be used to oxygenate the water column and promote mixing; e.g., wetlands could be modified with the use of sprinkler systems, waterfalls, and/or windmills. Other factors limiting treatment performance might include

1) short circuiting or stagnation,
2) reduced surface area, and
3) low temperatures (especially in northern areas).

Pond versus marsh

Wetlands may include both open-water (pond) areas, with water depths of greater than 1 m, and marshlike areas with shallow water and high densities of macrophytes. Both kinds of areas have advantages in terms of treatment performance and ecological characteristics. For example, open pond areas have been recommended to enhance nitrification of ammonia-ammonium, and this conceptual approach would likely be beneficial to other constructed wetlands as well (e.g., industrial wastes). Open areas could be created by either direct (e.g., harvesting) or indirect (e.g., increasing water depth) control of vegetation density. Experience with hydrocarbon contaminants has indicated that the dissolved oxygen concentrations in the open water column of a wetlands are greater and enhance breakdown of contaminants by increased decomposition. This breakdown can be severely depressed in vegetated areas due to the lack of wind or wave action, resulting in decreased treatment performance for some contaminants that require higher oxygen water-column content for degradation.

Pest control

Pest control may be required to satisfy public health or acceptability issues or to maintain the wetland ecosystem (e.g., reduce plant disease, minimize grazing by mammals).

Sediment or sludge removal

The removal of sediment or sludge may be required as a result of

1) an increase in toxic sediments, which may decrease treatment performance or create an unacceptable risk to the public and/or the environment, or
2) the buildup of sediments from routine processes of sedimentation, which ultimately could alter the depth of the water column and hence change habitat characteristics and/or treatment performance.

Vegetation

Management of vegetation may be required under the following circumstances

1) If a certain plant density is desired, the addition of fertilizers may be needed
2) if only selected plants are desired, then control procedures will be needed to inhibit colonization by other plants; and
3) if nutrient removal is an objective, then harvesting the plant crop may enhance treatment performance, but harvesting will result in soil disturbances.

Location

Management decisions related to location revolve around issues of

1) public access (is it desired?);
2) the geographical location of the wetland discharge to the receiving environment; and
3) the availability and cost of the required land area.

Contingencies

Because constructed wetlands are subject to many natural variables (e.g., plant diseases, predation by grazers, changes in temperature) that can be more controlled in engineered systems, system redundancies or contingencies are an important feature that should be incorporated if possible. In general, these might include

1) parallel treatment wetlands (to provide duplication) and/or
2) a series of treatment wetlands to accommodate events such as the shock loadings of contaminants or the need to remove sediment from selected sections to improve their hydrology.

Treatment Performance versus Ecological Acceptability

The need for ecological assessment to evaluate if the habitat quality of the constructed wetland is comparable to that of nearby natural wetlands must consider the intended role of the wetland. For those applications where wetland rehabilitation is being implemented, a complete site-specific ecological risk assessment may be required. A beneficial consequence of constructed wetland development may be enhancement of wildlife in an otherwise unattractive area. Where wildlife interfaces with the wetland, ecological risk assessment may play an important role in determining the value of the project. Constructed wetland applications that focus the treatment system approach, rather than on wildlife or habitat enhancement, may require little ecological risk assessment to determine the appropriateness of the project.

In most cases, the principal objective of constructed wetlands is to reduce point and nonpoint chemical and nonchemical stressors and to achieve low-cost treatment performance. In systems with little or no relation to the landscape ecology and which are solely treatment units with no wildlife enhancement, design considerations regarding the ecological acceptability or habitat quality of constructed wetlands may be negligible, or at least of secondary importance. Indeed, if a maximum level of ecological acceptability was an absolute criterion, then these constructed wetlands may, by definition, be incapable of functioning. This is because the input of contaminants into constructed wetlands may inevitably result in dissimilar ecological characteristics compared with uncontaminated natural wetlands (Friend 1985). For example, different bacterial and fungal communities will develop in response to inputs of biodegradable hydrocarbons compared with populations of these microorganisms in a natural wetlands that presumably does not receive these inputs. The transformation and/or physical treatment of inorganic compounds (e.g., phosphorus, metals) also will inevitably alter the micro- (e.g., sediment redox) or macro- (e.g., water depth) environment such that some effects on habitat quality, perhaps subtle, will occur.

Notwithstanding this primary objective of constructed wetlands (e.g., the removal of contaminants), habitat quality may or may not become a design issue. This need to address ecological/habitat quality issues results from a fundamental difference between conventional waste treatment systems and constructed wetlands: constructed wetlands may be exposed to the external environment and hence may be utilized or colonized by a variety of plants and/or animals (unless measures are taken to exclude their access). For the same reason, constructed wetlands are also more exposed to public scrutiny compared with conventional waste treatment systems (especially those wetlands treating nonpoint sources such as urban runoff). As a result of this exposure to both the environment and the public, and the possibility that habitat quality may be an important secondary objective of some wetlands (e.g., restoration or rehabilitation of damaged water or terrestrial systems), the ecological characteristics of selected constructed wetlands will likely become increasingly important as the size of the total treatment area increases and/or with its degree of permanency as part of the overall landscape.

If the constructed wetland objectives specifically exclude habitat enhancement and actions are taken to minimize attractiveness to wildlife, the wetland will operate solely as a treatment unit. However, if there is habitat enhancement, an ecological risk assessment is recommended. In this application, where the wetland may produce habitat and increase the wildlife community, the relationship between treatment performance and ecological acceptability must be determined. Under conditions of negligible treatment performance, a high quality of habitat can be achieved. However, as treatment performance increases (e.g., contaminant input and removal), a decrease in ecological quality of the wetland compared to nearby natural wetlands may result. As treatment performance increases to a maximum (then decreases due to contaminant overloading), ecological acceptability is likely to continue to decrease. In those wetlands where habitat is a valued component of the design function, the challenge will be to establish and meet criteria for both performance and ecological acceptability.

Regulatory Context for Constructed Wetlands

The primary law affecting constructed wetlands is the 1972 Federal Water Pollution Control Act (PL500-30), as amended, otherwise known as the Clean Water Act (CWA). Three sections in the CWA are especially applicable: §§401, 402, and 404. Section 402 regulates point source discharges through the issuance of NPDES permits. Criteria for permit issuance are chemistry, toxicity, and ecological health of the receiving body. The chemistry criteria take the form of ambient water quality criteria, which generally may not be exceeded in the effluent discharge. Mixing in the receiving body may or may not be considered in the evaluation of compliance. Toxicity is evaluated with effluent toxicity bioassays. Biocriteria are used to evaluate the ecological health of the receiving body. Section 402 has been used primarily to regulate point discharges from industrial and municipal sources. Most states have permit authority with USEPA oversight. The primary technical support document is USEPA's Technical Support Document for Water Quality Permitting.

Section 404 of the CWA regulates the discharge of dredge and fill material into the waters of the U.S. This program is administered by the U.S. Army Corps of Engineers (USACOE) in conjunction with the USEPA. The USACOE issues §404 permits using criteria developed by the USEPA. The permit applicant or the USACOE in the case of a federal action, must demonstrate that no practicable alternatives exist and that the project will not significantly degrade the environment. Obviously, these criteria are much more vague than those found in §402. The permit applicant must, under all circumstances, meet mitigation criteria. That is, they must provide compensation through restoration for lost or degraded wetlands. Finally, applicants must comply with other applicable laws and criteria (e.g., state laws, Endangered Species Act). The USEPA has veto authority under §404(c) for permits issued by the USACOE. However, this authority has been used rarely. Between 1979 and 1995, the USEPA has completed only 11 veto actions out of an estimated 150,000 permit actions (less than 1%).

Section 401 authorizes the states to review, approve, condition, or deny permits or licenses that might result in a discharge to state waters, including wetlands. This action often takes the form of a state water quality certification. In some instances, the state and federal offices have closely coordinated the permit review process so that the state review may be invisible to the applicant. Because §401 is a state action, evaluative criteria are state-specific and vary considerably.

The regulatory context for NPS pollution is much less clear than for point sources (§402) and discharge from dredge and fill (§404). Recent revisions of the CWA (§319) established a grants program for best management practices designed to protect or restore wetlands and riparian habitats from the adverse effects of runoff. Perhaps the clearest example is the use of buffer zones composed of wetlands between agricultural fields and adjacent aquatic habitats. Wetlands in these buffer zones "treat" NPS agricultural runoff in a manner analogous to primary (solids removal) and secondary (biodegradation) treatment in sewage treatment plants.

NPS pollution is also addressed in §6217 of the Coastal Zone Act Reauthorization Amendments of 1990. Under this section, the USEPA and National Oceanic Atmospheric Administration (NOAA) developed guidance for managing NPS that affect coastal waters. That guidance includes a chapter regarding the protection and restoration of wetlands and riparian areas and the use of vegetated treatment programs. The coastal states are implementing this program.

How do these laws and implementing regulations affect constructed wetlands? The answer is, "That depends." The complexity of most constructed wetland projects clouds the regulatory context. Clearly, if there is discharge to U.S. waters or if a discrete point discharge exists, §404 and §402 criteria predominate. As discussed above, criteria for the 2 programs differ substantively and substantially. One could imagine constructing settling basins with overflows in existing wetlands to control agricultural runoff. Would this construction be regulated from a point source or an NPS perspective? How would degradation of organophosphate pesticides in the settling basin affect that perspective?

Risk Assessment for Constructed Wetlands

Risk is the probability of an adverse event. For constructed wetlands, major adverse events include

1) impacts to ecologically important species,
2) human exposure to water and/or contaminated food, and
3) failure to meet treatment performance criteria.

Risk to ecological receptors is a function of chemical toxicity and exposure potential. Chemical-specific toxicity can be expressed as a threshold concentration in media (soil, sediment, water, or food chain biota), as an ingestion rate, or as a threshold body burden. Toxicity can also be expressed as a percent of the contaminated media (e.g., % treated effluent). The domain of ecotoxicological threshold values is small relative to those for human health, especially because the values may vary from species to species. Extrapolations increase the uncertainty associated with the toxicity assessment. An important axiom to remember is that chemical risks are not managed by altering toxicity. Toxicity is fixed. Rather, it is the reduction or elimination of chemical exposure that decreases risk.

Exposure is a function of the spatial or temporal distribution of contaminants *vis a vis* the receptor of concern. Managing risks involves reducing spatial or temporal exposures. For constructed wetlands, an important consideration is the temporal distribution of receptors of concern. Receptors may be permanent, temporary (seasonal), or transient residents of the constructed wetlands. Concern for permanent residents is generally low in wetlands constructed for treatment purposes. In fact, some residents (e.g., microorganisms, vegetation) may be essential to the successful treatment of chemicals. Exposure of temporary or transient visitors, however, may represent unacceptable ecological risks. Whether these risks are important will be driven by site-specific concerns. Prescriptive guidance for evaluating ecological risks does not exist; however, general guidance is available (USEPA 1998).

Human health risks at constructed wetlands may arise from consumption of contaminated drinking water (surface or ground water) or ingestion of contaminated food (fish, shellfish, and avian species). Standard procedures are available for evaluating human health risks and would be applicable to constructed wetlands.

Failure to meet treatment performance criteria is an engineering risk associated with all constructed wetlands. Successful system performance is a function of the many engineering and operational features included in the wetland design. There is a certain confidence associated with the performance of each feature. For example, design criteria may require an HRT of 3 days. Confidence surrounding this design specification is a function of

1) the quality of the hydraulic model,
2) the accuracy of data inputs to the model, and
3) stochasticity or natural variability (e.g., rainfall events).

To the degree that HRT can be predicted accurately, risk can be avoided. If predictive confidence is low, one must engineer conservatively to reduce risk. Because constructing wetlands for the treatment of contaminated effluents is an emerging technology, predictive confidence in treatment performance is generally low. Consequently, these systems generally must be designed and engineered conservatively.

By definition, all risk has uncertainty. All risk assessments, therefore, must address this uncertainty explicitly. The uncertainty analysis (UA) should convey to the risk manager the limits and level of confidence associated with the technical results. Uncertainty analysis can be quantitative, qualitative, or both. Qualitative UA can be as simple as a list of assumptions made during the risk assessment and discussion of how they may affect the conclusions. This type of UA is cost-effective and often more easily understood by the risk manager and the public than traditional quantitative UA. Quantitative UA permits a numerical estimate of the uncertainty associated with estimates of risk. This type of UA is much more data- and model-intensive and thus more expensive.

Risk Management for Constructed Wetlands

Risk management is the suite of proactive steps taken to reduce the probability of the adverse event to acceptable levels. Risk management must be consistent with the applicable regulatory context. The primary concern for wetlands constructed to treat chemical wastes may be chemical exposure of invasive organisms. For wetlands constructed for habitat restoration or rehabilitation, the concern is to manage ecological function so that the desired wetland value is realized. Constructed wetlands can serve the dual purpose of chemical treatment and habitat restoration or rehabilitation.

An approach for design, construction, and operation of constructed wetlands to treat wastewater is shown in Figure 10-2. Embedded in this diagram are major risk management decision points. The first decision is to determine the goal and objectives of the constructed wetlands. The second is whether to proceed with the constructed wetlands approach or consider another alternative (e.g., trickling filter). The third decision point is selection of appropriate ecological characteristics of the wetland to achieve the project goal but minimize risk. The fourth risk management decision is a cost consideration: capital, operational, and monitoring. The final decision occurs after start-up. One must decide whether to gear up for full-scale operations.

Success Criteria for Constructed Wetland Treatment

Successful wetland treatment can be measured in a number of ways. It may be directly related to a standard set by the CWA in terms of a technically achievable water standard for variables like O_2, pH, NH_4-N, or metals, etc., or it may be based on state, regional, or federal water quality standards. A primary objective of the act is to ensure that designated instream uses and natural processes are maintained and protected. Waters and wetlands in the U.S. under current law cannot be degraded by a wastewater discharge. Both systems must be considered as receiving systems and not as treatment systems. Each discharger of wastes to surface waters is required to obtain an NPDES permit, which specifies the allowable pollutant load. Effluent limitations contained in NPDES permits are either technically and economically achievable or water quality-based, reflecting treatment levels required to protect water quality standards as noted in the ambient water criteria (USEPA 1986). In

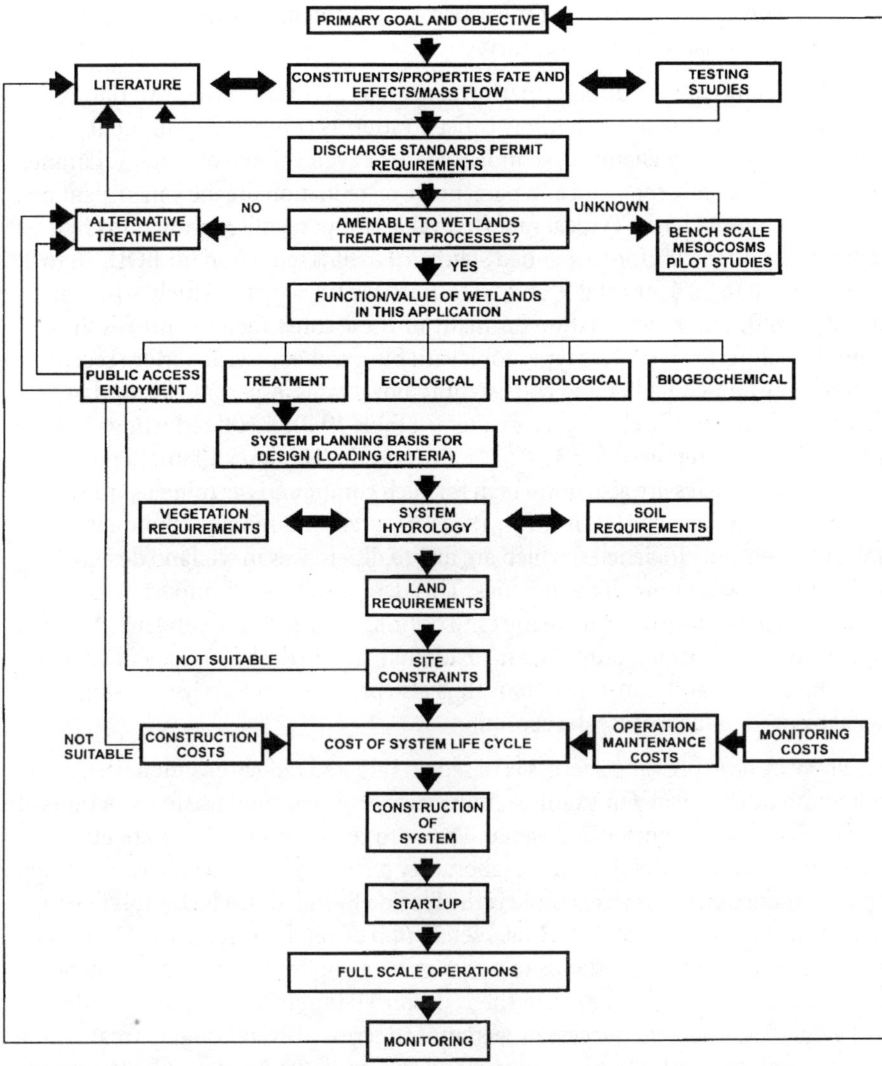

Figure 10-2 Guidelines for the selection and design of constructed wetlands for wastewater treatment

addition, many states have set technology-based limits (e.g., secondary treatment for municipal wastewater) for wetland dischargers because there is no proven method of predicting wastewater assimilation in wetlands to serve as a basis for setting water quality-based limits. This approach is currently changing with new information on predicting assimilative capacity for wetlands based on an analysis of the North American database for wastewater in wetlands and as more constructed wetlands are successfully utilized for wastewater treatment (Richardson et al. 1997).

Currently, constructed wetlands for wastewater treatment may not be included as part of the national wetland inventory.

Foremost in any consideration of performance success in wastewater wetlands treatment is the reduction in outflow concentration as compared to influent concentration for any chemical, sediment load, or even volume of water (Hammer 1989). This is usually reported as a percentage of reduction for the constituent on a monthly or annual basis. Typical reported values for percentage reductions by wetlands are 60 to 90% for suspended solids, 70 to 95% reduction for BOD, 10 to 90% for total N, 10 to 90% for total P, and 20 to 100% for trace metals (Richardson and Nichols 1985). The wide variation for many of these constituents is the result of comparing different wetlands types for a variable number of years. More recent case studies report much higher and consistent removal rates, especially for wetlands constructed for specific chemical treatments (Table 10-2). Metal reductions in excess of 90% have been reported for Al, Cd, Cr, Cu, and Zn (Hammer 1989). Reported retention efficiencies are also quite high for such compounds as toluene, p-xylene, chloroform, and benzene (Wolverton 1987). Several contaminants show a wide range of retention efficiencies, which are due to differences in wetland design, loadings, and water flow characteristics. This demonstrates the importance of building a wetland with design features to optimize biotic and abiotic mechanisms (e.g., absorption sedimentation, metal oxidation, and hydrolysis) that enhance removal, storage, and transformations. It is also prudent not to rely on a single mechanism to remove or treat a contaminant.

Another way of expressing success is based on targeted reductions for a specific compound or chemical. For example, industries or agricultural waste reductions are agreed upon for the constructed wetland prior to construction. These are often based on predicted reductions from laboratory tests or models, which can be used to estimate reductions. A case example is the Florida Everglades. The Everglades Forever Act (1994; 373.4592 Fla. Stat.) set 50 ppb of total phosphorus (TP) as the interim standard for the wetlands to be constructed on former agricultural lands. This is nearly a 67% reduction from the 150-ppb TP inputs from agricultural lands to the Everglades. Thus, the success of wetlands in terms of water quality treatment is measured on the basis of agreed-upon standards or government-regulated concentrations.

Synthesis and Summary

We are concerned about effects of chemical stressors in natural and constructed wetlands, but it is clear that wetlands have assimilative capacity for treatment of many chemicals. In constructed wetlands, the potential for ecological risks is highly variable, ranging from those wetlands that strictly serve for wastewater treatment to those that serve for wildlife habitat and other public uses. We developed a decision-support system or guidance framework for selection, design, and implementation of constructed wetlands for wastewater treatment (Figure 10-2). This decision-support system can serve to aid selection and decisions regarding constructed wetlands.

Research Needs

It was concluded by this workgroup that there are many research needs in the area of constructed wetlands. It was decided that the following research categories and corresponding specific areas are in need of technical information.

Microbial ecology

- Biodegradation of single compounds and mixtures
- Decomposer response to compounds-toxic/biostatic
- Population dynamics and nutrient cycling
    - Metal cycling of sulfur
    - Nitrification/denitrification

Hydrology

- Hydrodynamic models
- Fate-and-transport models
- Evapotranspiration
- Micrometeorological effects
- Groundwater recharge, self-clogging, groundwater mounding

Vector control

- Mosquito population dynamics
- Role of wildlife
- Role of fish
- Role of insects: life stages
- Natural larvicides
- Role of plants

Vegetation

- Hydroperiod: Plant community development
- Vegetation planting and management techniques
- Role of plants supporting microbial ecology
- Role of plants in nutrient cycling
- Role of plants: litter, detritus, carbon cycling, particulization
- Accretion rate of recalcitrant plant material
- Role of plants in determining capacity of treatment effectiveness
- Community structure, vertical and horizontal, and impact on velocity fields
- Role of periphyton in biogeochemical cycling

Sediments, soils, suspended solids

- Particle size characterization distribution, impact on removal, accumulation amount, distribution, and redistribution
- Metal or soil binding and fate
- Soil and plant community development

References

Armstrong W. 1978. Root aeration in the wetland environment. In: Hook DD, Crawford RR, editors. Plant life in anaerobic environments. Ann Arbor MI: Ann Arbor Science. p 269–297.

Armstrong W, Armstrong J, Beckett PM. 1990. Measurement and modeling of oxygen release from roots of *Phragmites australis*. In: Cooper PF, Findlater BC, editors. Constructed wetlands in water pollution control. Oxford UK: Pergamon p 41–52.

Baker LA. 1992. Introduction to nonpoint source pollution in the United States and prospects for wetland use. *Ecol Eng* 1:1–26.

Bastian RK, Shanaghan PE, Thompson BP. 1989. Use of wetlands for municipal wastewater treatment and disposal-regulatory issues and EPA policies. In: Hammer DA, editor. Constructed wetlands for wastewater treatment: municipal, industrial, and agricultural. Chelsea MI: Lewis. p 265–278.

Batcherer A, Scott WE, Wood A. 1990. Constructed wetland research program in South Africa. In: Cooper PF, Findlater BC, editors. Constructed wetlands in water pollution control. Oxford UK: Pergamon p 373–382.

Birkbeck A-E, Reil D, Hunter R. 1990. Application of natural and engineered wetlands for treatment of low-strength leachate. In: Cooper PF, Findlater BC, editors. Constructed wetlands in water pollution control. Oxford UK: Pergamon p 411–418.

Brix H. 1990. Gas exchange through the soil-atmosphere interphase and through dead culms of *Phragmites australis* in a constructed reed bed receiving domestic sewage. *Water Res* 24(2):259–266.

Brix H. 1993. Macrophyte-mediated oxygen transfer in wetlands: transport mechanisms and rates. In: Moshiri GA, editor. Constructed wetlands for water quality improvement. Boca Raton FL: Lewis. p 391–398.

Brix H, Schierup H. 1990. Soil oxygenation in constructed reed beds: the role of macrophyte and soil-atmosphere interface oxygen transport. In: Cooper PF, Findlater BC, editors. Constructed wetlands in water pollution control. Oxford UK: Pergamon p 53–66.

CH2M Hill. 1986. Boggy gut wetland treated effluent disposal system Hilton Head Island, South Carolina. Final status report prepared for Sea Pines Public Service District.

CH2M Hill. 1987. Central wastewater treatment plant wetlands discharge first annual report. June 1986–June 1987. Paper prepared for Grand Strand Water and Sewer Authority.

Cooper PF, Findlater BC. 1990. Constructed wetlands in water pollution control. Oxford UK: Pergamon 605 p.

Craft CB, Richardson CJ. 1993. Peat accretion and N, P, and organic C accumulation in nutrient-enriched and unenriched Everglades peatlands. *Ecologic Appl* 3(3):446–458.

Daukas P, Lowry D, Walker WW. 1988. Design of a wet detention basin and constructed wetlands for treatment of stormwater runoff from a regional shopping mall in Massachusetts. Proceedings from the First International Conference on Constructed Wetlands for Wastewater Treatment; 13–17 Jun 1988; Chattanooga TN.

Dunbabin JS, Browner KH. 1992. Potential use of constructed wetlands for treatment of industrial wastewaters containing metals. *Sci Total Environ* (2–3):151–168.

Eger P, Melchert G, Antonson D, Wagner J. 1993. The use of wetland treatment to remove trace metals from mine drainage. In: Moshiri GA, editor. Constructed wetlands for water quality improvement. Boca Raton FL: Lewis. p 283–292.

Eger P, Lapakko K. 1988. Nickel and copper removal from mine drainage by a natural wetland. In: Metal mining and the environment bibliography. Pittsburgh PA: U.S. Dept. of the Interior, Bureau of Mines. p 301–309.

Faulkner SP, Richardson CJ. 1989. Physical and chemical characteristics of freshwater wetland soils. In: Hammer DA. Constructed wetlands for wastewater treatment: municipal, industrial, and agricultural. Chelsea MI: Lewis. p 41–72.

Friend M. 1985. Wildlife health implications of sewage disposal in wetlands. In: Godfrey PJ, Kaynor ER, Pelczanski S, Benforado J, editors. Ecological considerations in wetlands treatment of municipal wastewaters. New York: Van Nostrand Reinhold. p 262–269.

Giblin AE. 1985. Comparisons of the processing of elements by ecosystems. II: metals. In: Godfrey PJ, Kaynor ER, Pelczarski S, Benforado J, editors. Ecological considerations in wetlands treatment of municipal wastewaters. New York: Van Nostrand Reinhold. p 158–179.

Girts MA. 1988. Operational optimization. International Conference on Constructed Wetlands for Wastewater Treatment; 1988 June; Chattanooga TN.

Godfrey PJ, Kaynor ER, Pelczarski S, Benforado J. 1985. Ecological considerations in wetlands treatment of municipal wastewaters. New York: Van Nostrand Reinhold 473 p.

Greeson PE, Clark JR, Clark JE, editors. 1978. Wetland functions and values: state of our understanding. Minneapolis MI: American Water Resources Association.

Hammer DA. 1989. Constructed wetlands for wastewater treatment. Municipal, industrial, and agricultural. Chelsea MI: Lewis.

Kadlec RH. 1988. Denitrification in wetlands treatment system. *J Water Pollut Control Fed* 60:

Kadlec RH, Knight RL. 1996. Treatment wetlands. Boca Raton, FL: Lewis. 893 p.

Kusler JA, Brooks G. 1988. Proceedings of the national wetland symposium: wetland hydrology. Berne NY: Association of State Wetland Managers.

Litchfield DK. 1993. Constructed wetlands for wastewater treatment at Amoco Oil Company's Mandan, ND refinery. In: Moshiri GA, editor. Constructed wetlands for water quality improvement. Chelsea MI: Lewis. p 485–488.

Machemer SD, Lemke PR, Wildeman TR, Cohen RR, Klusman RW, Emerick JC, Bates ER. 1990. Passive treatment of metals mine drainage through use of a constructed wetland. Washington DC: USEPA. EPA/600/9-90037.

Mitsch WJ, Gosselink JG. 1993. Wetlands. 2nd ed. New York: Van Nostrand Reinhold.

Morea SC, Olsen RL, Chappell RW. 1989. Assessment of a passive treatment system for acid mine drainage at a Colorado Superfund site. 62nd Annual Conference Water Pollution Control Federation; October 1989; San Francisco CA.

Moshiri GA. 1993. Constructed wetlands for water quality improvement. Boca Raton FL: Lewis.

Reddy KR, Smith WH. 1987. Aquatic plants for water treatment and resource recovery. Orlando FL: Magnolia Publishing.

Richardson CJ. 1989. Freshwater wetlands: transformers, filters, or sinks? In: Sharitz RR, Gibbons JW, editors. Freshwater wetlands and wildlife. Oak Ridge TN: U.S. Department of Energy. CONF-8603101.

Richardson CJ, Craft CB. 1993. Effective phosphorus retention in wetlands: fact or fiction? In: Moshiri GA, editor. Constructed wetlands for water quality improvement. Boca Raton FL: Lewis. p 271–282.

Richardson CJ, Kadlec JA, Wentz WA, Chamie JPM, Kadlec RH. 1976. Background ecology and the effects of nutrient additions on a central Michigan wetland. In: Lefor MW, Kennard WC,

Helfgott TB, editors. Proceedings: Third Wetlands Conference. Storrs CT: Institute of Water Resources No. 26. p 34–74.

Richardson CJ, Nichols DS. 1985. Ecological analysis of wastewater management criteria in wetland ecosystems. In: Godfrey PJ, Kaynor ER, Pelczarski S, Benforado J, editors. Ecological considerations in wetlands treatment of municipal wastewaters. New York: Van Nostrand Reinhold. p 351–391.

Richardson CJ, Qian S, Craft CB. 1997. Predictive models for phosphorus retention in wetlands. *Wetlands Ecology and Management* 4:159–175.

Sanford WE, Kopka RJ, Steenhuis TS, Surface JM, Lavine MJ. 1990. An investigation into the use of subsurface rock-reed filters for the treatment of leachate from a solid waste landfill. Water Pollution Control Federation Specialty Conference, Water Quality Management of Landfills; 15–18 Jul 1990; Chicago IL.

Shea-Albin VR. 1992. Abatement of manganese in coal mine drainages through use of constructed wetlands. Denver CO: U.S. Bureau of Mines. Interim Report: FY 1992. Federal Research in Progress.

Sinicrope TL, Langis R, Gersberg RM, Busanardo MJ, Zedler JB. 1992. Metal removed by wetland mesocosms subjected to different hydroperiods. *Ecol Eng* 1(4):309–322.

Spangler FL, Fetter Jr CW, Sloey WE. 1976. Artificial and natural marshes as wastewater treatment systems in Wisconsin. In: Tilton DL, Kadlec RH, Richardson CJ, editors. Freshwater wetlands and sewage effluent. Ann Arbor MI: Univ Michigan. p 215–240.

Spangler FL, Sloey WE, Fetter Jr CW. 1976. Wastewater treatment by natural and artificial marshes. Report to the Robert S. Kerr Environmental Research Laboratory, Ada, OK. EPA/600/2-76-207.

Tilton DL, Kadlec RH, Richardson CJ, editors. 1976. Freshwater wetlands and sewage effluent disposal. Ann Arbor MI: Univ Michigan. NTIS PB259305.

Tourbier J, Pierson Jr RW. 1976. Biological control of water pollution. Philadelphia PA: Univ Pennsylvania Pr.

[USEPA] U.S. Environmental Protection Agency. 1986. Quality criteria for water 1986. Washington DC: USEPA Office of Water. EPA/440/5-86-001.

[USEPA] U.S. Environmental Protection Agency. 1988. Design manual. Constructed wetlands and aquatic plant systems for municipal wastewater treatment. Cincinnati OH: USEPA Office of Research and Development. EPA/625/1-88/022.

[USEPA] U.S. Environmental Protection Agency. 1998. Guidelines for ecological risk assessment. Washington DC: USEPA Risk Assessment Forum. EPA/630/R-95/002F.

Watson JT. 1990. Design and performance of the constructed wetlands wastewater treatment system at Phillips High School at Bear Creek, Alabama. Chattanooga TN: Tennessee Valley Authority. TVA/WR/WQ-90/5.

Watson JT, Danzig AJ. 1993. Pilot-scale nitrification studies using vertical-flow- and shallow-horizontal-flow-constructed wetland cells. In: Moshiri GA, editor. Constructed wetlands for water quality improvement. Boca Raton FL: Lewis. p 301–313.

Wetzel RG. 1975. Limnology. Philadelphia PA: W.B. Saunders.

Wildeman TR, Machemer SD, Klusman RW, Cohen RRH, Lemke P. 1990. Metal removal efficiencies from acid mine drainage in the Big Five constructed wetland. 1990 Mining and Reclamation Conference; 1990 Apr 23–26; Charleston WV. p 417–424.

Wolverton BC. 1987. Artificial marshes. In: Reedy KR, Smith WH, editors. Aquatic plants for water treatment and resource recovery. Orlando FL: Magnolia Publishing.

Wolverton BC, McDonald RC, Duffer WR. 1983. Microorganisms and higher plants for wastewater treatment. *J Environ Qual* 12(2):236–242.

CHAPTER 11

Summary of Workshop Sessions

Marcia K. Nelson, chair
Foster L. Mayer, Mary G. Henry

Important aspects of the effect of contaminants on wetland ecological structure and function, in both natural and constructed systems, were reviewed and evaluated in a Society of Environmental Toxicology and Chemistry (SETAC) Workshop, Ecotoxicology and Risk Assessment for Wetlands, held 30 July–3 August 1995. Experts from many disciplines in the scientific community examined influences of chemical and nonchemical stressors on wetland ecosystems, as well as wetland processes that affect contaminant fate and effects. This special publication summarizes the accomplishments of the workshop and represents an up-to-date compilation of information about several types of wetlands, focusing on identifying creative contaminant treatment solutions, critical issues regarding the fate and effect of contaminants with associated risk, and areas for future research and development.

CHAPTER PREVIEW

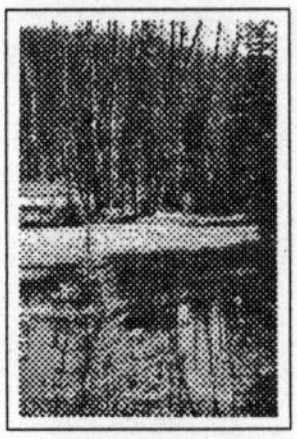

Ecotoxicology and Risk Assessment for Wetlands. Michael A. Lewis et al., editors.

Workgroup sessions included discussions of biogeochemical processes of wetlands; fate and effect of contaminants in freshwater, coastal, and estuarine wetlands; regulatory issues and risk assessment; and constructed wetlands as a risk mitigation alternative. In addition to the workgroup sessions, prominent case studies were presented on contaminant problems that affect the nation's wetland resources, including Se contamination and remediation of the Kesterson National Wildlife Refuge in California, agricultural nonpoint-source runoff in the Everglades National Park and South Carolina near-coastal areas, and the Milltown Reservoir Wetlands of the Clark Fork River in Montana. The overall workshop objectives were to discuss

1) current scientific information and the uncertainties concerning the basic types of wetlands and their ecologies and geochemistries;
2) the extent of damage to wetland biota from specific contaminants;
3) current laboratory and field methodologies used to assess the effects of toxicants, nutrients, and nonchemical stressors on wetland organisms;
4) site-specific examples of wetland risk assessments;
5) regulations and regulatory issues concerning wetlands and assessment of current guidelines used in risk assessment;
6) risk mitigation processes utilizing wetlands as wastewater treatment facilities; and
7) key areas where new information is needed, along with recommended mechanisms for obtaining the information.

Workgroup I: Biogeochemical Processes

Biogeochemical processes are directly relevant to issues in wetland ecotoxicology because the deposition, fate, and effects of contaminants are influenced by the ecosystem components of sediment, biota, and water, which in turn are affected by the presence of the contaminants. The principal objectives of the Biogeochemistry Workgroup were to review and provide recommendations for further study on the following issues:

1) effects of contaminants and nonchemical stressors on biogeochemical processes in wetlands,
2) relationships of these stressors to the ecological functioning of wetlands and connecting watersheds,
3) linkages between sediment–plant processes and ecological functioning of wetlands,
4) analytical and conceptual techniques for integrating ecological processes, and
5) experimental and analytical techniques for monitoring process outputs from wetlands and evaluating significant changes that may result from contamination.

Throughout this session, the spatial and temporal importance of biogeochemical processes on wetland structure and function were emphasized. A critical assessment of the relevance of microcosm and mesocosm experimental results to ecological process endpoints was conducted. Finally, the integrated information on ecological processes and contaminant fate and effects was evaluated within the watershed and landscape perspective. Important fate and transport processes for toxic organics in wetlands systems were outlined, and biogeochemical indicators were evaluated in relation to the effects of contaminants on water quality and biological productivity. The biogeochemical functions of wetlands used as indicators were divided into microbial processes, physicochemical processes, and transport processes.

Critical issues:

- Flow and transformation rates of elements and energy that are functionally unchanged from effects of stressors because functionally equivalent species can replace those removed or impaired.
- Experimental designs to explicitly address sources of variation in complex systems and the analytical approach used to express the data.
- Consideration of oxidation-reduction potential (Eh) as an integrating or "master" variable in many sediment–water systems, and its usefulness as a functional indicator in wetlands ecosystems.
- Effects of surfacewater runoff on contaminant flux in seasonally or periodically flooded and drained contaminated wetlands.

Research needs:

- The relationship between measured Eh values and the chemistry of dissolved constituents in situ is uncertain.
- Studies are needed to encompass larger scales (watershed) and more complex interactions.
- Humification or polymerization of organics in wetland sediments needs to be related to contaminant fate.
- Analytical approaches need to be applied that accommodate a large number of correlated values, i.e., the simultaneous estimation of a series of dependence relationships.

Workgroup II: Contaminant Fate and Effects in Freshwater Wetlands

The main objectives of the Freshwater Workgroup were to provide a critical review, propose new approaches, and recommend future research needs for the following:

1) hazard assessment approaches to wetland ecotoxicology and risk assessment;
2) an ecosystem approach to integrating ecology, hydrology, geomorphology, and wetland soils;

3) application of the ecosystem approach to wetland-specific risk assessment; and
4) evaluation of case studies using the ecosystem approach.

In order to adequately characterize the fate and effects of contaminants in freshwater wetlands, several issues had to be considered. Most fundamental was the recognition that much of the remaining freshwater wetlands in the U.S. have been altered from their natural state through changes in hydrology and surrounding land use. In addition, it was necessary to place the risk assessment process into an ecological context for the evaluation of those remaining wetlands. This involved identifying and integrating the principal ecosystem processes (ecology, hydrology, geomorphology, soils) that serve to structure wetlands and determine contaminant transport, chemical speciation, and biological exposure and effects.

The proposed ecosystem approach for risk assessments uses hydrogeomorphic characterization and wetland functions to establish transport, fate, and effects of chemical and nonchemical stressors. Coupled with toxicity assessments at 4 organizational levels, organism, population, community, and ecosystem, this new approach to risk assessment may be used to describe exposure and effects of stressors in freshwater wetlands. Results of these assessments can be used as a predictive tool for management purposes and, in addition, characterization of existing conditions. The major research needs identified in this session centered around the development of "tools" that can be used to deal with integration and analysis of complex ecosystem interactions and to characterize temporal and spatial variability.

Critical issues:

- Integration of principal ecosystem processes (ecology, hydrology, geomorphology, soils) into the risk assessment process.
- Better integration of wetland science into the risk assessment process.
- Enlistment of the requisite disciplines and expertise in the risk assessment process.
- Consideration of problems at watershed, landscape, and ecosystem scales.

Research needs:

- Determine whether contaminant effects measured by surrogate species toxicity tests are representative of all wetland organisms.
- Determine whether laboratory-to-field extrapolations from single-species toxicity tests could be better estimated if ecologically relevant wetland species were used as test organisms and if a battery of tests were conducted representing various levels of taxonomic complexity.
- Examine the benefits and practical application of an ecosystem-based approach for evaluating impacts and risks from chemical, biological, and physical stressors.

Workgroup III: Contaminant Fate and Effects in Coastal and Estuarine Wetlands

The primary objectives of this workgroup were to review the effects and fate of contaminants in wetlands, to examine the current scientific knowledge, and to recommend needed research. The primary discussion topics were the characteristics and processes that are unique or of unusual importance in coastal and estuarine wetlands. Existing information does not adequately detail the magnitude of changes in species diversity and density that are due to contaminant stresses or the relevance of current diagnostic tools used to monitor the changes. In addition, there is a lack of understanding of the magnitude of change required to result in an ecosystem effect. Unlike freshwater wetlands, the complexity of the biota, the influence of salinity, and tidal magnitude complicate current scientific understanding of toxicant impacts in estuarine wetlands.

It was concluded that existing information concerning the fate and effects of contaminants in coastal wetlands is insufficient to determine current impacts, and the complexity of the biota and influence of environmental modifying factors complicate the interpretation of existing data.

Critical issues:

- Fate and effects of contaminants in relatively poorly studied coastal wetlands, including mangrove swamps, tidal freshwater marshes, and subarctic salt marshes.
- Reference conditions for coastal and estuarine wetlands.
- Effects of changing environmental conditions (e.g., freshwater inflow and eutrophication) on the storage, bioavailability, and release of contaminants (particularly chlorinated hydrocarbons and other persistent organics), including assimilative capacity and desorption from sediment sequestration.

Research needs:

- Develop a framework for reference conditions in salt marshes, brackish marshes, and mangroves based on comparative synthesis that includes the natural variability of those physicochemical conditions.
- Determine the effects of contaminants on physical, chemical, and biological processes of wetland soil formation and remineralization processes.
- Characterize contaminant exposure and effects on populations of important resident and migratory species.
- Characterize the effects of environmental factors on storage, release, and bioavailability of contaminants in coastal and estuarine wetlands.
- Identify salt-tolerant vascular plants suitable for use in toxicity testing and the development of additional phytotoxicity test methods.
- Develop models and other methods to evaluate the changes in coastal wetlands on various spatial scales, from site-specific wetland types to re-

gional, national, and global perspectives, to determine the significance of locally observed changes as well as to allow extrapolation of results.

- Develop interpretive models to translate results of contaminant fate and effects to population, community, and ecosystem levels, and develop methods to validate these models in the field.

Workgroup IV: Regulatory Issues and Risk Assessment

The objectives of this workgroup were to discuss current regulatory expectations related to wetlands and to evaluate the strengths and limitations of wetland risk assessment procedures. Discussions by the Regulatory Issues Workgroup first centered on identifying regulations pertaining to wetlands and providing a brief explanation of each. The USEPA's Framework for Ecological Risk Assessment (1992) was then reviewed in relation to unique aspects of wetlands. Issues regarding problem formulation, identification of assessment and measurement endpoints, and development of a conceptual model were discussed. Analysis of exposure to estimate or measure the distribution and magnitude of a stressor and analysis of effects to identify and quantify the adverse effects resulting from exposure to a stressor were covered, with emphasis on the uniqueness of wetland characteristics. The risk characterization phase, which integrates the results of the exposure and effects analysis, was discussed, along with the ecological significance of the risk findings. Chemical stressors were the focus of this workgroup; however, the group recognized the importance of nontoxicant stressors and the difficulty in separating the effects caused by multiple stressors. Finally, examples of how the risk assessment thought process could be used in Superfund (CERCLA) assessments; permitting programs under Section 404 of the Clean Water Act; registration and regulation of pesticides under the Federal Insecticide, Fungicide, and Rodenticide Act (FIFRA); and establishment of water quality standards were discussed. (Editorial note: Since the workshop was held, additional regulatory guidance has been published [USEPA 1997, 1998]).

Critical issues:

- Relevance of the results of current standardized toxicity tests to wetland flora and fauna.
- Significance of biotic indices and community profiles as related to ecosystem fitness.
- Reference site selection and characterizations for different wetland types.
- Relative impact and integrative effects of toxic and nontoxic stressors.
- Water and sediment quality criteria specific to wetlands.

Research needs:

- Understand how hydrological, biogeochemical, and biological functions affect contaminant bioavailability.

- Understand the effects of stressors on wetland-specific organisms, the extrapolation of laboratory tests to field situations, and the impact of one stressed species on the rest of the wetland ecosystem.
- Develop contaminant transport and fate models that accurately predict movement within a wetland.
- Clarify issues surrounding the identification and use of reference sites as the basis for ecological risk assessments.
- Integrate sociological aspects into the problem formulation phase of ecological risk assessments to minimize inadequate or incomplete characterization of risk.

Workgroup V: Constructed Wetlands as a Risk Mitigation Alternative

The primary objectives of this workgroup were to discuss

1) the application of constructed wetlands to treating point and nonpoint sources,
2) the creation of a decision support system to aid in implementing constructed wetlands and dealing with risk management issues, and
3) case studies delineating the performance and feasibility of constructed wetlands.

Detailed discussion points included a history of wetlands used in a wastewater treatment context and why there is a movement from natural to constructed wetlands for this purpose. Design issues surrounding construction of wetlands include hydrological considerations, scale, site selection, cost, maintenance, longevity, capacity, and success criteria. The engineering solutions (size, capacity) and biological aspects (compatibility of emergent, submerged, and woody vegetation; microbial community issues) must be collectively examined and assessed for long-term success of constructed wetlands.

Critical issues:

- Treatment performance versus ecological compatibility and acceptability.
- Wetlands functions and values that should be optimized and made self-sustainable.
- Contaminant removal.
- Regulatory context for dealing with constructed wetlands, along with risk assessment and risk management aspects.

Research needs:

- Conduct demonstration studies on pesticide classes with local or regional major crop-use patterns in relation to exceedance of drinking water or environmental standards or criteria.

- Conduct small-scale, controlled studies to address fundamental design and effectiveness questions.
- Develop real-world, small-scale watershed demonstration projects to assess the life span and effectiveness of constructed wetlands.

Workshop Summary Needs

The workshop attendees stressed the need for basic knowledge of wetland ecology and water quality functions. However, this need should be balanced with wetland management requirements in the near future. Overall areas of recommended research follow:

- Determine which wetland types are at risk from specific types of stressors (wastewater, runoff, irrigation, etc).
- Identify chemicals of concern (single and mixtures) that will have an effect on wetlands, and determine relevant assessment strategies for wetland flora and fauna.
- Determine which wetland functions (e.g., fish nurseries, primary productivity, wildlife habitat) are most likely to be affected by nutrients and toxics.
- Develop predictive capabilities for the capacity of wetlands to retain and export contaminants, and assess sediment processes as they relate to the fate of contaminants in denitrification, nutrient uptake, and heavy metal mobilization.
- Develop relevant water and sediment quality criteria to protect wetland biota, and implement programs to ensure their effectiveness to maintain wetland structure and function.
- Link watershed activities and water use with wetland water quality, hydrology, and ecological processes.

References

[USEPA] U.S. Environmental Protection Agency. 1992. Framework for ecological risk assessment. Washington DC: Risk Assessment Forum, USEPA. EPA/630/R-92/001.

[USEPA] U.S. Environmental Protection Agency. 1997. Ecological risk assessment guidance for Superfund: process for designing and conducting ecological risk assessments. Washington DC: Office of Solid Waste and Emergency Response. EPA/540/R-97/006.

[USEPA] U.S. Environmental Protection Agency. 1998. Guidelines for ecological risk assessment. Washington DC: Risk Assessment Forum. EPA/630/R-95/002F.

Abbreviations

AC-1	Alston Creek-1 site (South Carolina)
AC-2	Alston Creek-2 site (South Carolina)
AChE	Acetylcholinesterase
AEC	Anion exchange complex
AFDM	Ash-free dry mass
ANOVA	Analysis of variance
AOSA	Association of Official Seed Analysts
ARAMDG	Aquatic Risk Assessment and Mitigation Dialogue Group
ARAR	Applicable or relevant and appropriate requirements
AREM	Avian richness evaluation method
ASTM	American Society for Testing and Materials
ATP	Adenosine triphosphate
AVS	Acid-volatile sulfide
AWIS	Area-wide wetland impact study
BMP	Best management practices
BOD	Biological/biochemical oxygen demand
CC-GC	Capillary column gas chromatography
CERCLA	Comprehensive Environmental Response, Compensation, and Liability Act
CDF	Confined disposal facility
CEC	Cation exchange complex or cation exchange capacity
CEQ	Council on Environmental Quality
CFR	Clark Fork River (Montana)
COD	Chemical oxygen demand
COPEC	Contaminant of potential ecological concern
CTL	Control (reference site)
CVP	Central Valley Project (California)
CWA	Clean Water Act

Ecotoxicology and Risk Assessment for Wetlands. Michael A. Lewis et al., editors.

DBOFBP	Dibromooctafluorobiphenyl
DDD	1,1-dichloro-2,2-bis(p-chlorophenyl)ethane
DDE	1,1-dichloro-2,2-bis(p-chlorophenyl)ethylene or dicholordiphenyldichloroethylene
DDT	1,1,1-trichloro-2,2-bis-(p-chlorophenyl)ethane or dichlorodiphenyl-trichloroethane
DIC	Dissolved inorganic compound
dl	Detection limit
DO	Dissolved oxygen
DOC	Dissolved organic carbon
DOM	Dissolved organic matter
DTPA	Diethylenetriaminepentaacetic acid
dw	Dry weight
ECD	Electron capture detector
EEC	Estimated environmental concentration
EIA	Environmental impact assessment
ERL	Effects range low
ET	Evapotranspiration
FAA	Flame atomic absorption
FCI	Functional capacity index
FCU	Functional capacity unit
FDER	Florida Department of Environmental Regulation
FETAX	Frog embryo teratogenesis assay Xenopus
FICWD	Federal Interagency Committee for Wetland Delineation
FIFRA	Federal Insecticide, Fungicide, and Rodenticide Act
FTE	Full time equivalent
GC-ECD	Gas chromatography–electron capture detection
GFAA	Graphite furnace atomic absorption
GC-ITMS	Gas chromatography–ion trap mass spectrometry
GIS	Geographical information systems

GLEAMS	Groundwater loading effects of agricultural management systems
GPC	Gel permeation chromatography
HCB	Hexachlorobenzene
HDPE	High-density polyethylene
HEP	Habitat evaluation procedure
HGM	Hydrogeomorphic
HP-GPC	High-performance gel permeation chromatography
HPLC	High-performance liquid chromatography
HRT	Hydraulic retention time
HSI	Habitat suitability index
HSPF	Hydrological simulation program Fortran
IBI	Index of biotic/biological integrity
IDP	Interagency Drainage Program (San Joaquin Valley, California)
IPM	Integrated pest management
KWA	Kiawah (South Carolina) watershed site
LC50	Lethal concentration to 50% population
LISREL	Linear structural relations
LOC	Level of concern
MDL	Method detection limit
mer	Mercury resistance
MI	Murrells Inlet (South Carolina)
MIF	Murrells Inlet Flo's Restaurant site
MRW	Milltown Reservoir Wetlands (Montana)
NCP	National Contingency Plan/National Comprehensive Plan
NEC	No-effects concentration
NEPA	National Policy Act of 1969

NI	North Inlet Estuary
NIOL	North Inlet site (South Carolina)
NIST	National Institute of Standards and Technology
NMFS	National Marine Fisheries Service
NOAA	National Oceanic and Atmospheric Administration
NOAEL	No-observed-adverse-effects level
NOEC	No-observed-effects concentration
NPD	Nitrogen phosphorus detector
NPDES	National Pollutant Discharge Elimination System
NPS	Nonpoint source
NRDA	Natural resources damage assessment
NWR	National Wildlife Refuge
OC-6	Oak Creek site (South Carolina)
OECD	Organization for Economic Cooperation and Development
OM	Organic material
OPA	Oil Pollution Act of 1990
OPP	Office of Pesticide Programs
PAH	Polycyclic aromatic hydrocarbon
PCB	Polychlorinated biphenyl
PE	Perkin-Elmer
POM	Particulate organic matter
ppm	Parts per million
PS-3	Parson Creek site (South Carolina)
PVC	Polyvinyl chloride
RCRA	Resource Conservation and Recovery Act
RI/FS	Remedial investigation and feasibility study
RO	Reverse osmosis
RP	Oxidation-reduction "redox" potential (Chapters 3 and 4)

RP	Retention pond (Chapter 8)
SARA	Superfund Amendments and Reauthorization Act
SCE	Saturated calomel electrode
SCS	Soil Conservation Service
SDWA	Safe Drinking Water Act
SEM	Simultaneously extracted metal (Chapter 5)
SEM	Structural equation modeling (Chapter 3)
SPE	Solid-phase extraction
TOC	Total organic compound
TP-1	Trailer Park-1 site (South Carolina)
TRT	Treatment watershed site
TSCA	Toxic Substances Control Act of 1976
TSD	Technical support document
UA	Uncertainty analysis
USACOE	U.S. Army Corps of Engineers
USBR	U.S. Bureau of Reclamation
USDOI	U.S. Department of the Interior
USEPA	U.S. Environmental Protection Agency
USFWS	U.S. Fish and Wildlife Service
USGAO	U.S. General Accounting Office
UV	Ultraviolet
WES	Waterways Experiment Station (USACOE)
WET	Wetland evaluation technique

Index

A

Ecotoxicology and Risk Assessment for Wetlands. Michael A. Lewis et al., editors.
© 1999 Society of Environmental Toxicology and Chemistry (SETAC). ISBN 1-880611-16-3

C

D

I

J

K

L

M

N

O

P

R

T

U

V

W

X

Z

SETAC

A Professional Society for Environmental Scientists and Engineers and Related Disciplines Concerned with Environmental Quality

The Society of Environmental Toxicology and Chemistry (SETAC), with offices currently in North America and Europe, is a nonprofit, professional society established to provide a forum for individuals and institutions engaged in the study of environmental problems, management and regulation of natural resources, education, research and development, and manufacturing and distribution.

Specific goals of the society are:

- Promote research, education and training in the environmental sciences.
- Promote the systematic application of all relevant scientific disciplines to the evaluation of chemical hazards.
- Participate in the scientific interpretation of issues concerned with hazard assessment and risk analysis.
- Support the development of ecologically acceptable practices and principles.
- Provide a forum (meetings and publications) for communication among professionals in government, business, academia, and in other segments of society involved in the use, protection, and management of our environment.

These goals are pursued through the conduct of numerous activities which include:

- Hold annual meetings composed of study and workshop sessions, platform and poster papers, and presentation of achievement and merit awards.
- Sponsor a monthly scientific journal, a news letter, and special technical publications.
- Provide funds for education and training through the SETAC Scholarship/Fellowship Program.
- Organize and sponsor chapters to provide a forum for the presentation of scientific data and for the interchange and study of information about local concerns.
- Provide advice and counsel to technical and nontechnical persons about scientific issues through a number of standing and *ad hoc* committees.

SETAC membership is currently composed of nearly 6,000 individuals from government, academia, business, and public-interest groups with technical backgrounds of chemistry, toxicology, biology, ecology, atmospheric sciences, health sciences, earth sciences, and engineering.

If you have training in these or related disciplines and are engaged in the study, use, or management of environmental resources, SETAC can fulfill your professional affiliation needs.

All members receive a newsletter highlighting environmental topics and SETAC activities, and reduced fees for the Annual Meeting and SETAC special publications.

All members except Students and Senior Active Members receive monthly issues of *Environmental Toxicology and Chemistry* (ET&C), a peer-reviewed journal of the Society. Student and Senior Active Members may subscribe to the journal. Members may hold office and, with the Emeritus Members, constitute the voting membership.

If you desire further information, contact the appropriate SETAC office.

SETAC Office
1010 North 12th Avenue
Pensacola, FL 32501-3367
T 850 469 1500 F 850 469 9778 E setac@setac.org